S. Braun, H.-O. Kalinowski, S. Berger

100 and More Basic NMR Experiments

VCH

Related Titles from VCH:

H. Friebolin
Basic One- and Two-Dimensional NMR Spectroscopy
2nd ed., 1993. XXI, 368 pages with 161 figures and 48 tables.
Softcover. ISBN 3-527-29059

F.J.M. van de Ven
Multidimensional NMR in Liquids
1995. XVII, 382 pages with appendices, figures, and tables.
Hardcover. ISBN 1-56081-665-1

W. R. Croasmun, R. M. K. Carlson (Eds.)
Two-Dimensional NMR Spectroscopy
2nd ed., 1994. XX, 958 pages.
Hardcover. ISBN 1-56081-664-3

© VCH Verlagsgesellschaft mbH, D-69451 Weinheim (Federal Republic of Germany), 1996

Distribution:

VCH, P. O. Box 101161, D-69451 Weinheim (Federal Republic of Germany)

Switzerland: VCH, P. O. Box, CH-4020 Basel (Switzerland)

United Kingdom and Ireland: VCH (UK) Ltd., 8 Wellington Court,
    Cambridge CB1 1HZ (England)

USA and Canada: VCH, 220 East 23rd Street, New York, NY 10010–4606 (USA)

Japan: VCH, Eikow Building, 10-9 Hongo 1-chome, Bunkyo-ku, Tokyo 113 (Japan)

ISBN 3-527-29091-5

S. Braun, H.-O. Kalinowski, S. Berger

100 and More
Basic NMR Experiments

A Practical Course

Weinheim · New York
Basel · Cambridge · Tokyo

Siegmar Braun
Institut für Organische Chemie
Technische Hochschule Darmstadt
Petersenstraße 22
D-64287 Darmstadt

Hans-Otto Kalinowski
Institut für Organische Chemie
Justus-Liebig-Universität Gießen
Heinrich-Buff-Ring 58
D-35392 Gießen

Stefan Berger
Fachbereich Chemie
Philipps-Universität Marburg
Hans-Meerwein-Straße
D-35032 Marburg

Published jointly by
VCH Verlagsgesellschaft, Weinheim (Federal Republic of Germany)
VCH Publishers, New York, NY (USA)

korrigierter Nachdruck der 1. Auflage 1996

Editorial Director: Dr. Michael Bär
Production Manager: Dipl. Wirt.-Ing. (FH) Hans-Jochen Schmitt

Library of Congress Card No. applied for.

A catalogue record for this book is available from the British Library.

Die Deutsche Bibliothek – CIP-Einheitsaufnahme
Braun, Siegmar:
100 and more basic NMR experiments : a practical course / S. Braun ; H.-O. Kalinowski ; S. Berger. – Weinheim ; New York ; Basel ; Cambridge ; Tokyo : VCH, 1996
ISBN 3-527-29091-5
NE: Kalinowski, Hans-Otto:; Berger, Stefan:; Braun, Siegmar: Hundred and more basic NMR experiments; Kalinowski, Hans-Otto: Hundred and more basic NMR experiments; Berger, Stefan: Hundred and more basic NMR experiments

Preface

NMR spectroscopy is now 50 years old. It is fascinating how this method has grown and developed in these five decades, in how many branches of science it has entered, and how it is storming further ahead. The most important milestones on this way have unquestionably been the introduction of the pulsed Fourier transform technique and the idea and development of multidimensional methods.

In the field of structure elucidation of chemical, especially organic, compounds progress occurs in such large strides, new experiments and new pulse sequences are presented in such rapid succession, that a normal user or even an advanced practitioner may lose sight of the overall picture, and many a novice may give up in view of the overwhelming variety of methods.

It is therefore the aim of the book presented here to give a compass, a kind of Ariadne's thread, to enable the reader to chart a straightforward path through the field of NMR experiments for structure determination. It is a practical course from which the user can learn by doing. It originated from various educational and advanced training activities of the authors, all being in charge of NMR spectroscopy laboratories and familiar with the daily practice of such facilities.

An introductory chapter on the FT NMR spectrometer and on practical aspects such as probe-head tuning, lock operation, and shimming, is followed by a series of more than a hundred different experiments, mostly on ^1H and ^{13}C, arranged in chapters according to common features, each with a short survey at the beginning. The content ranges from pulse length determinations, routine spectra and test procedures through decoupling techniques, variable temperature and LIS measurements, to 1D multipulse sequences and the observation of heteronuclides such as ^6Li, ^{15}N and ^{17}O. More demanding experiments include those using selective pulses, introducing the second and third dimensions, and/or using field gradients for coherence selection.

The experiments have been selected primarily because of their importance and general applicability. All experiments have been specially performed for this book, exactly as described and depicted. Three compounds have been chosen as the main demonstration samples, namely chloroform, ethyl crotonate, and strychnine (the latter should be used as a sealed sample).

A standard scheme has been adopted for the detailed description of the experiments, organized in the following specific sections:

Purpose explains the idea and goal of an experiment and refers the user to related experiments.

Literature presents references to the original publication and to improvements and/or sections in monographs and reviews.

Pulse Scheme and Phase Cycle gives the pulse sequence in an instrument-independent graphic and self-explanatory form, and the phase cycles of the pulses and the receiver.

Acquisition is the main section with instructions on the sample to be used, the spectrometer configuration, the type of program, and finally the parameters necessary for the performance of the experiment.

Processing describes how to treat the time-domain data.

Results presents the spectrum obtained by following the procedure exactly, as well as some remarks concerning the interpretation.

Comments contains an explanation of the most important steps of the pulse sequence, sometimes with a description using the product operator formalism for which elementary rules are collected in the Appendix.

It is obvious that the acquisition program of a specific experiment cannot be given explicitly, since the languages of the various manufacturers are different. Moreover, since even one and the same manufacturer may have different dialects in use, an acquisition program is not necessarily transferable to another spectrometer of the same company. Corresponding to the spectrometers used by the authors, the nomenclature of the experimental parameters follows the Bruker notation; a glossary of abbreviations and symbols of different dialects and languages of other equally well-known manufacturers is given in the Appendix for comparison.

For some of the experiments, especially the newest ones, the manufacturer's software may not contain the specific acquisition program. In that case ask an application chemist of your manufacturer for support or, if you need the program for the particular instrument referred to in the experiment described here (AM-, AC-, AMX- or ARX-spectrometer), just send a fax or an e-mail to:

> Prof. Dr. Stefan Berger
> Fachbereich Chemie
> Philipps-Universität
> D-35032 Marburg
> Fax: +49..6421/288917
> e-mail: berger@ps1515.chemie.uni-marburg.de

In general the conditions for the experiments have not been optimized. In all cases the results are presented exactly as they were obtained, without cosmetic retouching; sometimes the samples used even show impurities.

Some recommendations regarding how best to use the collection presented here will help the user to get maximum benefit. In principle one could just jump into the chapter at the experiment one wants to perform, since each experiment is self-contained. However, the novice is recommended to first read Chapter 1 and the introductory remarks to Chapter 3 to perform the standard ^1H and ^{13}C experiments 3.1 and 3.2 (using the current settings of 90° pulse lengths etc. for the instrument being used). Then one should determine the pulses oneself, completing at least Experiments 2.1 to 2.3 before going on. In each case, whether a beginner or not, one should read the whole description first, including the "Comments". By doing so one will get information about the context, about essential prerequisites, and about possible problems. One will also find references to experiments which require less sophisticated equipment. When planning more advanced experiments one may start with an already known one near the level of the intended experiment, as a check and in order to get familiar with the notation used in the descriptions. It should be noted that no exhaustive theory is given; the references may serve as stimuli for further studies leading to a deeper insight and understanding.

The selection of the experiments is to some extent a matter of subjective preferences by the authors. If the reader fails to find his or her favorite experiment, he or she should not hesitate to notify the authors. They wish all users to gain maximum benefit from this learning medium, and will be grateful for comments, suggestions for improvements, or hints on mistakes and inconsistencies.

Finally, we would like to thank many colleagues for suggestions, our graduate students for helpful criticism, and Dr. J. K. Becconsall for proof reading and finishing the English text.

(October 1995)

S. Braun
H.-O. Kalinowski
S. Berger

Longum iter est per praecepta,

breve et efficax per exempla.

L. A. Seneca, *Ad Lucilium Epistulae Morales, VI*

Contents

Preface

Chapter 1 The NMR Spectrometer

1

1.1   Principles of an NMR Spectrometer   1
1.1.1   The Magnet   1
1.1.2   The Spectrometer Console   2
1.1.3   The Work-Station   3
1.1.4   Maintenance   3
1.2   Tuning a Probe-Head   3
1.2.1   Tuning and Matching with a Reflection Meter   3
1.2.2   Tuning and Matching with an R.F. Bridge and an Oscilloscope   4
1.2.3   Tuning and Matching with a Wobble Generator   5
1.3   The Lock Channel   6
1.4   The Art of Shimming   7
1.4.1   The Shim Gradients   8
1.4.2   The Shimming Procedure   9

Chapter 2 Determination of the Pulse-Length

13

Exp. 2.1:   Determination of the 90° ^{1}H Transmitter Pulse-Length   14
Exp. 2.2:   Determination of the 90° ^{13}C Transmitter Pulse-Length   17
Exp. 2.3:   Determination of the 90° ^{1}H Decoupler Pulse-Length   20
Exp. 2.4:   The 90° ^{1}H Pulse with Inverse Spectrometer Configuration   23
Exp. 2.5:   The 90°^{13}C Decoupler Pulse with Inverse Configuration   26
Exp. 2.6:   Determination of Radiofrequency Power   29

Chapter 3 Routine NMR Spectroscopy and Standard Tests

33

Exp. 3.1:   The Standard ^{1}H NMR Experiment   34
Exp. 3.2:   The Standard ^{13}C NMR Experiment   39
Exp. 3.3:   Line-Shape Test for ^{1}H NMR Spectroscopy   44
Exp. 3.4:   Resolution Test for ^{1}H NMR Spectroscopy   47
Exp. 3.5:   Sensitivity Test for ^{1}H NMR Spectroscopy   50
Exp. 3.6:   Line-Shape Test for ^{13}C NMR Spectroscopy   53
Exp. 3.7:   ASTM Sensitivity Test for ^{13}C NMR Spectroscopy   56
Exp. 3.8:   Sensitivity Test for ^{13}C NMR Spectroscopy   59
Exp. 3.9:   Quadrature Image Test   62
Exp. 3.10:   Dynamic Range Test for Signal Amplitudes   65

Chapter 4 Decoupling Techniques

68

Exp. 4.1:   Decoupler Calibration for Homonuclear Decoupling   69
Exp. 4.2:   Decoupler Calibration for Heteronuclear Decoupling   72
Exp. 4.3:   Low Power Calibration for Heteronuclear Decoupling   75

Exp. 4.4:   Homonuclear Decoupling   78
Exp. 4.5:   The Homonuclear SPT Experiment   81
Exp. 4.6:   The Heteronuclear SPT Experiment   84
Exp. 4.7:   1D Nuclear Overhauser Difference Spectroscopy   87
Exp. 4.8:   1D NOE Spectroscopy with Multiple Selective Irradiation   90
Exp. 4.9: ^{1}H Off-Resonance Decoupled ^{13}C NMR Spectra   93
Exp. 4.10:   The Gated ^{1}H-Decoupling Technique   96
Exp. 4.11:   The Inverse Gated ^{1}H-Decoupling Technique   99
Exp. 4.12: ^{1}H Single Frequency Decoupling of ^{13}C NMR Spectra   102
Exp. 4.13: ^{1}H Low-Power Decoupling of ^{13}C NMR Spectra   105
Exp. 4.14:   Measurement of the Heteronuclear Overhauser Effect   108

Chapter 5 Dynamic NMR Spectroscopy   111

Exp. 5.1:   Low Temperature Calibration with Methanol   112
Exp. 5.2:   High Temperature Calibration with 1,2-Ethanediol   115
Exp. 5.3:   Dynamic ^{1}H NMR Spectroscopy on Dimethylformamide   118
Exp. 5.4:   The Saturation Transfer Experiment   121

Chapter 6 1D Multipulse Sequences   124

Exp. 6.1:   Measurement of the Spin–Lattice Relaxation Time T_1 125
Exp. 6.2:   Measurement of the Spin–Spin Relaxation Time T_2 129
Exp. 6.3:   Editing ^{13}C NMR Spectra with SEFT   132
Exp. 6.4:   Editing ^{13}C NMR Spectra with APT   135
Exp. 6.5:   The Basic INEPT Technique   138
Exp. 6.6:   INEPT+   141
Exp. 6.7:   Refocused INEPT   144
Exp. 6.8:   Reverse INEPT   147
Exp. 6.9:   Editing ^{13}C NMR Spectra with DEPT   150
Exp. 6.10:   Editing ^{13}C NMR Spectra with PENDANT   154
Exp. 6.11:   1D-INADEQUATE   157
Exp. 6.12:   The BIRD Filter   161
Exp. 6.13:   TANGO   164
Exp. 6.14:   The Heteronuclear Double Quantum Filter   167
Exp. 6.15:   Water Suppression by Presaturation   170
Exp. 6.16:   Water Suppression by the Jump and Return Method   173

Chapter 7 NMR Spectroscopy with Selective Pulses   176

Exp. 7.1:   Determination of a Shaped 90° ^{1}H Transmitter Pulse   177
Exp. 7.2:   Determination of a Shaped 90° ^{1}H Decoupler Pulse   180
Exp. 7.3:   Determination of a Shaped 90° ^{13}C Decoupler Pulse   183
Exp. 7.4:   Selective Excitation with DANTE   186
Exp. 7.5:   Selective COSY   189
Exp. 7.6:   SELINCOR: Selective Inverse H,C Correlation via ^1J(C,H)   192
Exp. 7.7:   SELINQUATE   195

Exp. 7.8:   Selective TOCSY   199
Exp. 7.9:   INAPT   203
Exp. 7.10:   Determination of Long Range C,H Coupling Constants   206
Exp. 7.11:   SELRESOLV   209
Exp. 7.12:   SERF   212

Chapter 8 Auxiliary Reagents, Quantitative Determinations,   215
and Reaction Mechanism

Exp. 8.1:   Signal Separation Using a Lanthanide Shift Reagent   216
Exp. 8.2:   Signal Separation of Enantiomers Using a Chiral Shift Reagent   219
Exp. 8.3:   Signal Separation of Enantiomers Using a Chiral Solvating Agent   222
Exp. 8.4:   Determination of Enantiomeric Purity with Pirkle's Reagent   225
Exp. 8.5:   The Relaxation Reagent $Cr(acac)_3$ 228
Exp. 8.6:   Quantitative ^1H NMR Spectroscopy: Determination of the   231
             Alcohol Content of Polish Vodka
Exp. 8.7:   Quantitative ^{13}C NMR Spectroscopy with Inverse Gated   234
             ^1H-Decoupling
Exp. 8.8:   Determination of Paramagnetic Susceptibility by NMR   237
Exp. 8.9:   The CIDNP Effect   240

Chapter 9 Heteronuclear NMR Spectroscopy   243

Exp. 9.1: ^1H-Decoupled ^{15}N NMR Spectra with DEPT   248
Exp. 9.2: ^1H-Coupled ^{15}N NMR Spectra with DEPT   251
Exp. 9.3: ^{19}F NMR Spectroscopy   254
Exp. 9.4: ^{29}Si NMR Spectroscopy with DEPT   257
Exp. 9.5: ^{119}Sn NMR Spectroscopy   261
Exp. 9.6: ^2H NMR Spectroscopy   264
Exp. 9.7: ^{11}B NMR Spectroscopy   267
Exp. 9.8: ^{17}O NMR Spectroscopy with RIDE   270

Chapter 10 The Second Dimension   273

Exp. 10.1:   2D J-Resolved ^1H NMR Spectroscopy   277
Exp. 10.2:   2D J-Resolved ^{13}C NMR Spectroscopy   280
Exp. 10.3:   The Basic H,H-COSY Experiment   283
Exp. 10.4:   Long-Range COSY   286
Exp. 10.5:   Phase-Sensitive COSY   289
Exp. 10.6:   Phase-Sensitive COSY-45   292
Exp. 10.7:   Double Quantum Filtered COSY with Presaturation   295
Exp. 10.8:   C,H Correlation by Polarization Transfer (HETCOR)   299
Exp. 10.9:   Long-Range C,H Correlation by Polarization Transfer   302
Exp. 10.10: C,H Correlation via Long-Range Couplings (COLOC)   305
Exp. 10.11: The Basic HMQC Experiment   308
Exp. 10.12: Phase-Sensitive HMQC with BIRD Selection and   312
             GARP Decoupling

Exp. 10.13: Phase-Sensitive HMBC with BIRD Selection   315
Exp. 10.14: The Basic HSQC Experiment   318
Exp. 10.15: The HOHAHA or TOCSY Experiment   322
Exp. 10.16: The NOESY Experiment   326
Exp. 10.17: The CAMELSPIN or ROESY Experiment   330
Exp. 10.18: The HOESY Experiment   334
Exp. 10.19: 2D-INADEQUATE   337
Exp. 10.20: The EXSY Experiment   341

Chapter 11 NMR Spectroscopy with Pulsed Field Gradients 344

Exp. 11.1:   Calibration of Pulsed Field Gradients   346
Exp. 11.2:   The Pulsed Gradient Spin-Echo Experiment   349
Exp. 11.3:   Gradient-Selected H,H-COSY   352
Exp. 11.4:   Gradient-Selected Phase-Sensitive DQF COSY   356
Exp. 11.5:   Gradient-Selected HMQC   360
Exp. 11.6:   Gradient-Selected HMBC   364
Exp. 11.7:   Phase-Sensitive Gradient-Selected HSQC   368
Exp. 11.8:   Gradient-Selected TOCSY   372
Exp. 11.9:   Gradient-Selected HMQC-TOCSY   376
Exp. 11.10: Gradient-Selected ^{1}H-Detected 2D INEPT-INADEQUATE   380
Exp. 11.11: Gradient-Selected SELINCOR   384
Exp. 11.12: GRECCO   387
Exp. 11.13: WATERGATE   390

Chapter 12 The Third Dimension 393

Exp. 12.1:   3D HMQC-COSY   394
Exp. 12.2:   3D Gradient-Selected HSQC-TOCSY   398
Exp. 12.3:   3D H,C,P-Correlation   402

Appendix 1 405

Instrument Dialects   406

Appendix 2 409

Elementary Product Operator Formalism Rules   409

Glossary and Index 411

Chapter 1

The NMR Spectrometer

1.1 Principles of an NMR Spectrometer

1.1.1 The Magnet

In most current NMR spectrometers the magnetic field is generated by a superconducting magnet (Fig. 1.1). The first stage in reaching the very low temperature needed is an outer stainless steel or aluminum dewar which contains liquid nitrogen. Typically, this has to be refilled every ten days. In practice, it is advisable to do this refilling on a fixed day every week. An inner dewar contains the superconducting coil (4) immersed in liquid helium, which has to be refilled, depending on the construction, every two to four month. The *helium* refill should be carried out only by experienced people. A room-temperature bore is fitted with the shim coils (7), providing a room temperature homogeneity adjustment, and a spinner assembly (5), which contains the turbine system for spinning the NMR sample tube. The probe-head (8) is usually introduced into the magnet from the bottom. The probe-head is connected to at least three r.f. cables providing the ^{2}H lock, ^{1}H frequency, and one X-nucleus frequency. Additional devices to control temperature (heater, thermoelement, air, sometimes water to insulate the probehead from the magnet) are needed.

1 Ports for liquid N_2

2 Ports for liquid He

3 Superinsulation and
   high vacuum

4 Main magnet coils + liquid helium

5 Sample lift and spinner
   assembly

6 NMR tube

7 Shim assembly

8 Probe head

Fig. 1.1 Principles of a superconducting magnet

1.1.2 The Spectrometer Console

The spectrometer console provides at least three radiofrequency channels. Usually these frequencies are derived from digital frequency synthesizers which are phase-locked to a central quartz oscillator. These frequencies are controlled, amplified, pulsed, and transmitted to the probe-head. The various signals are preamplified, then mixed with the local oscillator frequency to yield the intermediate frequency (i.f.) The i.f. signal is further amplified, then in a second mixing stage the NMR audio signal is obtained after quadrature phase detection. The two signal components are digitized in the ADC and fed into the computer memory or, in the case of the lock signal, used for field/frequency regulation. Figures 1.2 and 1.3 show the principles of the system.

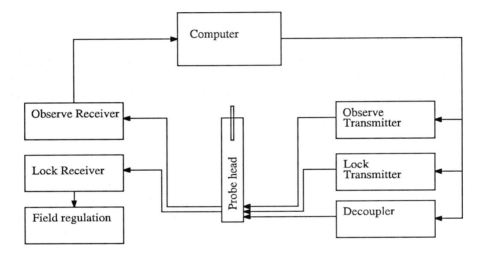

Fig. 1.2 Principles of an NMR spectrometer

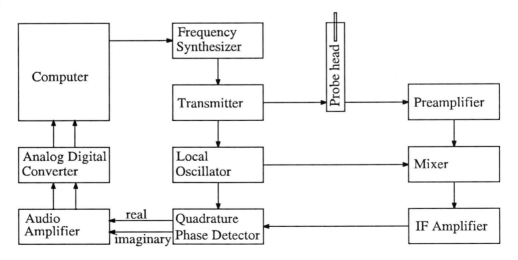

Fig. 1.3 Components of the observe channel

1.1.3 The Work Station

Modern NMR instruments are controlled by a work-station, commonly based on the UNIX operating system. In addition, one finds a process controller integrated into the spectrometer console. The computing system has, in principle, two different tasks. First, the process controller must have on line control of many spectrometer functions such as lock, generation and timing of r.f. pulses, digitization and accumulation of the NMR signal (FID, free induction decay). Less time demanding are the other, mainly graphic, tasks in the processing of the NMR spectra. However, the massive amount of data in modern two- or multidimensional NMR spectroscopy techniques requires high storage capacities both on disk and in RAM, and a very high speed of computing.

1.1.4 Maintenance

Although most parts of modern NMR spectrometers are more or less maintenance-free, it is the experience of the authors that careful and regular checking of several components can save considerable money and time. Most important is the regular checking of the cryogens, which should be replenished on a strict schedule. Of course all magnet openings equipped with O-rings have to be carefully monitored. This is especially important for very low temperature work which can lead to icing of the O-rings. Regular checking of several hidden fans within the spectrometer console is advisable.

1.2 Tuning a Probe-Head

With a high field superconducting NMR spectrometer it is essential for obtaining a good signal-to-noise ratio, and for some advanced experiments to get any meaningful results at all, that the probe-head should be correctly tuned to the observe frequency with the particular sample of interest. There can be a huge difference depending on whether a compound is dissolved in water or in an organic solvent.

Although the construction of the resonant circuits of different probe-heads may vary considerably one has in general two capacitors to adjust, one which tunes the circuit to the desired resonance frequency (tuning) and one which performs the necessary impedance matching of the network (matching). However, these are mutually interactive and therefore they have to be adjusted in turn.

There are at least three common procedures for obtaining a global best, both on tuning and matching, and these are described below.

1.2.1 Tuning and Matching with a Reflection Meter

The simplest procedure works with a reflection meter introduced into the signal path. A tuning file on the computer should provide uninterrupted rapid pulsing in order to obtain a steady signal at the reflection meter. Turn the spinner off to avoid mechanical interference. Typical NMR parameters are p1 = 40 µs, td = 1 k, sw = 20 kHz, and ns = 64 k, which provide an acquisition time aq and hence a repetition time of 0.0256 s. Be sure that all filter boxes and other unnecessary devices are removed from the signal path in order to tune only the probe-head itself.

The goal is to minimize the strength of the reflected signal at the reflection meter. The procedure has to be done for all frequencies of the probe head starting from the lowest frequency. Thus, in the usual dual probe heads (^{1}H and ^{13}C) adjust the ^{13}C coil first.

Typically, proceed as follows:

Obtain a first minimum on tuning and then on matching. Then alter the matching capacitor in one direction and check whether the tuning can be improved compared with the previous minimum. If yes, alter the matching further in the same direction as before and try to further improve the tuning. If not, alter the matching in the other direction and search for a better minimum, until a global minimum of both matching and tuning is obtained.

1.2.2 Tuning and Matching with an R.F. Bridge and an Oscilloscope

The probe-head is connected to an r.f. bridge and an oscilloscope as shown in Figure 1.4. The oscilloscope must be set to display the r.f . pulses. Tuning and matching is now adjusted as described above to obtain an oscilloscope pattern such that in the center of the pulse the r.f. amplitude is minimized, and only on the edges some signal is seen, as shown in Figure 1.5. The advantage of this method is that the tuning position can be found even in a grossly misadjusted probe-head. For experienced users this method is much more sensitive than using the reflection meter, but is more laborious.

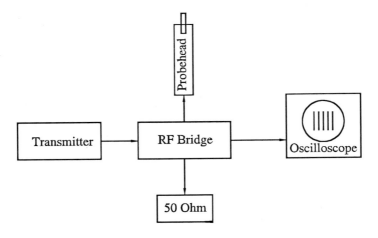

Fig. 1.4 R.f. bridge arrangement for probe-head tuning

Fig. 1.5 Oscilloscope pattern before and after tuning

1.2.3 Tuning and Matching with a Wobble Generator

Professionals tune the probe head with a wobble generator, which, in addition, provides a symmetry information of the frequency dependence of the tuning. In recently built NMR spectrometers wobbling functions are programmed in the software, thus making tuning and matching a very easy process which can be followed on the computer screen. One simply has to obtain the lowest point of the wobbling curve. Such a curve is shown in Figure 1.6.

Fig. 1.6 Wobbling curve during probe-head tuning

1.3   The Lock Channel

As neither magnetic fields nor frequencies derived from synthesizers are stable enough for a long period of time, high resolution NMR measurements require a special field/frequency stabilization to allow accumulation of signals, which may be separated by less than one Hz. The basic idea of this stabilization device, called the "lock", is to hold the resonance condition by a separate NMR experiment, which runs parallel to the one in the observe channel. As long as the lock signal is held in resonance the field/frequency relationship is defined also for the observe channel. Figure 1.7 shows the principles of the lock channel.

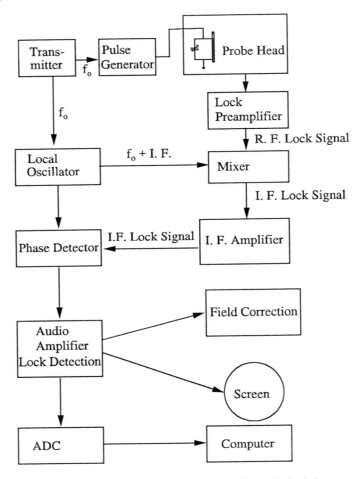

Figure 1.7 Schematic arrangement of the lock channel

Usually the ^2H resonance of the deuterated solvent is used to provide the NMR lock signal. Thus, an extra ^2H lock transmitter is needed, which transmits its frequency in pulsed form to the probe-head, in which the ^1H coil is often doubly tuned to both the ^1H and ^2H frequencies. The deuterium signal is preamplified and processed in the same way as the normal NMR signals in the observe channel. However, the final audio signal is used in dispersion mode to derive a negative or positive control voltage, which regulates the field position. Very recent developments employ a so-called digital lock, where the lock i.f. is fed directly into the ADC. The lock signal is displayed on the computer screen and provides a means of shimming the magnet. This is possible, because a narrower lock signal results in a higher d.c. voltage after rectification. Thus, by adjusting the various shim currents one aims for an optimum lock signal.

For special cases, e. g. for ^2H NMR spectroscopy, an ^{19}F lock is used instead of the ^2H resonance. The lock substance can be just the solvent, as described above, or may be provided within a capillary for chemical reasons. Special applications, such as probe-heads used as detectors for LC-NMR, use an external lock derived from an extra capillary within the probe-head.

On current NMR instruments, which are equipped with automatic sample changers, the lock capture and lock-in procedure is done by the instrument itself. However, any beginner in the NMR field should first learn how to do it manually. This is the basic start of any NMR experiment and a meaningful shimming procedure is only possible after having properly locked in.

There are several parameters which control the lock display on the computer screen. First, one needs a device to sweep the magnetic field (mostly forward and backward) over the lock resonance position, usually a sawtooth modulation. Its amplitude and sweep rate can be adjusted. Secondly, the position of the magnetic field must be adjusted to find the lock signal and to fix it at its lock-in position. The r.f. power of the lock transmitter, the gain of the lock receiver, and the phase and d.c. offset of the lock signal have to be correctly chosen. As for any NMR application, the lock transmitter power should not saturate the signal, and thus the lock transmitter must be sufficiently attenuated. The noise level of the receiver, however, should not be excessive. The lock-in procedure (i. e. pressing the "lock" button) automatically switches off the field sweep and holds the lock signal at its resonance position. After the lock-in procedure the operator should fine-adjust the magnetic field homogeneity by maximizing the lock signal level. Further attenuation adjustment of the transmitter power may be needed to ensure that the lock signal is not saturated.

If, for some reason, one wants to measure NMR spectra without the lock, one must turn off the field modulation manually; however, one has to be aware of the magnet field drift.

1.4 The Art of Shimming

The process of optimizing the magnetic field homogeneity for recording high resolution spectra is called "shimming" a magnet. Usually this is done by observing an NMR signal which has a natural line-width less than 0.1 Hz. This line-width corresponds to a homogeneity of the magnetic field better than 1 ppb for a 100 MHz spectrometer. Adjusting the homogeneity can be performed in different ways, by observing (i) a swept NMR signal (without lock), (ii) the lock level (with locking), or (iii) the FID or the area of the FID on the observe channel. The homogeneity is checked by the procedures described in Experiments 3.3, 3.4, and 3.6.

In the very first days of NMR spectroscopy shimming was performed mechanically (in the original meaning shims are small pieces of metal), but now an electronic device called the shim system is used for the shimming process. This device is essentially a set of coils causing very specific magnetic field contours. Because the homogeneity must be maintained over the total volume of NMR observation (probe coil), the shim system is installed in the room-temperature bore of the magnet and surrounds the probe-head and especially the sample region. The currents for the shim coils can create various gradients of any desired strength and shape and can be controlled separately by potentiometers from the spectrometer console. Table 1.1 shows the common room-temperature shims together with their specific functions and their interaction order. There is a second set of shims called cryoshims, which are adjusted during the installation of the magnet.

Table 1.1 Common room temperature shims with function and interaction order

Common Shim Name	Function	Gradient order	Inter-action order
Z0	1	0	0
Z1	z	1	0
Z2	$2z^2 - (x^2 + y^2)$	2	1
Z3	$z[2z^2 - 3(x^2 + y^2)]$	3	2
Z4	$8z^2[z^2 - 3(x^2 + y^2)] + 3(x^2 + y^2)^2$	4	2
Z5	$48z^3[z^2 - 5(x^2 + y^2)] + 90z(x^2 + y^2)^2$	5	2
X	x	1	0
Y	y	1	0
ZX	zx	2	2
ZY	zy	2	2
XY	xy	2	1
$X^2 - Y^2$	$x^2 - y^2$	2	1
Z^2X	$x[4z^2 - (x^2 + y^2)]$	3	2
Z^2Y	$y[4z^2 - (x^2 + y^2)]$	3	2
ZXY	zxy	3	2
$Z(X^2 - Y^2)$	$z(x^2 - y^2)$	3	2
X^3	$x(x^2 - 3y^2)$	3	1
Y^3	$y(3x^2 - y^2)$	3	1

1.4.1 The Shim Gradients

The different shims are also called shim gradients. One has to adjust the shim currents so that they cancel any gradients in the NMR sample as accurately as possible. There are two types of gradients: spinning ($Z0$–$Z5$) and non-spinning shims where z is the coordinate direction of the field B_0. Spinning the sample averages the field inhomogeneities along two axes but not along the axis about which the sample is spun. Therefore the shim procedure can be divided into two steps: shimming with and shimming without spinning the sample. Usually the sample spinning produces an amplitude modulation of the NMR signal, which gives rise to spinning sidebands on both sides of the signal. The spinning sidebands occur at integer multiples of the spinning frequency and become smaller as the homogeneity increases or the spinning rate is increased. Shimming is not a simple maximization process, because the shims have different gradient order and different interaction order (see Table 1.1). For the shim process you should use sample tubes with a filling height of 6 cm to avoid vortices. The following classification follows the gradient order. The total number of available shim gradients increases with the magnetic field strength of the magnet:

Zero order: The $Z0$ shim is the only zero order shim. This is the field position in most instruments.

First order: The $Z1$, X and Y shims are first order shims. These gradients produce a linear variation of magnetic field strength and have shapes like the p atomic orbitals. They are optimized by a simple maximization process; this corresponds to an interaction order of 0.

Second order: There are five second order shim gradients (see Table 1.1; on older instruments $Z2$ is called curvature), which have shapes like d atomic orbitals, e.g. $Z2$ corresponds to the d_{z^2} orbital. These gradients cause quadratic variations in field strength. For three of them the interaction order is 1, for the other two the interaction order is 2. First order interaction means that the shims are adjusted by an successive iterative process. After the adjustment of the complete set of shims, you have to readjust the first shim of the set and you will find a different optimum. Successive iterations will lead to smaller and smaller changes on readjustment until no further change is observed. A typical example is $Z1$ and $Z2$. After optimization of $Z1$ followed by $Z2$, you will find a new optimum for $Z1$ when readjusted. With an interaction order of 2 you have to change a given shim first and then adjust others before any improvement of the homogeneity can be observed. This means: change the shim a measured amount and optimize the other shims of the set. If this leads to a better response proceed to change the shim in the same direction another measured amount and repeat the process until the response (lock level or FID area) starts to decline. If the initial response is worse try the other direction.

Third order: The complete set of third order shims has seven different gradients corresponding to the shape of the seven f atomic orbitals. A complete set of these gradients is found on 600 and 750 MHz spectrometers. These gradients produce cubic variations of field strength. Usually there is only one 4th order and one 5th order shim gradient on high field instruments.

1.4.2 The Shimming Procedure

In the following shimming procedure, which is described very precisely by Conover [1], it is assumed that the sample is in the center of the shim-set. If this is not the case the center of the shim-set has to be located first. This is done by moving the sample with respect to the receiver coil. Usually the field centering has been performed by the manufacturer's engineer in the course of the installation of the magnet.

First Round

If the magnetic field is in a state of unknown homogeneity or is known to have poor homogeneity use the swept NMR signal, usually the deuterium lock signal, for the first steps in the shimming process. Otherwise proceed with the second round.

1. Spin the sample (20 to 30 Hz) and adjust the phase of the lock signal for absorption. The signal-to-noise ratio should be sufficient to allow height and the ring-down pattern (wiggles) to be observed. The ring down pattern can be used for the final adjustment. Adjust $Z1$ and $Z2$ interactively to produce the tallest swept signal (first order process).
2. Stop the spinner and adjust X and Y for the tallest swept signal response (first-order process).
3. Adjust X and ZX for the tallest swept signal (second-order process).
4. Adjust Y and ZY for the tallest swept signal (second-order process).
5. Adjust XY and $X2 - Y2$ for the tallest swept signal (first-order process)
6. If any large shim changes were observed in the above process than repeat the process from 1. The NMR spectrometer should now be capable of operating with a field-frequency lock.

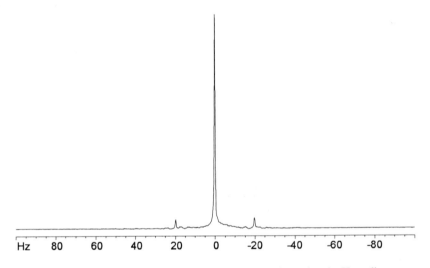

Fig. 1.8 Spinning sidebands obtained after incorrectly setting the X gradient

Second Round (Spinning Shims)

Spin the sample at 20 to 30 Hz, make sure that there is no vortex, especially if using a probe-head for 10 mm sample tubes. A vortex will lead to a false shim optimum, especially for $Z2$. If the lock signal is used for shimming, avoid saturation by using as low a lock power as possible. If the FID or FID area is used for shimming, use a pulse repetition time which is long enough for full relaxation; otherwise the NMR signal is saturated. The lock phase should be carefully adjusted and reexamined each time a large change is made to a shim with an even interaction order [$Z3$, $Z4$, $Z5$, ZX, ZY, Z^2X, Z^2Y, ZXY, $Z(X^2 - Y^2)$].

1. Optimize $Z1$ and $Z2$ (first order process).
2. Optimize $Z3$ (second order process). Note the setting of $Z3$ and the response. Change $Z3$ to degrade the response by 20–30%. Repeat the process in step 1. If

the new setting for Z3 has yielded a better response then continue in the same direction. If the new response is less then try the other direction for Z3.

3.   Optimize Z4 (second order process). Note the position of Z4 and the response. Change Z4 to degrade the response by 30–40%. Repeat the process in step 1. Adjust Z3 to provide the optimum response. If the Z3 shim change is considerable, then repeat step 1 again and readjust Z3 for maximum response. If, after optimizing Z3, Z2, and Z1, the new response is better than the previous one, continue in the same direction. If the response is worse then try the other direction.

4.   The Z5 shim normally needs to be adjusted only with wide-bore magnets and large-diameter sample tubes. Change Z5 enough to degrade the response by 30–50%. Repeat step 1 and reoptimize Z3. Adjust Z4 for maximum response. If either Z3 or Z4 changed by a considerable amount, repeat step 1 and reoptimize Z3 and Z4. If the new response obtained after this procedure is better than before, continue in the same direction. If the response is worse, try the other direction with Z5.

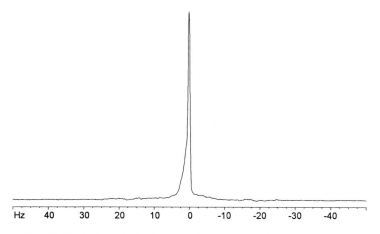

Fig. 1.9 Typical result obtained after incorrectly setting the Z4 gradient

Third Round (Non-spinning Shims)

This shim-set has to be adjusted while the sample is not spinning. Changing the shim gradients with Z-components causes changes in the spinning shim set. The spinning shim sequence should be repeated after completion of the non-spinning shim procedure, especially if one of the non-spinning shims changes significantly.

1.   Turn the spinner off. Adjust X and Y for maximum response (first-order process).

2.   Note the position of ZX and the response. Change ZX to degrade the response by 10% and adjust X for a maximum response. If the new response is better, continue in the same direction with ZX. If the response is less, try the opposite direction with ZX.

3.   Repeat step 2 but using the Y and ZY shims.

4.   Adjust XY and $X^2 - Y^2$ interactively (first-order process) for maximum response. If either XY or $X^2 - Y^2$ changed significantly then repeat steps 2 and 3.

5.   Adjust Z^2X (second-order process). Note the position of Z^2X and the response. Change Z^2X enough to degrade the response by 30%. Maximize the response with ZX. Optimize the response with X. If the new response is larger than the initial response continue with Z^2X in the same direction. If the response is less then try the other direction.

6.   Repeat step 5 but using Z^2Y, ZY and Y.

7.   Adjust ZXY (second-order process). Note the position of ZXY and the response. Change ZXY enough to degrade the response by 20%. Maximize the response with XY. If the new response is larger than the initial one, continue with ZXY in the same direction. If the response is less, try the other direction.

8.   Repeat step 7 but using $Z(X^2 - Y^2)$ and $X^2 - Y^2$.

9.   Adjust X^3 and X interactively for maximum response (first-order process).

10.   Adjust Y^3 and Y interactively for maximum response (first-order process).

11.   If the non-spinning shim settings have significantly changed, then repeat the second round. If there are significant changes in the spinning shims, repeat the non-spinning shim procedure also.

Final Round

After all spinning and non-spinning shim gradients have been optimized the NMR instrument should be delivering less than 0.5 Hz line-width with a good line-shape (see Exp. 3.3) and minimal spinning side bands.

Very recent developments use a probe-head with x, y, and z pulsed field gradients. With such a device it is in principle possible to record an image of the homogeneity. With that the computer calculates the required changes for good homogeneity and finds the optimum after a few iterations [3].

Literature

[1] W. W. Conover, *Top. Carbon-13 NMR Spectrosc.* **1983**, *4*, 37–51.

[2] *SAM 1.0, Shimming Simulation Software package for IBM-PC compatible Computers*, ACORN NMR, 46560 Fremont Blvd., Fremont, CA 94538-6482.

[3] J. Hu, T. Javaid, F. Arias-Mendoza, Z. Liu, R. McNamara, T. R. Brown, *J. Magn. Reson. Ser. B* **1995**, *108*, 213–219.

Chapter 2

Determination of the Pulse-Length

In pulsed Fourier transform NMR spectroscopy there is nothing more important than the use of correct radiofrequency pulses. This applies not only for advanced multipulse and multidimensional methods but for the most simple routine experiments as well. The use of a wrong excitation pulse can render all FT experiments insensitive and useless. Regular determinations of pulse-length (also often called pulse-width) are also necessary for instruments working in an automatic mode with a sample changer. Aging or malfunctioning components can increase the pulsewidth corresponding to the normal setting (e.g. 90°) and therefore degrade the performance of these spectrometers, if not corrected.

In this first experimental chapter we therefore provide five basic methods for measuring the pulse-width. First we describe the calibration of transmitter pulse-width both for ^1H and ^{13}C (Exps. 2.1–2.2) and of the ^1H decoupler pulse-width (Exp. 2.3). Corresponding experiments are then performed for the inverse mode of operation (Exps. 2.4–2.5). At the end of the chapter we show how the pulse-length is connected to radiofrequency power and the excitation bandwidth (Exp. 2.6). This provides important knowledge for the setting up more advanced experiments like those using spin-locks or selective pulses. The calibration of selective pulses is demonstrated in Chapter 7.

Literature

[1] A. E. Derome, *Modern NMR Techniques for Chemistry Research*, Pergamon, Oxford, **1987**, 67–77.
[2] E. Fukushima, S. B. W. Roeder, *Experimental Pulse NMR*, Addison Wesley, Reading, **1981**, 47–60.

Experiment 2.1

Determination of the 90° ^{1}H Transmitter Pulse-Length

1. Purpose

One of the basic requirements of NMR spectrometer operation is the knowledge of the 90° pulse-length. The 90° or $\pi/2$ pulse or in general the flip angle θ is important not only for routine operation, but also for 1D multipulse and multidimensional NMR experiments. The flip angle depends on the r.f. magnetic field strength B_1, the pulse-length p, and the gyromagnetic ratio γ of the nucleus under observation, as expressed in radians and in degrees by Equations (1) and (2).

$$\theta \, [\text{rad}] = \gamma B_1 \cdot p \tag{1}$$

$$\alpha \, [°] = (360/2\pi) \, \gamma B_1 \cdot p \tag{2}$$

Usually the 90° or $\pi/2$ pulse-length is determined by measuring the 180° (π) or 360° (2π) pulse-lengths since these pulses give a minimum signal. Here we present a description for the ^{1}H transmitter pulse calibration.

2. Literature

[1] J. K. M. Sanders, B. K. Hunter, *Modern NMR Spectroscopy*, 2nd Edition, Oxford University Press, Oxford,. **1993**, 33–34.
[2] D. Shaw, *Fourier Transform NMR Spectroscopy*, 2nd Edition, Elsevier, Amsterdam, New York, **1984**, Ch. 7.
[3] A. E. Derome, *Modern NMR Techniques for Chemistry Research*, Pergamon, Oxford, **1987**, 153–157.

3. Pulse Scheme and Phase Cycle

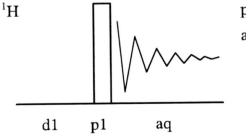

^{1}H

p1: x, x, -x, -x, y, y, -y, -y

aq: x, x, -x, -x, y, y, -y, -y

d1   p1   aq

4. Acquisition

Time requirement: 30 min

Sample: 10% CHCl₃ in [D₆]acetone; *do not use a degassed and sealed sample,* since that would make the relaxation time of the CHCl₃ protons exceedingly long.

The probe-head should be tuned to the sample. Load standard ¹H parameters, record a normal ¹H NMR spectrum and note the offset of CHCl₃. On older instruments change to the absolute intensity mode. You have to set:

> td: 4k
> sw: 500 Hz
> o1: on resonance of CHCl₃ signal
> p1: ¹H transmitter pulse, to be varied, 1 μs as initial value
> d1: 30 s
> rg: receiver gain for correct ADC input
> transmitter attenuation (3 dB)
> ns: 1

Increase p1 in 2 μs steps until the intensity of the processed signal begins to drop to nearly zero. Now use smaller steps in increasing p1, e.g. 0.1 μs, to find the minimum for the 180° pulse. With the determined pulse-length check the 90° pulse (maximum positive intensity), the 270° pulse (maximum negative intensity) and the 360° pulse (minimum intensity). If there are small deviations, calculate an average value for the 90° pulse-length. In case of large deviations repeat the procedure. If the deviations are still present, the probe-head may be arcing; increase the transmitter attenuation.

5. Processing

Use standard 1D processing (see Exp. 3.1) applying an exponential window with a line-broadening factor lb = 1 Hz. Adjust the phase of the first spectrum for pure absorption and always use the same phase correction.

6. Result

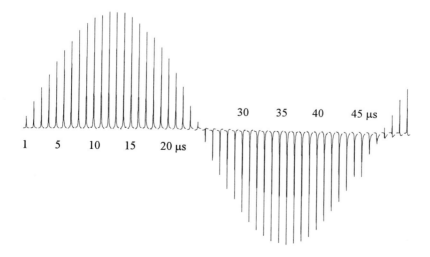

The figure on page 15 shows the full sinusoidal dependence of the signal intensity obtained on an AM-400 spectrometer with a 5 mm dual probe-head. The pulse-width was incremented in steps of 1 µs; the 90° pulse-length was determined as 12.5 µs.

7. Comments

It is important to avoid using too short a pulse repetition time. The delay between successive measurements should be 5 times T_1. Even for protons in small molecules like $CHCl_3$ this can pose a problem, if the sample is degassed. For nuclei with long relaxation times it is more convenient to measure the 360° pulse-length.

In the rotating frame the r.f. pulse rotates the magnetization vector $M_0 = M_z$, creating an observable transverse magnetization M_{xy}. After a 180° pulse M_{xy} is theoretically zero and $M_0 = -M_z$, but in practice residual signals caused by inhomogeneities in B_1 can be seen.

The typical pulse-length for all probe-heads should be recorded in the logbook of the instrument.

8. Own Observations

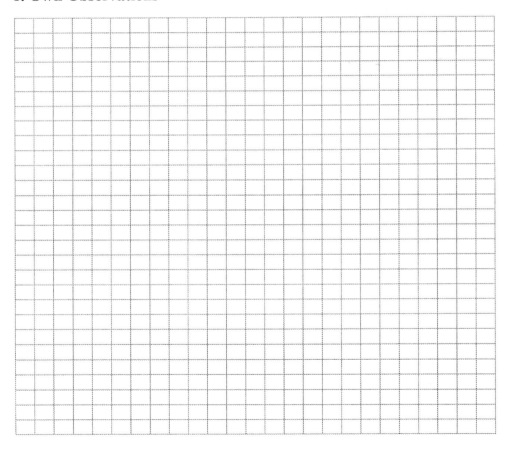

Experiment 2.2

Determination of the 90° ¹³C Transmitter Pulse-Length

1. Purpose

This experiment is very similar to Experiment 2.1. Here, however, the pulse width determination is decribed for the ^{13}C nucleus and has to be performed with broad band proton decoupling. Although the experiment could be performed exactly like exp. 2.1 we describe here a procedure given by [4] which yields the 90° pulse by just two measurements. This method is helpful for very slowly relaxing nuclei.

2. Literature

[1] J. K. M. Sanders, B. K. Hunter, *Modern NMR Spectroscopy,* 2nd Edition, Oxford University Press, Oxford, **1993**, 33–34.
[2] D. Shaw, *Fourier Transform NMR Spectroscopy,* 2nd Edition, Elsevier, Amsterdam, New York, 2.Edition **1984**, Ch. 7.
[3] A. E. Derome, *Modern NMR Techniques for Chemistry Research*, Pergamon, Oxford, **1987**, 153–157.
[4] E. Haupt, *J. Magn. Reson.* **1982**, *49*, 358–364.

3. Pulse Scheme and Phase Cycle

p1: x, x, -x, -x, y, y, -y, -y
aq: x, x, -x, -x, y, y, -y, -y

4. Acquisition

Time requirement: 15 min

Sample: 40% CHCl₃ in [D₆]acetone; *do not use a degassed and sealed sample,* since that would make the relaxation time of the CHCl₃ carbons exceedingly long.

The probe-head should be tuned to the sample. Load standard ^{13}C parameters with ^1H broad-band decoupling, record a normal ^{13}C NMR spectrum and note the offset of $CHCl_3$. On older instruments change to the absolute intensity mode. You have to set:

td: 4k
sw: 500 Hz
o1: on resonance of ^{13}C signal
o2: middle of ^1H NMR spectrum
p1: ^{13}C transmitter pulse, 7 µs for experiment a and 14 µs for experiment b
d1: 60 s
rg: receiver gain for correct ADC input
transmitter attenuation (3dB)
decoupler attenuation and 90° pulse for CPD
ns: 1

Record spectrum **a** with p1 = 7 µs and spectrum **b** with p1 = 14 µs. Note the heights I_1 and I_2 of the $CHCl_3$ signal in these two spectra. If the pulse-width in the second experiment is double that in the first experiment, Equation (1) holds, from which the pulse angle α_1 (in degrees) of the first experiment can be calculated:

$$\alpha_1 = \ \text{arccos} \ (0.5 \ I_2/I_1) \tag{1}$$

Using Equation (2) the 90° pulse-length p_{90} can be calculated, where p1 is the pulse-length of the *first* experiment. p_{90} should be checked by applying the corresponding 180° pulse.

$$p_{90} = 90 \ p1 \ / \ \alpha_1 \tag{2}$$

5. Processing

Use standard 1D processing (see Exp. 3.2) applying an exponential window with a line-broadening factor lb = 1 Hz. Adjust the phase of the first spectrum for absorption and use the same phase correction for the second experiment.

6. Result

The figure on page 18 shows the result obtained on an AM-400 spectrometer with a 5 mm dual probe-head. Spectrum **a** (p1: 7 μs) yielded $I_1 = 12.43$, spectrum **b** (p1: 14 μs) yielded $I_2 = 2.56$. According to Equation (1) α_1 is calculated to be 84°, and using Equation (2) gives p90 to be 7.5 μs. This was checked in **c** using p1 = 15 μs.

7. Comments

This procedure is very convenient if one does not know anything about the pulse-length, e.g. if one is using a probe-head for the very first time or studying a heteronuclide for the first time. The method works best if α_1 can be estimated to about 60°.

The pulse-width determinations in Experiments 2.1 and 2.2 use a narrow spectral width of only 500 Hz and the transmitter on resonance. Note that radiofrequency pulse-lengths are offset-dependent, the 180° pulse-length especially is quite different for signals with different offsets.

8. Own Observations

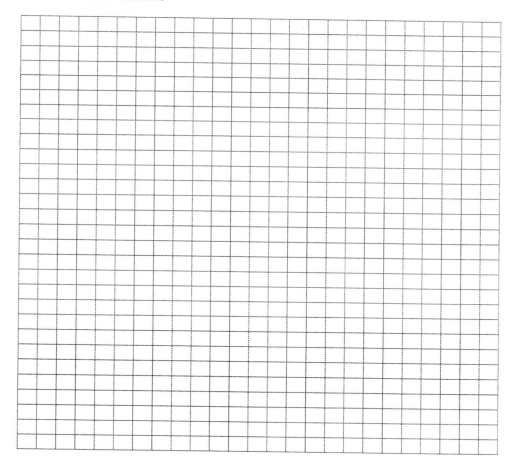

Experiment 2.3

Determination of the 90° ^{1}H Decoupler Pulse-Length

1. Purpose

Many 1D and 2D multipulse sequences use defined ^{1}H decoupling pulses. Without knowledge of these pulses some important experiments such as DEPT (Exp. 6.9) or HETCOR (Exp. 10.8) cannot be performed. Furthermore, the common broad-band decoupling technique for ^{13}C NMR spectroscopy, which uses composite pulses (CPD), fails if the decoupling pulse is wrong. This experiment has typically to be performed twice, once with low attenuation of the decoupler to calibrate the "hard" pulses which are used during a pulse sequence and once with high attenuation of the decoupler to define the pulses used for CPD.

2. Literature

[1] A. Bax, *J. Magn. Reson.* **1983**, *52*, 76–80.

3. Pulse Scheme and Phase Cycle

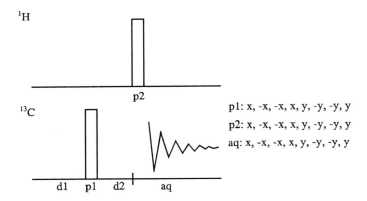

p1: x, -x, -x, x, y, -y, -y, y
p2: x, -x, -x, x, y, -y, -y, y
aq: x, -x, -x, x, y, -y, -y, y

4. Practical Procedure

Time requirement: 10 min

Sample: 50% CHCl$_3$ in [D$_6$]acetone, *do not use a degassed and sealed sample* since that would make the relaxation times of carbons and protons exceedingly long.

Obtain both offsets for the ^{1}H and ^{13}C signals of the sample. Load the pulse program for the sequence shown above. You have to set:

td: 4k
sw: 500 Hz

o1: on resonance of ^{13}C signal
o2: on resonance of ^{1}H signal
p1: 90° ^{13}C transmitter pulse (Exp. 2.2)
p2: ^{1}H decoupler pulse, 0 µs as starting value, to be varied
d1: 60 s
d2: 1/[2 J(C,H)] = 2.36 ms for ^{1}J(C,H) = 212 Hz
rg: receiver gain for correct ADC input
decoupler attenuation level
ns: 1

Record a first spectrum with p2 = 0 and adjust the doublet in antiphase. Then repeat the experiment with increasing pulse lengths p2 until the signals disappear, which corresponds to the 90° hard decoupler pulse.
    In a second set of experiments use high decoupler attenuation for CPD and vary it so that p2 is in the region of 100 µs.

5. Processing

Use standard 1D processing (see Exp. 3.2) applying an exponential window with a line-broadening factor lb = 2 Hz.

6. Result

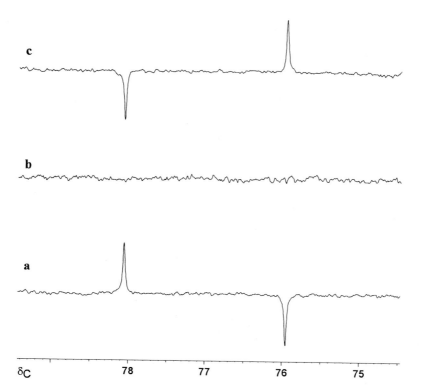

The figure on page 21 shows the result of a 0° decoupling pulse (**a**) and of a 90° de-coupling pulse (**b**) obtained on an AM-400 spectrometer with a 5mm dual probe-head. Note the disappearance of the signals in **b**. The spectrum **c** was obtained with a 180° pulse.

7. Comments

We consider a $^{13}C,^{1}H$ spin pair. The equilibrium magnetization is converted by the 90° ^{13}C pulse into a transverse ^{13}C magnetization as described by Equation (1).

$$I_{Cz} + I_{Hz} \xrightarrow{\quad 90°\ I_{Cx}\quad} -I_{Cy} + I_{Hz} \tag{1}$$

During the period $\tau = d2 = 1/2J$ spin–spin coupling between proton and ^{13}C evolves, as in Equation (2).

$$-I_{Cy} + I_{Hz} \xrightarrow{\quad \pi J\,\tau\,2I_{Hz}I_{Cz}\quad} 2I_{Cx}I_{Hz}\sin\pi J\tau - I_{Cy}\cos\pi J\tau + I_{Hz} \tag{2}$$

Since τ was set to $1/2J$, (2) simplifies to (3).

$$2I_{Cx}I_{Hz}\sin\pi J\tau - I_{Cy}\cos\pi J\tau + I_{Hz} \;=\; 2I_{Cx}I_{Hz} + I_{Hz} \tag{3}$$

A 90_x ^{1}H pulse converts $2I_{Cx}I_{Hz}$ into double quantum magnetization as in Equation (4), from which no observable ^{13}C signal can be generated. Thus, if the decoupling pulse is exactly 90°, the doublet disappears.

$$2I_{Cx}I_{Hz} + I_{Hz} \xrightarrow{\quad 90°\ I_{Hx}\quad} -2I_{Cx}I_{Hy} - I_{Hy} \tag{4}$$

Note that with this method, in contrast to Experiments 2.1 and 2.2, the 90° pulse yields a minimum signal, whereas the 180° pulse rotates the initial phases of the doublet.

8. Own Observations

Experiment 2.4

The 90° ¹H Pulse with Inverse Spectrometer Configuration

1. Purpose

In "inverse" experiments one observes protons and decouples heteronuclei X (e.g. ^{13}C, ^{15}N). On NMR instruments built later than 1991 the pulse-lengths in normal and inverse modes are usually quite similar. Older instruments, however, use different r.f. sources and signal routings in these two configurations. Therefore, before starting an inverse experiment, such as an HMQC experiment (Exp. 10.11), the pulse-lengths of protons and X nuclei have to be determined in this spectrometer configuration. This can be done exactly as described in Experiment 2.1. Here, however, we describe the 360° method.

2. Literature

[1] E. Fukushima, S. B. W. Roeder, *Experimental Pulse NMR* Addison Wesley, Reading, **1981**, 47–60.

3. Pulse Scheme and Phase Cycle

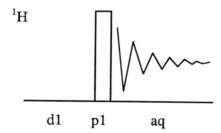

¹H

p1: x, x, -x, -x, y, y, -y, -y

aq: x, x, -x, -x, y, y, -y, -y

d1   p1   aq

4. Acquisition

Time requirement: 10 min

Sample: 3% CHCl₃ in [D₆]acetone, *do not use a degassed and sealed sample* since that would make the relaxation times of the protons exceedingly long.

An inverse probe-head (inner coil ¹H, outer coil ^{13}C or other heteronuclei) is placed into the magnet, both coils are tuned to the sample. On older instruments change to the inverse set-up. Since the inverse set-up varies widely depending on the year of spectrometer's construction it cannot be discussed here. Load the correct pulse program to obtain an inverse ¹H NMR spectrum. You have to set:

    td: 4k
    sw: 500 Hz

o1: 100 Hz towards higher frequency of $CHCl_3$ signal
p1: ^1H transmitter pulse, near 360° as starting value, to be varied
d1: 5 s
rg: receiver gain for correct ADC input
ns: 8

Set the pulse-width approximately to 360°, typically in the order of 40 µs, and record 8 transients. If the pulse-width is not exactly 360° a large FID signal will build up during the accumulation. Change the pulse-width until you observe a minimum FID signal. Divide the value by 4 and by 2 and check with the 90° and 180° pulses using one transient in each case.

5. Processing

No signal processing is required, since the FID is directly observed.

6. Result

The figure shows the result obtained on an AM-400 spectrometer in the inverse mode. In **a** p1 was 39 µs, in **b** 40 µs and in **c** 41 µs. Note how the signal area changes if the pulse-width is increased only by 1 µs, which corresponds to a change of 0.25 µs for the 90° pulse.

7. Comments

The advantage of the method is that no long waiting times are needed to allow spin–lattice relaxation. R.f. pulses which are close to 360° will change the magnetization vector only slightly. The method is very sensitive, since already small deviations from 360° will cause a large FID signal.

Inverse experiments can be performed in normal probe-heads as well. As an exercise you may measure the pulse-length using a standard dual probe-head.

8. Own Observations

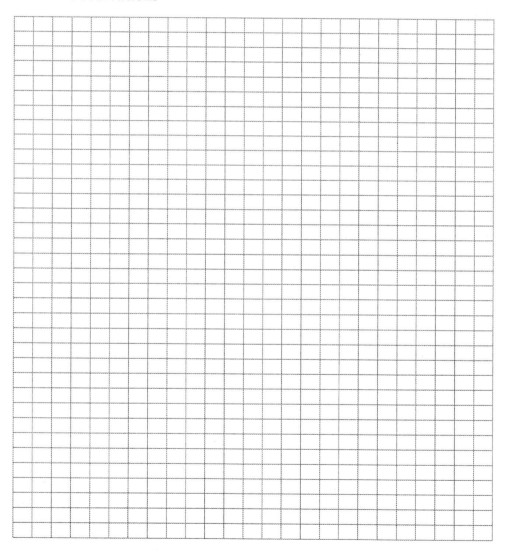

Experiment 2.5

The 90° 13C Decoupler Pulse with Inverse Configuration

1. Purpose

In "inverse" experiments one observes protons and decouples heteronuclei X (e.g. ^{13}C, ^{15}N). On NMR instruments built later than 1991 the pulse-lengths in normal and inverse set-up are usually quite similar. Older instruments, however, use quite different signal routings and r.f. sources in these two configurations. Therefore, before starting an inverse experiment, such as an HMQC experiment (Exp. 10.11), the pulse-lengths have to be determined in this spectrometer configuration. Here the ^{13}C decoupling pulse is determined; prior to this experiment you have to perform Experiment 2.4. Depending on the attenuation of the decoupler the pulse-lengths are quite different. Short ("hard") pulses with low decoupler attenuation are used for 90° or 180° pulses during a pulse sequence, whereas long pulses with high decoupler attenuation are needed for composite pulse decoupling such as GARP during acquisition. Thus, this experiment has typically to be performed twice, once with low and once with high attenuation of the decoupler.

2. Literature

[1] A. Bax, *J. Magn. Reson.* **1983**, *52*, 76–80.

3. Pulse Scheme and Phase Cycle

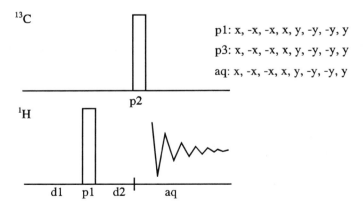

p1: x, -x, -x, x, y, -y, -y, y
p3: x, -x, -x, x, y, -y, -y, y
aq: x, -x, -x, x, y, -y, -y, y

4. Acquisition

Time requirement: 10 min

Sample: 10% $CHCl_3$ in [D_6]acetone, *do not use a degassed and sealed sample* since that would make the relaxation times of carbons and protons exceedingly long.

Obtain both offsets for the ^1H and ^{13}C signals of the sample with the spectrometer in the normal mode and tune both coils to the sample. Older spectrometers are then changed to inverse set-up, and an inverse probe-head (inner coil ^1H, outer coil ^{13}C) is placed into the magnet. Since the inverse set-up varies widely dependent on the year of spectrometer's construction it cannot be discussed here. Load the correct pulse program to obtain an inverse ^1H NMR spectrum with ^{13}C decoupling. You have to set:

    td: 4k
    sw: 500 Hz
    o1: on resonance of ^1H signal
    o2: on resonance of ^{13}C signal
    p1: 90° ^1H transmitter pulse in inverse configuration (Exp. 2.4)
    p2: ^{13}C decoupler pulse in inverse configuration, 0 µs as starting value, to be varied
    d1: 20 s
    d2: $1/[2\,J(C,H)] = 2.33$ ms for $^1J(C,H) = 215$ Hz
    rg: receiver gain for correct ADC input
    ^{13}C decoupler attenuation
    ns: 1

Record a first spectrum with p2 = 0 and adjust the phase of the big signal stemming from the protons bound to ^{12}C in dispersion; look for a clean anti phase pattern of the ^{13}C satellites. Then repeat the experiment with increasing pulse-lengths p2 until you get a zero for the satellites, which corresponds to the 90° decoupler pulse.

    In a second set of experiments use a high decoupler attenuation for GARP and vary it so that p2 is in the region of 70 µs.

5. Processing

Use standard 1D processing (see Exp. 3.1) applying an exponential window with a line-broadening factor lb = 1 Hz.

6. Result

The figure on page 28 shows the results of a 0° decoupling pulse (**a**) and of a 90° decoupling pulse (**b**) obtained on an AMX-500 spectrometer with an inverse probe-head. Note the disappearance of the satellites in (**b**).

7. Comments

The product operator formalism is exactly the same as given in Experiment 2.3, only the notation for C and H spins has to be interchanged. If this method is used to determine ^{13}C decoupler pulses for GARP decoupling, be sure that the chosen ^{13}C offset is correct.

    Inverse experiments can be performed in normal probe-heads as well. As an exercise you may measure the pulse-length using a standard dual probe-head.

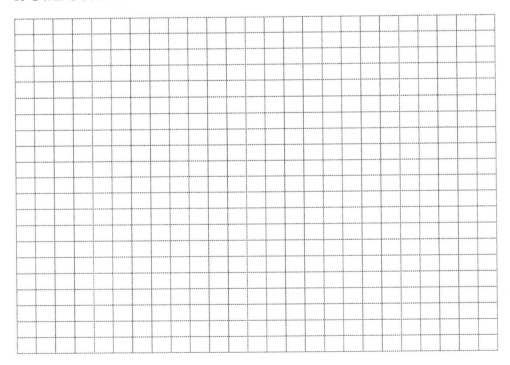

8. Own Observations

Experiment 2.6

Determination of Radiofrequency Power

1. Purpose

In many experiments the transmitter or decoupler power is attenuated to produce a radiofrequency field of a certain strength. This is needed e.g. for presaturation to suppress water signals (Exp. 6.15), for SPT investigations (Exp. 4.5), for TOCSY (Exp. 10.15), or for ROESY (Exp 10.17) experiments. The NMR literature uses a variety of measures to describe the power of a frequency source. In the experiment described here the fundamental parameters 90° pulse-width [µs], transmitter attenuation [dB], transmitter power [W], radiofrequency field strength [Hz] and peak to peak voltage [V] are measured and interrelated in a tabular form. The example is chosen from ^{1}H NMR spectroscopy, but the procedure can be used for any nucleus. In addition to a deeper understanding of the function of a frequency source, this experiment provides a check on the performance of the transmitter and the attenuators.

2. Literature

[1] M. L. Martin, J. J. Delpuech and G. J. Martin, *Practical NMR Spectroscopy*, Heyden, London, **1980**, p. 100–101.

3. Pulsescheme and Phase Cycle

^{1}H

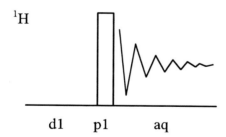

d1   p1   aq

p1: x, x, -x, -x, y, y, -y, -y

aq: x, x, -x, -x, y, y, -y, -y

4. Acquisition

Time requirement: 2 h

Sample 10% CHCl$_3$ in [D$_6$]acetone

Experimentally, this is a 90° pulse-width determination (actually performed by finding the 180° pulse), exactly as described in Experiment 2.1. However, in addition, we vary the transmitter attenuation and determine the pulse-width as a function of transmitter attenuation. On older instruments which do not allow variation of the transmitter power, the experiment can be performed in the inverse mode using the decoupler as the frequency source (Exp. 2.4). Load standard ^{1}H NMR parameters, record a normal ^{1}H NMR spectrum, and note the offset of CHCl$_3$. You have to set:

td: 4k
sw: 500 Hz
o1: on resonance of ^{1}H signal
p1: 90° ^{1}H transmitter pulse, to be determined for each attenuation level
d1: 60 s
ns: 1
transmitter attenuation: 0 dB initial value, to be increased in 3 dB steps

Determine the 90° pulse-width at 0 dB attenuation. Then change the attenuation in 3 dB steps and redetermine the 90° pulse width for each attenuation level by varying p1. If available, measure with an oscilloscope the peak-to-peak voltage of your pulse (for this set ns to 64k, d1 to 10 ms, p1 to 40 µs and td to 256 points in order to obtain rapid pulsing; connect the transmitter cable to an external attenuator and an oscilloscope with 50 Ω impedance).

5. Processing

Use standard 1D processing (see Exp. 3.1) applying an exponential window with a line-broadening factor lb = 1 Hz. From the 90° pulse-width calculate the radiofrequency field using Equation (3). Verify that the expected values correspond to the attenuation. Note the large power range, from 0 to 90 dB, required in different types of NMR experiments.

6. Result

The table lists results obtained with an ARX-200 spectrometer.

Attenuation [dB]	90°Pulse width [µs]	γB_1 [Hz]	U_{pp} [V]	P [W]
0	7.8	32051	107	28.6
3	10.3	24271	82	16.8
6	13	19230	59	8.7
9	19.5	12820	41	4.2
12	27.5	9090	29	2.1
15	39.5	6329	20	1.
18	55	4545	15	0.56
21	75	3333	11	0.30
24	105	2380	7.9	0.16
27	145	1724	5.9	0.087
30	200	1250	4.3	0.046
33	290	862	3.3	0.027
36	425	588	2.2	0.012
39	600	416	1.6	0.0064
42	825	303	1.3	0.0042

45	1100	227	1	0.0025
48	1600	156	0.74	0.0014
51	2400	104	0.46	0.00053
54	3500	71	0.33	0.00027
57	5000	50	0.23	0.00013
60	6800	37	0.17	0.000072
63	9000	28	0.13	0.000042
66	12500	20	0.099	0.000024
69	19000	13	0.073	0.000013
72	28500	9	0.054	0.0000073
75	41000	6	0.043	0.0000046
78	55600	4.5	*	
81	80000	3	*	
84	110000	2.3	*	
87	145000	1.7	*	
90	200000	1.25	*	

* oscilloscope used not sensitive enough

7. Comments

The magnetization vector precesses around the radiofrequency field B_1 according to Equation (1).

$$\omega = 2\pi v = \gamma B_1 \tag{1}$$

The angle of precession θ, measured in radians, is proportional to the pulse-width p and is given by Equation (2). For a 90° pulse ($\theta = \pi/2$) Equation (3) follows from (1) and (2).

$$\theta = \gamma B_1 \cdot p \tag{2}$$

$$\gamma B_1 = \frac{1}{4p} \tag{3}$$

Thus, knowing the pulse-width of a 90° pulse at a certain transmitter attenuation, we can estimate the radiofrequency field strength γB_1 measured in Hz from the simple relationship in Equation (3).

The dB unit used on NMR instruments is defined by Equation (4).

$$dB \equiv 10 \log (P/P_0) \tag{4}$$

Thus, attenuation by 3 dB means, that the ratio P/P_0 decreases by a factor of 2. The power P of a transmitter measured in watt is given by Equation (5).

$$P = \frac{U_{\text{eff}}^2}{R} \tag{5}$$

U_{eff} is the effective voltage, which is equal to $\dfrac{U_{\text{pp}}}{2\sqrt{2}}$, and R is the load resistance. By measuring the peak to peak voltage U_{pp} on a 50 ohm load one can calculate the transmitter power in watt. The strength of the radiofrequency field is proportional to the square root of the transmitter power, as evident from Equation (6), and is therefore proportional to the peak to peak voltage measured with an oscilloscope. It can be calculated in tesla (SI magnetic field unit) from equation (6) if the quality factor Q, the frequency v, and the volume V of the NMR coil are known.

$$B_1 = 3 \cdot 10^{-4} \sqrt{\frac{PQ}{vV}} \tag{6}$$

On recent NMR instruments one also finds the unit dBm. Whereas dB is a relative unit, dBm refers to a P_0 of 1 mW, as given in Equation (7).

$$\text{dBm} = 10 \log(P/\ 1 \text{ mW}) \tag{7}$$

Thus, the power of 1 mW corresponds to a dBm value of 0, 1 W corresponds to 30 dBm and 1 µW to −30 dBm.

8. Own Observations

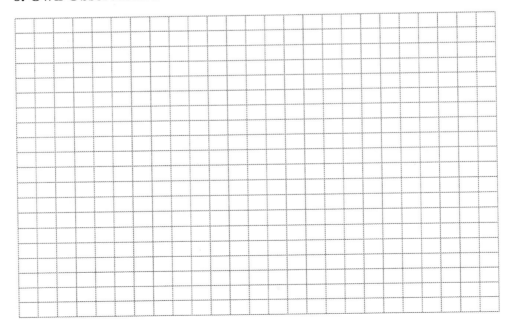

Chapter 3

Routine NMR Spectroscopy and Standard Tests

This chapter begins by describing how to record standard ^1H and ^{13}C NMR spectra. These descriptions are somewhat detailed, so that a beginner in this field should find sufficient advice. Furthermore, we describe in this chapter several important test procedures which are essential for the maintenance of instruments getting on in years. Performed regularly they give an early indication of developing problems.

Since a great variety of spectrometers and, much more important, of field strengths exists, one should have in mind all the possible consequences thereof when performing the experiments at a field strength different from that used here and comparing the results. These include the following:

1. The experimental time given depends on the acquisition time, since it is determined by the spectral width, entered in Hz and thus depending on field strength (and sometimes on the way the data are transferred to disk). It should be mentioned here that the time given for each experiment only roughly represents the time from the starting command just to the last acquisition step; preparations, setting-up, processing and output are not included.

2. At different field strength the appearance of a spectrum may change due to differences in the extent of signal overlap and to higher-order effects in spectra of spin-coupled nuclei.

3. The field strength also affects the digital resolution (for a given spectral width and time-domain data file); the data file and/or the processing parameters may be changed accordingly

4. At other field strengths the relaxation behaviour may be different, with consequences for the line-widths.

5. The signal-to-noise ratio depends on field strength (also, for example, on the probe-head used and on its tuning).

Literature

[1] M. L. Martin, J. J. Delpuech, G. J. Martin, *Practical NMR Spectroscopy*, Heyden, London, **1980**.
[2] A. E. Derome, *Modern NMR Techniques for Chemistry Research*, Pergamon, Oxford, **1987**.
[3] E. Fukushima, S. B. W. Roeder, *Experimental Pulse NMR*, Addison-Wesley, Reading, **1981**.

Experiment 3.1

The Standard ^{1}H NMR Experiment

1. Purpose

The aim of the standard ^{1}H NMR Experiment is to record a routine proton NMR spectrum in order to get structure-related information for the protons of the sample, i.e. chemical shifts, spin–spin couplings, and intensities. Here we apply this standard procedure to ethyl crotonate.

2. Literature

[1] A. E. Derome, *Modern NMR Techniques for Chemistry Research*, Pergamon, Oxford, **1987**.
[2] K. K. M. Sanders, B. K. Hunter, *Modern NMR Spectroscopy*, 2nd Edition, Oxford University Press, Oxford, **1993**.
[3] H. P. Friebolin, *Basic One- and Two- Dimensional NMR Spectroscopy*, 2nd Edition, VCH, Weinheim, **1993**.
[4] H. Günther, *NMR Spectroscopy*, 2nd Edition, Wiley, Chichester, **1995**.

3. Pulse Scheme and Phase Cycle

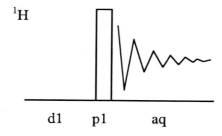

^{1}H

p1: x, x, -x, -x, y, y, -y, -y

aq: x, x, -x, -x, y, y, -y, -y

d1   p1   aq

4. Acquisition

Time requirement: 5 min

Sample: 5% ethyl crotonate in CDCl$_3$ with TMS as standard

For sample preparation fill a clean and dry 5 mm sample tube with 0.7 ml CDCl$_3$ (5 cm filling height), 40 µl ethyl crotonate, and few drops of a solution of 3% TMS in CDCl$_3$ (for easier dosage). Clean the tube outside, close it with a cap, mark it (do not use a flag-like label which hinders rotation) and put it into the spinner turbine. Be sure that it is tight, but not too tight in the spinner, and adjust the depth of the tube using the depth gauge.

Put the tube into the magnet by means of the air lift, adjust the rotation frequency (20 Hz), and display the lock signal on the screen. Perform the lock procedure and optimize the field homogeneity (see Ch. 1, Section 1.4).

The spectrometer is to be adjusted for ¹H observation in quadrature detection mode. Load the ¹H acquisition program, which comprises the following basic commands: zero memory, set the relaxation delay, set the excitation pulse, perform acquisition, and write the data on file.

For acquisition the following parameters have to be set:

td: 32 k

td (time domain) is the number of points at which the free induction decay (FID) is sampled and the data stored. This parameter has to be chosen according to the desired digital resolution of the FID, which in turn depends on the spectral width sw. The settings of td and sw determine the acquisition time aq.

sw: 20 ppm

sw, the spectral width, has to be chosen so that all types of protons are within this spectral window; otherwise folding occurs. Folding of noise is prevented by appropriate filters which are set by the software corresponding to sw. The settings of sw and td determine the *acquisition time* aq, the time during which the FID data are acquired. The relationship between these three parameters, where aq is usually the dependent variable and sw has to be expressed in Hz, is described by the following fundamental equation (1):

$$aq = td/(2 \text{ sw}) \tag{1}$$

Thus, with the above settings at 300 MHz, the acquisition time is 2.7 s.

o1: frequency (offset) *of the r.f. pulse at the center of the ¹H NMR spectrum:*
In quadrature detection mode the frequency of the exciting r.f. pulse (often called transmitter offset) is positioned in the center of sw, e.g. at about $\delta_H = 7$. On older instruments without digital lock, o1 depends on the field position of the deuterium lock and thus on the deuterated solvent used.

p1: 30°

p1, the ¹H transmitter pulse, creates an observable x,y-magnetization by tipping the magnetization vector towards the $-y$-axis through an angle α, determined by Equation (2):

$$\alpha = (360/2\pi) \gamma B_1 \cdot p \tag{2}$$

where γ is the proton gyromagnetic ratio, γB_1 the field strength of the radiofrequency field, and p the duration of the pulse. Since p1 is known for a flip angle $\alpha = 90°$ (see exp. 2.1), the duration of p1 corresponding to 30° is easily obtained.

Although a 90° pulse gives maximum signal intensity (Exp. 2.1), a shorter pulse-length of about 30° is used for routine work with data accumulation in order to avoid a long pulse repetition time of 5 T_1, which is necessary after a 90° pulse (see d1).

It should be mentioned here that between the irradiating pulse and the opening of the detector a *preacquisition delay* is introduced. It prevents the break-through of the transmitter pulse into the detector, is in the order of 10 to 100 µs, and is automatically calculated and set by the software.

d1: 0.1 s

d1, the relaxation delay, is introduced in order to establish thermal equilibrium of the spin system before the excitation pulse is applied. In routine ^{1}H NMR work with small flip angles and relatively long acquisition times, this delay may be short, especially for larger molecules with short T_1-values, since it is the *pulse repetition time*, the sum of aq and d1, which serves for spin–lattice relaxation.

ns: 8

ns, the number of "scans" (individual FIDs), is chosen so that a reasonable signal-to-noise ratio is obtained in the final spectrum. Because of phase cycling a multiple of 8 and a minimum of 4 is advisable.

rg:

rg, the receiver gain, has to be carefully adjusted so that the incoming FID does not exceed the ADC input limits. Otherwise signal distortions at the baseline will occur after Fourier transformation.

5. Processing

After data acquisition you have to process the data. Perform the following steps using the given settings:

size of the processed real data file: set **si = 16 k**. Normally si corresponds to td/2 (see acquisition), since, after Fourier transformation, half of the td data adresses contain the real part of the spectrum. This gives a digital resolution (Hz/data point) after Fourier transformation of 2 sw/td. (Note that on the older Bruker instrument series the parameter SI corresponds to 2 si of the newer ones.)

However, si may be set to a value greater than td/2, e.g. si = 32 k; this procedure is termed "zero filling" and leads, according to Equation (3) for the general case, to a higher digital resolution:

$$\text{digital resolution} = \text{sw/si} \tag{3}$$

With the above data, the digital resolution is 0.37 Hz/point, a reasonable value in comparison to the line-width usually obtained for a non-degassed sample. If a higher digital resolution is desired, one may optimize sw, increase td, or perform zero filling.

baseline correction: perform this correction on the *FID* in order to eliminate the d.c. offset between the two channels used in quadrature detection mode.

digital filtering: for standard applications use as window function an exponential window on the FID, characterized by the line-broadening factor lb; here set **lb = 0.1 Hz**. This type of digital filtering generally improves the signal-to-noise ratio, but at the cost of resolution. Here a very mild filtering is used since there is no signal-to-noise problem. On the other hand, by applying a Lorentz–Gauss multiplication, a resolution enhancement may be achieved; here one has to pay with a reduction of the signal-to-noise ratio.

Fourier transformation: use the correct type in accordance with the simultaneous or sequential quadrature acquisition mode.

phase correction: adjust to achieve pure absorption mode signals.

baseline correction: perform this correction on the *spectrum* in order to remove baseline rolling.

referencing: set the TMS signal to $\delta_H = 0$.

peak picking: choose the desired level.

integration: carefully generate the integrals.

plot: set parameters and plot spectrum, including integrals, peak picking, and the relevant acquisition and processing parameters.

6. Result

The figure shows the 300 MHz ¹H NMR spectrum of ethyl crotonate recorded on an ARX-300 spectrometer equipped with a dual probe-head; the region $\delta_H = -0.5$ to 7.5 including the integrals is displayed. The insert contains an expansion of the signal at ca. $\delta_H = 7$ (H-3) so that the coupling constants can be determined.

A closer inspection of the integrals reveals that those of H-2 and H-3 are too small as compared to the integrals of the two methyl groups. This may be due to the fact that the T_1 values of the protons of ethyl crotonate are relatively long *and* somewhat shorter for the two CH₃ groups than for H-2 and H-3. As an exercise you should perform the experiment with d1 = 3 s, corresponding to a pulse repetition time of nearly 6 s. (Concerning the determination of T_1 values see Exp. 6.1).

7. Comments

The excitation pulse p1 converts the equilibrium magnetization I_{Hz} of the ^1H nuclei into a transverse magnetization $-I_{Hy}$ as shown in Equation (1). During the acquisition time chemical shifts and spin–spin couplings develop in the x,y plane, as shown separately in Equations (2) and (3) and are detected by the receiver in the x,y plane in quadrature mode.

$$I_{Hz} \xrightarrow{\quad 90°\, I_x \quad} -I_{Hy} \tag{1}$$

$$-I_{Hy} \xrightarrow{\quad \Omega I_z t \quad} -I_{Hy}\cos\Omega t + I_{Hx}\sin\Omega t \tag{2}$$

$$-I_{Hy} \xrightarrow{\quad \pi J\, 2I_{1z}I_{2z} t \quad} -I_{Hy}\cos\pi J t + 2I_{Hx}I_{Hz}\sin\pi J t \tag{3}$$

8. Own Observations

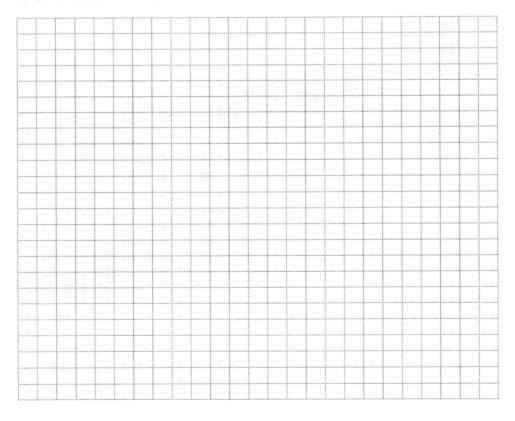

Experiment 3.2

The Standard 13C NMR Experiment

1. Purpose

The aim of the standard 13C NMR experiment is to record a 13C NMR spectrum with proton broad-band decoupling and data accumulation in order to get chemical shift information for structure determination. Here we apply this standard procedure to ethyl crotonate.

2. Literature

[1] H.-O. Kalinowski, S. Berger, S. Braun, *Carbon-13 NMR Spectroscopy*, Wiley, Chichester, **1988.**
[2] A. E. Derome, *Modern NMR Techniques for Chemistry Research*, Pergamon, Oxford, **1987.**
[3] K. K. M. Sanders, B. K. Hunter, *Modern NMR Spectroscopy*, 2nd Edition, Oxford University Press, Oxford, **1993.**

3. Pulse Scheme and Phase Cycle

¹H

composite pulse decoupling

¹³C

p1: x, x, -x, -x, y, y, -y, -y
aq: x, x, -x, -x, y, y, -y, -y

d1   p1   aq

4. Acquisition

Time requirement: 5 min

Sample: 20% ethyl crotonate in CDCl₃ with TMS as standard.

For sample preparation fill a clean and dry 5 mm sample tube of a quality appropriate to the spectrometer frequency with 0.7 ml CDCl₃ (5 cm filling height), 150 μl ethyl crotonate, and one drop of TMS. Clean the tube outside, close it with a cap, mark it (do not use a flag-like label which hinders rotation) and put it into the spinner turbine. Be sure that it is tight, but not too tight in the spinner, and adjust the depth of the tube using the depth gauge.

Put the tube into the magnet by means of the air lift, adjust the rotation frequency (about 20 Hz), and display the lock signal on the screen. Perform the lock procedure and optimize the field homogeneity (see Ch. 1, Section 1.4).

The spectrometer is to be adjusted for ^{13}C observation in quadrature detection mode. Load the ^{13}C acquisition program which comprises the following basic commands: zero memory, set ^{1}H broad-band decoupling (CPD-mode), set the relaxation delay, set the excitation pulse, perform acquisition, and write the data on file.

For acquisition the following parameters have to be set:

td: 32 k

td (time domain) is the number of points at which the free induction decay (FID) is sampled and the data stored. This parameter has to be chosen according to the desired digital resolution, which in turn depends on the spectral width sw. The settings of td and sw determine the acquisition time aq.

sw: 250 ppm

sw, the spectral width, has to be chosen so that the resonance frequencies of all types of ^{13}C nuclei are within this spectral window; otherwise folding occurs. Folding of noise is prevented by appropriate filters which are set by the software corresponding to sw. The settings of sw and td determine the *acquisition time* aq, the time during which the FID data are acquired. The relationship between these three parameters, where aq is usually the dependent variable and sw has to be expressed in Hz, is described by the following fundamental equation (1):

$$aq = td/(2\ sw) \tag{1}$$

Thus, with the above settings and a ^{13}C resonance frequency of 75 MHz, the acquisition time is 0.9 s.

o1: frequency (offset) *of the r.f. pulse at the center of the ^{13}C NMR spectrum:*
In quadrature detection mode the frequency of the exciting r.f. pulse (often called transmitter offset) is positioned in the center of sw, e.g. at about $\delta_C = 120$. On older instruments without digital lock, o1 depends on the field position of the deuterium lock and thus on the deuterated solvent used.

o2: frequency (offset) *of the decoupler at the center of the ^{1}H NMR spectrum:*
The frequency of the decoupling r.f. pulse (often called decoupler offset) is positioned in the center of the ^{1}H NMR spectrum, e.g. about $\delta_H = 7$. On older instruments without digital lock, o2 depends on the field position of the deuterium lock and thus on the deuterated solvent used.

p1: 30°
p1, the ^{13}C transmitter pulse, creates an observable *x,y*-magnetization by tipping the magnetization vector towards the −y-axis through an angle α, determined by eq. (32:

$$\alpha = (360/2\pi)\ \gamma B_1 \cdot p \tag{2}$$

where γ is the gyromagnetioc ratio for ^{13}C, γB_1 the strength of the radiofrequency field, and *p* the duration of the pulse. Since p1 is known for $\alpha = 90°$ (see Exp. 2.2), the duration of p1 for a flip angle of 30° is easily obtained. Although a 90° pulse gives maximum signal intensity (Exp. 2.2), a shorter pulse-length of about 30° is used for routine work with data accumulation; thus the long pulse repetition time of $5T_1$, which is necessary after a 90° pulse, may be reduced (see d1, where the term pulse repetition time is also explained).

It should be mentioned here that between the irradiating pulse and the opening of the detector a *preacquisition delay* (de) is introduced. It prevents the break through of the transmitter pulse into the detector, is in the order of 10 to 100 μs and is normally set by the computer.

d1: 0.4 s

d1, the relaxation delay, is introduced in order to establish thermal equilibrium of the spin system before the excitation pulse is applied. However, in routine ^{13}C NMR spectroscopy with long relaxation times, especially those of quaternary carbon nuclei, one accepts reduced intensities of their signals and uses a short d1 for time saving reasons. Often, especially for smaller molecules with longer T_1 values, thermal equilibrium is not reestablished; instead there is a steady state, reached initially by the introduction of a few dummy scans (ds) at the beginning of the experiment.

decoupler attenuation and 90° pulse-width for CPD

In routine work proton broad-band decoupling is usually performed by CPD (composite pulse decoupling), for which the 90° decoupler pulse and the attenuation have to be known (see Exp. 2.3).

ds: 2

ds, dummy scans, are inserted before accumulation starts in order to establish a steady state.

ns: 128

ns, the number of "scans" (individual FIDs), is chosen so that a reasonable signal-to-ratio is obtained in the final spectrum. Because of phase cycling a multiple of 8 is advisable.

rg:

rg, the receiver gain, has to be carefully adjusted so that the incoming FID does not exceed the ADC input limits. Otherwise signal distortions at the baseline will occur after Fourier transformation.

5. Processing

After data acquisition you have to process the data. Perform the following steps using the given settings:

size of the processed real data file: set **si = 16 k**. Normally si corresponds to td/2 (see acquisition), since, after Fourier transformation, half of the td data adresses contain the real part of the spectrum. This gives a digital resolution (Hz/data point) after Fourier transformation of 2 sw/td. (Note that on the older Bruker instrument series the parameter SI corresponds to 2 si of the newer ones.)

However, si may be set to a value greater than td/2, e.g. si = 32 k; this procedure is termed zero-filling and leads, according to Equation (3) for the general case, to a higher digital resolution:

digital resolution = sw/si   (3)

With the above data and at 75 MHz, the digital resolution is 1.1 Hz/point, a reasonable value in comparison to the line-width and peak separations normally encountered in

^{13}C NMR spectroscopy. If a higher digital resolution is desired, one may optimize sw, increase td, or perform zero-filling.

baseline correction: perform this correction on the *FID* in order to eliminate the dc offset between the two channels used in quadrature detection mode

digital filtering: for standard applications use as window function an exponential window function on the FID, characterized by the line broadening parameter lb; here set **lb = 2 Hz.**
This type of digital filtering generally improves the signal to-noise-ratio, but at the cost of resolution. Usually a value equal to the line-width obtained without application of an exponential multiplication is used.

Fourier transformation: use the correct type in accordance with the simultaneous or sequential quadrature acquisition mode.

phase correction: adjust to achieve pure absorption mode signals.

baseline correction: perform this correction on the *spectrum* in order to remove baseline rolling.

referencing: set the TMS signal to $\delta_C = 0$.

peak picking: choose the desired level.

plot: set parameters and plot spectrum, including integrals, peak picking, and the relevant acquisition and processing parameters.

6. Result

The figure on page 42 shows the ^1H broad-band decoupled ^{13}C NMR spectrum of ethyl crotonate as obtained on an ARX-300 spectrometer using a dual probe-head (region $\delta_C = -5$ to 180). Note that as usual no integration is performed, since under routine conditions the signal areas are not necessarily proportional to the number of ^{13}C nuclei giving rise to that signal (see especially the signal of the quaternary carbon C-1).

7. Comments

The excitation pulse p1 converts the equilibrium magnetization I_{Cz} of the ^{13}C nuclei to transverse magnetization $-I_{Cy}$ as shown in Equation (1). During the acquisition time the chemical shift develops in the x,y-plane as shown in Equation (2), and the resulting magnetization is detected by the receiver in the x,y-plane in quadrature mode.

$$I_{Cz} \xrightarrow{\quad 90° \ I_x \quad} -I_{Cy} \tag{1}$$

$$-I_{Cy} \xrightarrow{\quad \Omega I_z t \quad} -I_{Cy}\cos\Omega t + I_{Cx}\sin\Omega t \tag{2}$$

8. Own Observations

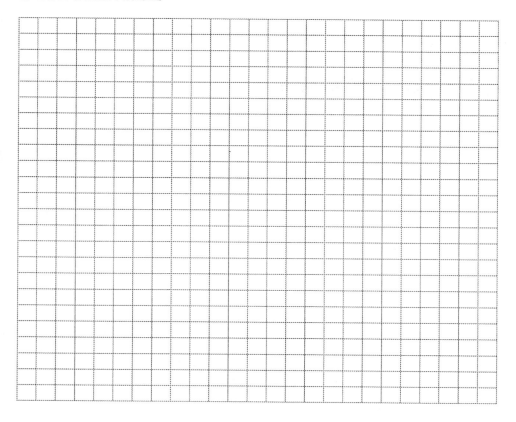

Experiment 3.3

Line-Shape Test for ^{1}H NMR Spectroscopy

1. Purpose

A good lineshape, as well as high resolution and high sensitivity, are the most important features for the performance of an NMR spectrometer (Exps. 3.3–3.8). In the line-shape test, also often called the hump test, the ^{1}H NMR signal of $CHCl_3$ is tested with regard to its line-width by measuring not only the width at half height (50%), but also at the height of the ^{13}C satellites (0.55%) and at 1/5 of this height (0.11%). NMR signals should have a Lorentzian line-shape. Therefore the widths at the latter two heights should be 13.5 and 30 times the half-height line-width $\Delta v_{1/2}$ (e.g. for $\Delta v_{1/2} = 0.2$ Hz these "hump" values are calculated to be 2.7 and 6 Hz). Deviations from these ratios indicate a non-Lorentzian line-shape; such a situation should be avoided, even if the measured values are smaller than the calculated ones.

2. Literature

[1] A. E. Derome, *Modern NMR Techniques for Chemistry Research*, Pergamon, Oxford, **1987**, 38–42.
[2] *SAM 1.0, Shimming Simulation Software package for IBM-PC compatible Computers*, ACORN NMR, 46560 Fremont Blvd., Fremont, CA 94538-6482.
[3] C. Anklin, D. v. Ow, H. Ruegger, *Standard Test Procedures for Supercon Systems*, Spectrospin AG, Fällanden, **1988**.

3. Pulse Scheme and Phase Cycle

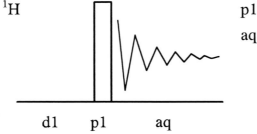

^{1}H

p1: x, x, -x, -x, y, y, -y, -y

aq: x, x, -x, -x, y, y, -y, -y

d1   p1   aq

4. Acquisition

Time requirement: approx. 1 h, very dependent on the skill of the operator and the state of the system

Sample: 10% $CHCl_3$ in [D_6] acetone, *degassed and sealed*

The magnet is shimmed as well as possible (see Ch. 1, Section 1.4). Record a normal ¹H NMR spectrum (see Exp. 3.1) and note the offset of the CHCl₃ signal. You have to set:

> spinning rate: 20 Hz
> td: 32 k
> sw: 500 Hz
> o1: on resonance of ¹H signal
> p1: 90⁰ ¹H transmitter pulse
> d1: 60 s
> rg: receiver gain for correct ADC input
> ns: 1

5. Processing

Use standard 1D processing with zero-filling to 32 k and no window multiplication. Set the intensity of the main signal to 1000 and check whether the satellites have a height of 5.5. Measure the line-width at half height, at the height of the satellites, and at 1/5 of their height.

6. Result

The figure shows the result obtained with a 5 mm dual probe-head on an ARX-200 spectrometer. Note that no spinning sidebands can be seen. The line-shape test is also a test for spinning sidebands, which must not exceed the height of the ¹³C satellites.

7. Comments

The protons bound to ^{13}C have a shorter relaxation time than those producing the main signal. Therefore a "good" but false hump test result may be obtained if too short a relaxation delay d1 is used. A bad hump results in a severe loss of sensitivity, since the main part of the signal intensity lies in the foot of the signal. The hump test should be performed regularly for all probe-heads available and recorded in the log-book of the instrument.

8. Own Observations

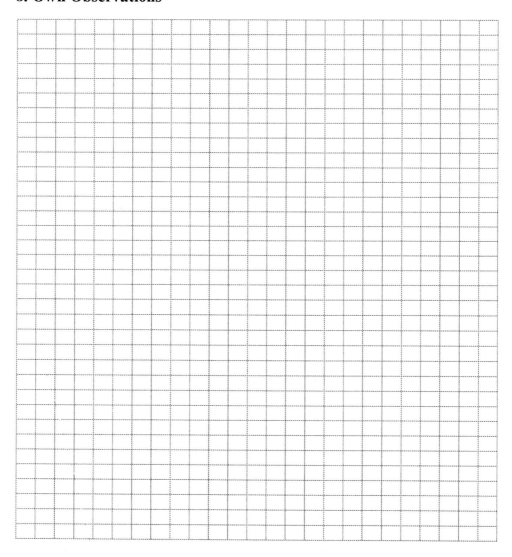

Experiment 3.4

Resolution Test for ^1H NMR Spectroscopy

1. Purpose

Resolution is the ability of an NMR spectrometer to observe resonance lines which are very close together as separate lines. This ability is measured by the line-width at half height, $\Delta\nu_{1/2}$, which is usually greater than the natural line-width. The experimental line-width $\Delta\nu_{1/2}$ is determined by the homogeneity of the magnetic field. For the standard ^1H NMR resolution test *ortho*-dichlorobenzene (ODCB) which gives an AA'BB' pattern, is used. Usually the eighth line from the left is used for resolution measurement.

2. Literature

[1] A. E. Derome, *Modern NMR Techniques for Chemistry Research*, Pergamon, Oxford, **1987**, 38–42.
[2] *SAM 1.0, Shimming Simulation Software package for IBM-PC compatible Computers*, ACORN NMR, 46560 Fremont Blvd., Fremont, CA 94538-6482.
[3] C. Anklin, D. v. Ow, H. Ruegger, *Standard Test Procedures for Supercon Systems*, Spectrospin AG, Fällanden, **1988**.

3. Pulse Scheme and Phase Cycle

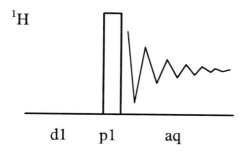

p1: x, x, -x, -x, y, y, -y, -y

aq: x, x, -x, -x, y, y, -y, -y

d1   p1   aq

4. Acquisition

Time requirement: approx. 1 h, very dependent on the skill of the operator and the state of the system

Sample: 10% *ortho*-dichlorobenzene in [D_6]acetone, *degassed and sealed*

The magnet is shimmed as well as possible (see Ch. 1, Section 1.4). Record a normal ^1H NMR spectrum (see Exp. 3.1) and note the offset of the center of the ODCB multiplet. You have to set:

spinning rate: 20 Hz
td: 32 k
sw: 1 ppm
o1: center of ODCB multiplet
p1: 90⁰ ^{1}H transmitter pulse
d1: 1 s
rg: receiver gain for correct ADC input
ns: 1

5. Processing

Use standard 1D processing as described in Experiment 3.1 with zero-filling to 32 k and no window multiplication.

6. Result

The figure shows the result (only the left half of the full AA'BB' pattern) obtained with a 5 mm probe-head on an ARX-200 spectrometer. The line-width at half-height measured on the eighth signal from the left was 0.07 Hz.

7. Comments

Note that the AA'BB' pattern is field dependent and slightly different splittings can be observed at higher field strength. The hump should not exceed 50% of the small inner signals (at 0 Hz above), indicated by the dotted line in the figure on page 48. The ODCB test should be performed regularly and the results should be recorded in the log-book of the instrument. Compared with the line-shape test in Experiment 3.3 the resolution test can be more rapidly achieved in practice.

8. Own Observations

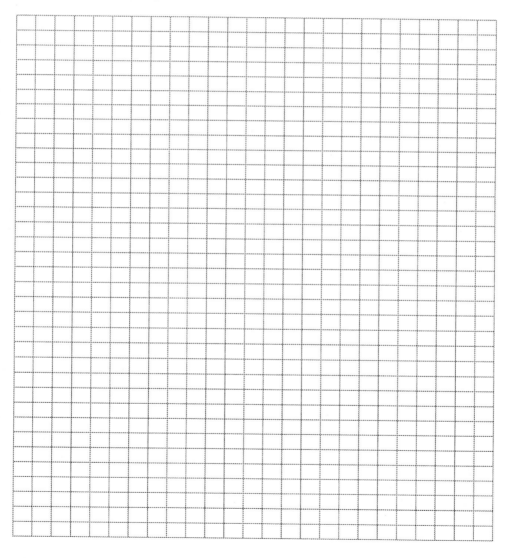

Experiment 3.5

Sensitivity Test for ^{1}H NMR Spectroscopy

1. Purpose

Sensitivity is one of the most debated points between manufacturers and customers buying new NMR instruments. Furthermore, sensitivity plays a central role concerning the performance of an NMR instrument in its everyday use. Therefore standardized tests have been developed which must be critically and honestly performed to yield meaningful results. In this experiment we describe the standard ^{1}H sensitivity test using ethyl benzene.

2. Literature

[1] A. E. Derome, *Modern NMR Techniques for Chemistry Research*, Pergamon, Oxford, **1987**, 50–56.
[2] C. Anklin, D. v. Ow, H. Ruegger, *Standard Test Procedures for Supercon Systems*, Spectrospin AG, Fällanden, **1988**.

3. Pulse Scheme and Phase Cycle

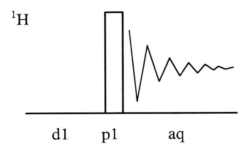

^{1}H

p1: x, x, -x, -x, y, y, -y, -y

aq: x, x, -x, -x, y, y, -y, -y

d1   p1   aq

4. Acquisition

Time requirement: 10 min

Sample: 0.1% ethyl benzene in CDCl$_3$, *degassed and sealed*

The magnet is shimmed as well as possible (see Ch. 1, Section 1.4). For a meaningful sensitivity test, the line-shape and resolution tests (Exps. 3.3 and 3.4) should be satisfactory. Load standard ^{1}H NMR parameters. You have to set:

td: 32 k
sw: 10 ppm
o1: middle of ^{1}H NMR spectrum
p1: 90^0 ^{1}H transmitter pulse

d1: 60 s
rg: receiver gain for correct ADC input
ns: 1

5. Processing

Apply standard 1D processing (see Exp. 3.1); zero filling to 32 k and an exponential window with lb = 1 Hz should be used. The full spectrum should be plotted and the noise between δ_H = 3 and 5 enlarged to allow a correct peak to peak noise measurement.

6. Result

The figure shows the result obtained on an ARX-200 spectrometer with a 5 mm dual probe-head. The signal height of the CH_2 group (largest quartet line) was measured to be 29 mm, and the 16 times enlarged peak-to-peak noise was 25 mm. From these numbers a signal to rms noise ratio of 46:1 is calculated.

7. Comments

One usually divides the peak-to-peak noise by a factor of 2.5 yielding the rms noise, thus the signal-to-noise ratio is given by equation (1), where S_H is the signal height and N_{pp} the the peak-to-peak noise amplitude.

$$S/N = 2.5\, S_H / N_{pp} \tag{1}$$

There are many "dirty tricks" to increase S/N ratios during instrument demonstrations; however, the only meaningful results are those which you can reproduce readily in your laboratory. Although current software allows calculation of the S/N ratio this parameter is still traditionally evaluated on paper with a ruler using the "spectroscopic eye". If the sensitivity of the instrument falls one can take as a rule of thumb that a factor of 2 may be due to bad resolution, whereas larger factors indicate hardware failures. Sensitivity tests should be performed regularly and the results should be recorded in the log-book of the instrument.

8. Own Observations

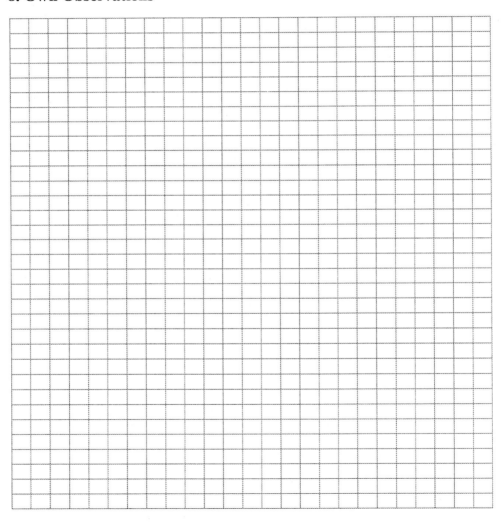

Experiment 3.6

Line-Shape Test for ^{13}C NMR Spectroscopy

1. Purpose

In this line-shape test, also often called the hump test, the ^{13}C NMR signal of benzene is tested with regard to its line-width by measuring not only the width at half height (50%), but also at the height of 0.55% and 0.11%. NMR signals should have a Lorentzian line-shape. Therefore the widths at the latter two heights should be 13.5 and 30 times the half-height line-width $\Delta v_{1/2}$. Deviations from these ratios indicate a non-Lorentzian line-shape: such a situation should be avoided. The ^{13}C line-shape test not only detects bad shimming or a defective probe-head but also checks for sufficient ^{1}H decoupling power.

2. Literature

[1] A. E. Derome, *Modern NMR Techniques for Chemistry Research*, Pergamon, Oxford, **1987**, 38–42.
[2] C. Anklin, D. v. Ow, H. Ruegger, *Standard Test Procedures for Supercon Systems*, Spectrospin AG, Fällanden, **1988**.

3. Pulse Scheme and Phase Cycle

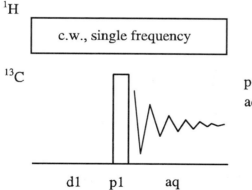

^{1}H — c.w., single frequency

^{13}C

p1: x, x, -x, -x, y, y, -y, -y
aq: x, x, -x, -x, y, y, -y, -y

d1   p1   aq

4. Acquisition

Time requirement: approx. 1 h, very dependent on the skill of the operator and the state of the system

Sample: 80% benzene in [D$_6$]acetone, *degassed and sealed*

The magnet is shimmed as well as possible (see Ch. 1, Section 1.4). Record normal ^1H and ^{13}C NMR spectra (see Exp. 3.1 and 3.2) and note the offsets of the benzene signals. You have to set:

> spinning rate: 20 Hz
> td: 16 k
> sw: 200 Hz
> o1: on resonance of ^{13}C signal
> o2: on resonance of ^1H signal
> p1: $90°$ ^{13}C transmitter pulse
> d1: 1 s
> decoupler attenuation for continous wave decoupling (see Exp. 4.2)
> rg: receiver gain for correct ADC input
> ns: 1

5. Processing

Use standard 1D processing with zero-filling to 16 k and no window multiplication. Set the intensity of the main signal to 1000 and check the line-width at heights 500, 5.5, and 1.1.

6. Result

The figure on page 54 shows the result obtained on an ARX-200 spectrometer with a 5 mm dual probe-haed. The small signals towards lower frequency from the main signal arise from benzene isotopomers which contain two ^{13}C nuclei.

7. Comments

A bad hump results in a severe loss of sensitivity, since the main part of the signal intensity lies in the foot of the signal. For this test on-resonance c.w. decoupling rather than the usual broad-band CPD decoupling technique is used, since the former is superior if only one signal has to be decoupled. The hump test should be performed regularly and recorded in the log-book of the instrument.

8. Own Observations

Experiment 3.7

ASTM Sensitivity Test for ^{13}C NMR Spectroscopy

1. Purpose

Good ^{13}C sensitivity is one of the most important points concerning the performance of any routine NMR service instrument in its everyday use. Therefore standardized tests have been developed which must be very critically and honestly performed to yield meaningful results. For ^{13}C two different tests are in common use. The ASTM (American Society for Testing and Materials) procedure using [D$_6$]benzene in dioxane described here checks only the ^{13}C performance on the transmitter channel, whereas the sensitivity test with ethyl benzene (Exp. 3.8) also tests the ^{1}H decoupling efficiency at the same time.

2. Literature

[1] *Standard Practice for Data Presentation Relating to High Resolution NMR Spectroscopy*, American Society for Testing and Materials, Designation E 386-90, Annual Book of ASTM Standards, Philadelphia, **1990**; reprinted in: H. Günther, *Nuclear Magnetic Resonance*, Wiley, Chichester, **1993**.
[2] A. E. Derome, *Modern NMR Techniques for Chemistry Research*, Pergamon, Oxford, **1987**, 50–56.
[3] C. Anklin, D. v. Ow, H. Ruegger, *Standard Test Procedures for Supercon Systems*, Spectrospin AG, Fällanden, **1988**.

3. Pulse Scheme and Phase Cycle

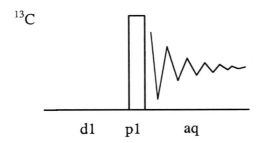

^{13}C

p1: x, x, -x, -x, y, y, -y, -y
aq: x, x, -x, -x, y, y, -y, -y

d1   p1   aq

4. Acquisition

Time requirement: 10 min

Sample: 60% [D$_6$]benzene in 1,4-dioxane, *degassed and sealed*

The magnet is shimmed as well as possible (see Ch. 1, Section 1.4). For a meaningful sensitivity test, the ^{13}C line-shape test (Exp. 3.6) should be satisfactory. Load standard ^{13}C NMR parameters. You have to set:

> td: 32 k
> sw: 200 ppm
> o1: middle of ^{13}C NMR spectrum
> p1: 90° ^{13}C transmitter pulse
> d1: 300 s
> rg: receiver gain for correct ADC input
> decoupler off
> ns: 1

5. Processing

Apply standard 1D processing (see Exp. 3.2); zero filling to 64 k and an exponential window with lb = 3.5 Hz should be used. The full spectrum should be plotted and the noise between δ_C = 120 and 80 enlarged to allow a correct peak-to-peak noise measurement.

6. Result

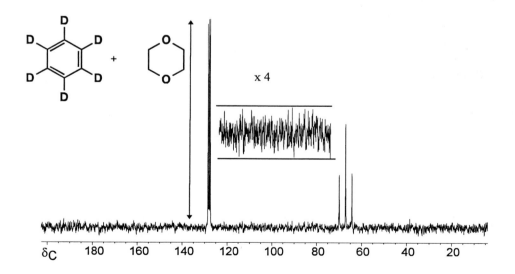

The figure shows the result obtained with a 5 mm probe-head on an ARX-200 spectrometer. The signal height of the benzene triplet was measured to be 70 mm, and the 4 times enlarged peak-to-peak noise was 17.5 mm. From these numbers a signal to rms noise ratio of 40:1 is calculated.

7. Comments

One usually divides the peak-to-peak noise by a factor of 2.5 yielding the rms noise, thus the signal-to-noise ratio is given by Equation (1), where S_H is the signal height and N_{pp} the height of the peak-to-peak noise.

$$S/N = 2.5\, S_H / N_{pp} \tag{1}$$

The resolution can be checked in this test by the splitting of the triplet of benzene which should be visible down to at least 10% of the signal height. If an instrument performs well the ASTM test but badly the ^{13}C sensitivity test with ethyl benzene, check the decoupler settings.

8. Own Observations

Experiment 3.8

Sensitivity Test for ^{13}C NMR Spectroscopy

1. Purpose

Good ^{13}C sensitivity is one of the most important points concerning the performance of any routine NMR service instrument in its everyday use. Therefore standardized tests have been developed which, to yield meaningful results, must be very critically and honestly performed. For ^{13}C two different tests are in common use. The sensitivity test with ethyl benzene shown here tests the spectrometer performance on both the ^{13}C transmitter and the ^{1}H decoupler channel. In comparison, the ASTM procedure (Exp. 3.7) checks only the ^{13}C performance on the transmitter channel.

2. Literature

[1] A. E. Derome, *Modern NMR Technique for Chemistry Research*, Pergamon, Oxford, **1987**, 50–56.
[2] C. Anklin, D. v. Ow, H. Ruegger, *Standard Test Procedures for Supercon Systems*, Spectrospin AG, Fällanden, **1988**.

3. Pulse Scheme and Phase Cycle

p1: x, x, -x, -x, y, y, -y, -y
aq: x, x, -x, -x, y, y, -y, -y

4. Acquisition

Time requirement: 10 min

Sample: 10% ethyl benzene in CDCl$_3$, *degassed and sealed*

The magnet is shimmed as well as possible (see Ch. 1, Section 1.4). For a meaningful sensitivity test, the ^{13}C line-shape test (Exp. 3.6) should be satisfactory. The CPD pulses for the decoupler should be recalibrated (Exp. 2.3). Load standard ^{13}C NMR parameters. You have to set:

td: 64 k
sw: 200 ppm
o1: middle of ^{13}C NMR spectrum
o2: middle of ^{1}H NMR spectrum
p1: 90° ^{13}C transmitter pulse
d1: 300 s
rg: receiver gain for correct ADC input
decoupler attenuation and pulse width for CPD
ns: 1

5. Processing

Apply standard 1D processing (see exp. 3.2); zero filling to 64 k and an exponential window with lb = 0.3 Hz should be used. The full spectrum should be plotted and the noise between δ_C = 120 and 80 enlarged to allow a correct peak to peak noise measurement.

6. Result

The figure shows the result obtained with a 5 mm dual probehead on an ARX-200 spectrometer. The signal intensity of the ortho and meta CH groups was measured to be 54 mm, and the 4 times enlarged peak-to-peak noise was 15 mm. From these numbers a signal to rms noise ratio of 36:1 is calculated.

7. Comments

One usually divides the peak-to-peak noise by a factor of 2.5 yielding the rms noise, thus the signal-to-noise ratio is given by Equation (1), where S_H is the signal height and N_{pp} the height of the peak-to-peak noise.

$$S/N = 2.5 \, S_H / N_{pp} \tag{1}$$

There are many factors such as decoupler offset, number of time domain data points, audio filter width, and selection of noise area which influence the result from the ethyl benzene sensitivity test. Very often so-called "optimum conditions" are obtained during an instrument demonstration. For meaningful comparisons keep a test file on the disk of your instrument and perform this test regularly. The results should be recorded in the log-book of the instrument.

8. Own Observations

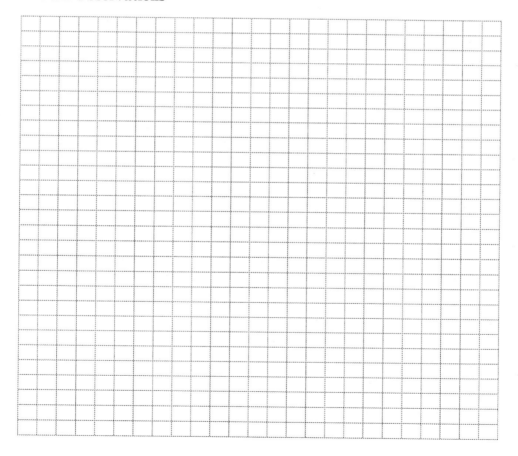

Experiment 3.9

Quadrature Image Test

1. Purpose

NMR signals are usually detected in quadrature mode with two phase detectors which are 90° out of phase (see Ch. 1, Section 1.1.2). These two audio signals are amplified and digitized either sequentially or simultaneously, then stored in different parts of the computer memory. This elegant scheme has many advantages. However, a drawback is that all components of the two channels involved must work identically. Failures which are often encountered include a d.c. offset between the two channels, wrong phase angle difference, and different amplification. Although small deviations can be eliminated by the usual quadrature phase cycle and by applying a baseline correction on the FID, it is important to know how well the two channels are matched to each other. The quadrature image test shown here gives a rapid indication of wrong adjustment.

2. Literature

[1] E. O. Stejskal, J. Schaefer, *J. Magn. Reson.* **1974**, *14*, 160–169.
[2] A. E. Derome, *Modern NMR Techniques for Chemistry Research*, Pergamon, Oxford, **1987**, 77–83.
[3] C. Anklin, D. v. Ow, H. Ruegger, *Standard Test Procedures for Supercon Systems*, Spectrospin AG, Fällanden, **1988**.

3. Pulse Scheme and Phase Cycle

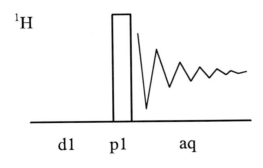

p1: x, x, -x, -x, y, y, -y, -y

aq: x, x, -x, -x, y, y, -y, -y

d1   p1   aq

4. Acquisition

Time requirement: 10 min

Sample: 10% $CHCl_3$ in [D_6]acetone

Record a normal ^{1}H NMR spectrum (see Exp. 3.1) and note the offset of the CHCl$_3$ signal. You have to set:

    td: 8 k
    sw: 1000 Hz
    o1: 250 Hz towards high frequency of CHCl$_3$ signal
    p1: 90^0 ^{1}H transmitter pulse
    d1: 1 s
    rg: receiver gain for correct ADC input
    ns: 1

5. Processing

Use standard 1D processing and exponential window multiplication with lb = 1 Hz. Set the intensity of the CHCl$_3$ signal to 1000 and enlarge the quadrature image signal, which is found 250 Hz towards higher frequencies from the offset position. This signal should be less than 1% of the main signal after one FID. As an exercise you may perform the experiment with ns = 8. Under these conditions the quadrature image signal should be significantly reduced by the quadrature phase cycle.

6. Result

The figure shows the result obtained on an AMX-500 spectrometer. The intensity of the quadrature image peak was 0.4 % of the main signal.

7. Comments

If the quadrature image peak exceeds the 1% limit you can try to correct the problem by adjusting the appropriate potentiometers or capacitors of the phase detection and audio amplification unit. Refer to the schematics provided by the manufacturer. However, these adjustments are bit tricky and should be performed by experienced personnel only. On very recent instruments a digital quadrature detection has been introduced.

8. Own Observations

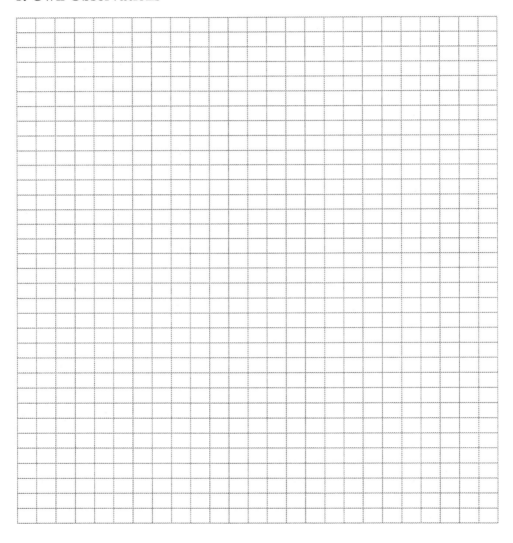

Experiment 3.10

Dynamic Range Test for Signal Amplitudes

1. Purpose

Very often it is necessary to measure rather weak NMR signals in the presence of other strong signals. One example is the detection of the ^{1}H signals of proteins in normal water. It is therefore useful to check the dynamic range performance of the spectrometer with a standard sample in order to know to what extent small signals can be detected in the presence of a strong signal without distortion.

2. Literature

[1] M. L. Martin, J. J. Delpuech, G. J. Martin, *Practical NMR Spectroscopy* Heyden, London , **1980**, 122–124.
[2] A. E. Derome, *Modern NMR Techniques for Chemistry Research*, Pergamon, Oxford, **1987**, 58–61.

3. Pulse Scheme and Phase Cycle

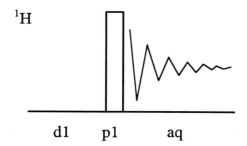

p1: x, x, -x, -x, y, y, -y, -y

aq: x, x, -x, -x, y, y, -y, -y

d1   p1   aq

4. Acquisition

Time requirement: 15 min

Sample: 90% H_2O, 1.056% CH_3OH, 0.136% CH_3CN, 0.008% $(CH_3)_3COH$, 8.8% D_2O (for lock) giving ^{1}H signal intensity ratios of 10000:100:10:1

Tune the probe-head to the water sample and obtain good shim settings. Load standard ^{1}H NMR parameters and very carefully adjust the receiver gain to give the optimum input for the analog-to-digital converter. You have to set:

td: 32 k
sw: 10 ppm
o1: middle of the ^{1}H NMR spectrum
p1: 90° ^{1}H transmitter pulse
d1: 5 s
ns: 1

5. Processing

Use standard 1D processing with an exponential weighting (lb = 0.2 Hz), carefully correct the phase of the water signal, try to detect the very small signal of *t*-butanol at δ_H = 1.28, and adjust the phase of this signal as well. Integrate the four relevant signals and check the integrals for consistency with the molar ratios of the four compounds in the sample.

6. Result

The figure shows the result obtained on a AMX-500 spectrometer equipped with a 16-bit digitizer. Besides some impurities of the sample, the resonances at δ_H = 4.8 (water), δ_H= 3.39 (methanol), and, after enlargement by a factor of 32, at δ_H = 2.1 (acetonitrile) and δ_H = 1.28 (*t*-butanol) can be seen.

7. Comments

The dynamic range is mainly dependent on the digitizer word length and, after accumulation, on the computer word length. The dynamic range behavior of all amplifiers and filter units also comes into account. Contrary to the common belief of many chemists, it does not make sense to accumulate signals endlessly, and newer software even sets a limit which is dependent on the difference between the computer and digitizer word lengths.

8. Own Observations

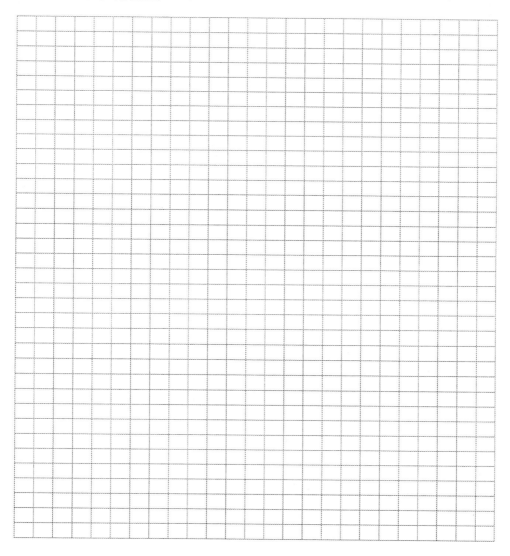

Chapter 4

Decoupling Techniques

In this chapter several basic 1D techniques are described which all use the proton decoupler (^{1}H broad-band decoupling using CPD is already shown in Exp. 2.3 and Exp. 3.2). Decoupling experiments are among the earliest techniques of NMR spectroscopy, and therefore some of the review literature cited is rather old but is still valid. One can distinguish between *homonuclear* and *heteronuclear* decoupling experiments. In the latter the observing channel is tuned to a heteronuclide X.

For both kinds of experiments it is essential to know the bandwidth of the decoupler for different attenuations. Therefore we provide three introductory experiments to calibrate the decoupler attenuation. It cannot be stressed enough that these experiments should be performed prior to any advanced application. With two exceptions (SPT experiments) the decoupler is used in such a way that no defined short decoupler pulses are required; therefore the experiments described in this chapter can be performed on any older instrument.

The homonuclear decoupling experiments described comprise the basic spin decoupling of protons, the SPT experiment and two variants of NOE difference spectroscopy. These are representative of the experiments which are most often performed in the routine service applications of any NMR laboratory.

The heteronuclear examples show the different decoupling techniques used in ^{13}C NMR spectroscopy before the advent of multipulse editing sequences and 2D spectroscopy. However, the gated decoupling and inverse gated decoupling experiments are still in routine use, and even the somewhat outdated off-resonance decoupling experiment is of some value in those cases where more modern methods fail.

Many of the 1D experiments described in this chapter have 2D equivalents and these are mentioned in the relevant paragraphs. However, the 1D experiments may provide a quicker answer if only one or two questions are outstanding in the course of a molecular structure determination.

Literature

[1] S. Forsén, R. A. Hoffmann, *Prog. NMR Spectrosc.* **1966**, *1*, 15–204.
[2] J. D. Baldeschwieler, E. W. Randall, *Chem. Rev.* **1963**, *63*, 81–110.
[3] W. McFarlane, *Ann. Rep. NMR Spectrosc.* **1972**, *5A*, 353–393.
[4] W. v. Philipsborn, *Angew. Chem. Int. Ed. Engl.* **1971**, *10*, 472–490.
[5] M. H. Levitt, R. Freeman, T. Frenkiel, *Adv. Magn. Reson.* **1983**, *11*, 47–110.
[6] A. J. Shaka, J. Keeler, *Progr. NMR Spectrosc.* **1987**, *19*, 47–129.

Experiment 4.1

Decoupler Calibration for Homonuclear Decoupling

1. Purpose

In this experiment the decoupler attenuation for homonuclear decoupling is calibrated. In homonuclear decoupling a certain proton signal is irradiated, and the change of the signal patterns of the coupled protons gives structural information immediately. For this experiment the decoupler bandwidth as a function of the decoupler attenuation has to be known. This calibration experiment gives the necessary data to enable the operator to perform a selective decoupling experiment with sufficient decoupler power both for standard homonuclear decoupling and for SPT experiments (see Exp. 4.5). The calibration routine described relies on the Bloch–Siegert shift [2].

2. Literature

[1] M. L. Martin, J.-J. Delpuech, G. J. Martin, *Practical NMR Spectroscopy*, Heyden, London, **1980**, 203–206.
[2] F. Bloch, A. Siegert, *Phys. Rev.* **1940**, *57*, 522–527.

3. Pulse Scheme and Phase Cycle

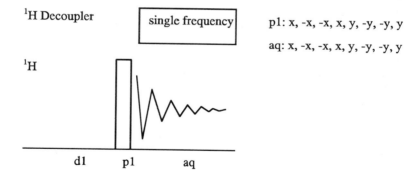

p1: x, -x, -x, x, y, -y, -y, y

aq: x, -x, -x, x, y, -y, -y, y

4. Acquisition

Time requirement: 30 min

Sample: 10% $CHCl_3$ in [D_6]acetone

The probe-head should be tuned to the sample. Load standard ^1H parameters, record a normal ^1H NMR spectrum and note the offset of $CHCl_3$. Reference the signal to 0 Hz. Switch to the homonuclear decoupling mode of the instrument, adjust the decoupler offset 50 Hz from the $CHCl_3$ signal, and record spectra with different decoupler attenuations. You have to set:

td: 4 k
sw: 500 Hz
o1: on resonance of ^{1}H signal
o2: 50 Hz towards lower frequency from o1
p1: 45° ^{1}H transmitter pulse
d1: 2 s
decoupler attenuation, to be varied

Measure the displacement of the signal and calculate the decoupler field strength γB_2 [Hz] from Equation (1)

$$\gamma B_2 = [2(\nu_A - \nu_2)(\nu_{obs} - \nu_A)]^{1/2} \tag{1}$$

where ν_A is the unperturbed resonance frequency, ν_2 the decoupler frequency and $\nu_{obs} - \nu_A$ the observed Bloch–Siegert shift. Note that Equation (1) is only valid if Equation (2) holds.

$$(\gamma B_2)^2 \ll (\nu_A - \nu_2)^2. \tag{2}$$

Repeat the experiment for different decoupler offsets.

5. Processing

Use standard 1D processing as described in Experiment 3.1, and use zero-filling to ensure enough data points for the relatively small Bloch–Siegert shifts.

6. Result

A typical set of values for $\nu_A - \nu_2 = 50$ Hz obtained on an ARX-200 spectrometer is given below, from which the graph on page 71 was calculated:

Dec. att. [dB]	70	67	64	61	58	55	52	49	46
$\nu_{obs} - \nu_A$ [Hz]	0.07	0.12	0.24	0.44	0.79	1.5	3.4	8.7	15.7

7. Comments

The calibration curve shown is dependent on the probe-head used. It should be determined for all the available probe-heads and documented in the log-book of the instrument. Note that homonuclear decoupling on FT instruments with probe-heads in a single coil arrangement requires a special decoupler mode, since the preamplifier must be protected against the decoupler r.f. power. This is usually done by applying the decoupling power only between the digitization points of the ADC with the preamplifier temporarily blanked.

8. Own Observations

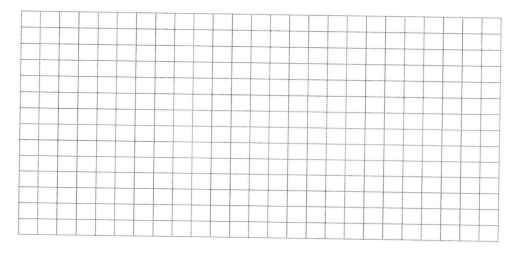

Experiment 4.2

Decoupler Calibration for Heteronuclear Decoupling

1. Purpose

Instead of using 2D NMR techniques such as HETCOR (see Exp. 10.8) it is sometimes more convenient to perform a heteronuclear decoupling experiment. A certain proton signal is irradiated, so that the connected carbon nucleus in the ^{13}C spectrum becomes decoupled. All other carbon signals are in the off-resonance decoupling situation. For this experiment the decoupler bandwidth as a function of the decoupler attenuation has to be known. The calibration experiment gives the necessary data to enable the operator to perform a selective decoupling experiment with the correct power to eliminate $^1J(C,H)$ spin couplings. The experiment also gives information about the decoupler bandwidth under normal broad-band decoupling settings.

2. Literature

[1] S. D. Simova, *J. Magn. Reson.* **1985**, *63*, 583–586.

3. Pulse Scheme and Phase Cycle

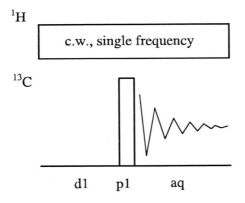

p1: x, x, -x, -x, y, y, -y, -y
aq: x, x, -x, -x, y, y, -y, -y

4. Acquisition

Time requirement: 30 min

Sample: 10% $CHCl_3$ in [D_6]acetone

The probe-head should be tuned to the sample. Record a normal ^1H NMR spectrum and note the offset of $CHCl_3$. Then load standard ^{13}C parameters with ^1H broad-band decoupling, record a normal ^{13}C NMR spectrum and note the offset of $CHCl_3$. Switch the instrument to c.w. decoupling. You have to set:

td: 4 k
sw: 500 Hz
o1: on resonance of ^{13}C signal
o2: 50 Hz offset from the ^1H signal
p1: 45° ^{13}C transmitter pulse
d1: 2 s
decoupler attenuation, to be varied
ns: 1

Record the ^{13}C doublet of CHCl3 using 500 Hz spectral width and the transmitter off-set adjusted directly on resonance; the decoupler should be switched off for the first experiment. Measure the spin coupling constant from the separation of the two doublet lines. Adjust the decoupler offset 50 Hz from the chloroform ^1H resonance and record the ^{13}C spectra with different decoupler attenuations. For certain decoupler offsets and attenuations you will obtain inner and outer doublets; the outer ones have a larger splitting than the normal CHCl3 doublet. Measure the residual splitting within the outer or inner doublet and from this calculate the decoupler field strength γB_2 [Hz] using the Equation (1).

$$\gamma B_2 = [(J \, \Delta/J_R)^2 + 0.25 \, (J_R^2 - J^2) - \Delta^2]^{1/2} \tag{1}$$

where J is the unperturbed spin coupling constant (214.8 Hz), J_R the residual splitting of the inner or outer doublett and Δ the offset of the decoupler frequency from the ^1H resonance. As an exercise perform the experiment with different decoupler offsets.

5. Processing

Use standard 1D processing as described in Experiment 3.2; use zero-filling to ensure enough data points to obtain accurate values for the residual splittings.

6. Result

A typical set of values for $\Delta = 50$ Hz obtained on an ARX-200 spectrometer is given below, from which the graph on page 74 was calculated:

Dec. att. [dB]	62	59	56	53	50	47	44	41	38
J_R [Hz]	91	90	84	77	61	50	38	29	21

7. Comments

For every probe-head available in the laboratory a corresponding figure should be determined and documented in the log-book of the instrument. Note that for water solutions the tuning of the probe-head might be quite different. Formic acid may be used as a calibration sample for water solutions.

8. Own Observations

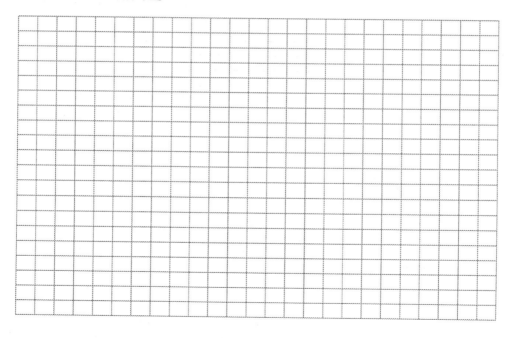

Experiment 4.3

Low Power Calibration for Heteronuclear Decoupling

1. Purpose

For certain applications it is necessary to irradiate a proton resonance with so little power that only the long-range spin couplings to ^{13}C are removed. As in Exp. 4.2 the decoupler bandwidth as a function of the decoupler attenuation has to be known, but in this case the calibration curve should cover γB_2-values from 1 to 40 Hz. Thus, the calibration experiment gives the necessary data to enable the operator to perform such a selective decoupling experiment. Accordingly, instead of $CHCl_3$, acetic acid is used as a calibration sample, where the effect of the decoupler in apparently reducing the $^2J(C,H)$ spin coupling constant is measured. The experiment also gives the necessary information to perform a heteronuclear SPT experiment (see Exp. 4.6).

2. Literature

[1] S. D. Simova, *J. Magn. Reson.* **1985**, *63*, 583–586.

3. Pulse Scheme and Phase Cycle

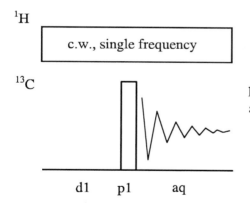

p1: x, x, -x, -x, y, y, -y, -y

aq: x, x, -x, -x, y, y, -y, -y

4. Acquisition

Time requirement: 30 min

Sample: 30% acetic acid in D_2O

The probe-head should be tuned to the sample. Record a normal ^1H NMR spectrum and note the offset of the methyl group signal of acetic acid. Then load standard ^{13}C parameters with ^1H broad-band decoupling, record a normal ^{13}C NMR spectrum, and note the offset of the carboxyl nucleus signal of acetic acid. Switch the instrument to c.w. decoupling. You have to set:

td: 2 k
sw: 100 Hz
o1: on resonance for carboxyl ^{13}C nucleus of acetic acid
o2: 25 Hz offset from the ^1H resonance of the CH_3 group of acetic acid
p1: 45° ^{13}C transmitter pulse
d1: 2 s
decoupler attenuation, to be varied
ns: 1

Record the ^{13}C quartet of the carboxyl signal of acetic acid using 100 Hz spectral width and the transmitter offset directly on resonance; the decoupler should be off for the first experiment. Measure the spin coupling constant from the separation of the two inner lines of the quartet. Adjust the decoupler offset to 25 Hz from the ^1H resonance of the methyl group of acetic acid and record the ^{13}C spectra with different decoupler attenuations. Measure the separation of the two inner lines of the quartet and from this calculate the decoupler field strength γB_2 [Hz] using Equation (1)

$$\gamma B_2 = [(J \, \Delta/J_R)^2 + 0.25 \, (J_R^2 - J^2) - \Delta^2]^{1/2} \tag{1}$$

where J is the unperturbed spin coupling constant (6.63 Hz), J_R the reduced splitting of the inner lines of the quartet and Δ the offset of the decoupler frequency from the ^1H resonance.

5. Processing

Use standard 1D processing as described in Experiment 3.2, with lb = 0.3 Hz, use zero-filling to ensure enough data points for the reduced splittings.

6. Result

A typical set of values for $\Delta = 25$ Hz obtained on an ARX-200 spectrometer is given below, from which the graph on page 77 was calculated:

Dec. att. [dB]	80	77	74	71	68	65	62	59
J_R [Hz]		6.6	6.54	6.4	6.2	5.65	5.05	4.45	3.48

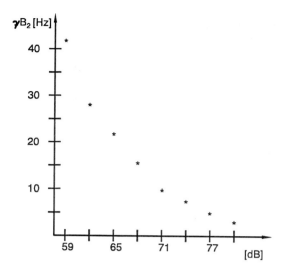

7. Comments

With the sample used here the calibration relates, of course, to a probe-head which was tuned to a sample containing water and thus might be quite different from a typical application with an organic solvent. For these you may use *t*-butyl acetate in CDCl$_3$ or similar compounds. A calibration curve for every probe-head present in the laboratory should be available in the log-book of the instrument.

8. Own Observations

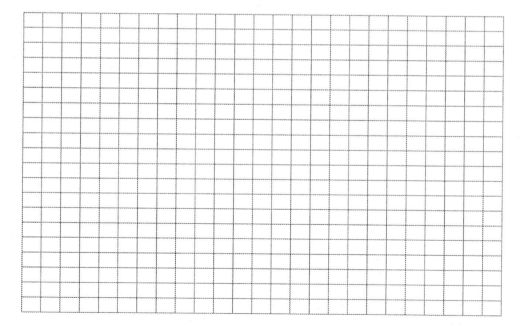

Experiment 4.4

Homonuclear Decoupling

1. Purpose

Complex spin systems can be simplified by homonuclear decoupling. By this technique residual multiplets are obtained in which the spin coupling to the irradiated proton is missing. The signal of the irradiated proton itself cannot be observed during decoupling. From a comparison with the undisturbed multiplet the relevant spin coupling constant can be evaluated. Similar information can also be obtained with the selective COSY technique (Exp. 7.5). Here we show a homonuclear decoupling experiment on ethyl crotonate.

2. Literature

[1] W. A. Anderson, R. Freeman, *J. Chem. Phys.* **1962**, *37*, 85–103.
[2] J. P. Jesson, P. Meakin, G. Kneissel, *J. Am. Chem. Soc.* **1973**, *95*, 618–620.
[3] M. L. Martin, J.-J. Delpuech, G. J. Martin, *Practical NMR Spectroscopy*, Heyden, London, **1980**, 203–206.
[4] J. D. Baldeschwieler, E. W. Randall, *Chem. Rev.* **1963**, *63*, 81–110.

3. Pulse Scheme and Phase Cycle

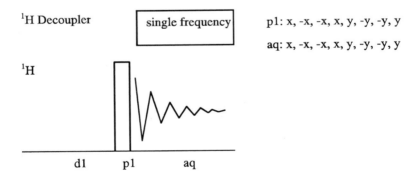

p1: x, -x, -x, x, y, -y, -y, y

aq: x, -x, -x, x, y, -y, -y, y

4. Acquisition

Time requirement: 20 min

Sample: 5% ethyl crotonate in $CDCl_3$

On some instruments you have to connect a directional coupler in order to feed the decoupler frequency into the transmitter line. Load standard ^1H parameters, record a normal ^1H NMR spectrum, and note the offsets of the signals to be irradiated. Change to the homonuclear decoupling mode of the spectrometer and adjust the decoupling power according to the width of the multiplet (see Exp. 4.1). You have to set:

td : 32 k
sw: 10 ppm
o1: middle of ^{1}H NMR spectrum
o2: on resonance of irradiated proton
p1: 45° ^{1}H transmitter pulse
d1: 1 s
ns: 8
decoupler attenuation for homonuclear decoupling

5. Processing

Use standard 1D processing as described in Exp. 3.1 with exponential multiplication (lb = 0.3 Hz).

6. Result

The figure shows the result for ethyl crotonate obtained on an AM-400 spectrometer. The signal region for the olefinic protons is shown in **a** (not decoupled), while **b** shows the result obtained by irradiation of the methyl group protons H-4 and **c** the result with irradiation of olefinic proton H-2. Note that in **c** some residual splitting is observed.

7. Comments

On FT instruments with a single coil probe-head homonuclear decoupling requires a special mode in order to avoid damage to the preamplifier. Thus the decoupling energy is applied in a pulsed mode within the duty cycle of the dwell time and the preamplifier is switched off during the decoupler pulses [2]. Note that homonuclear decoupling causes Bloch–Siegert shifts which can displace the residual multiplets from their original position. Bloch–Siegert shifts also affect the irradiated resonance, so that the best irradiation position is not the center of the unperturbed resonance.

8. Own Observations

Experiment 4.5

The Homonuclear SPT Experiment

1. Purpose

Spin coupling constants can have either sign, for example, the coupling constant $^2J(H,H)$ between two diastereotopic methylene hydrogen nuclei is usually negative. A sign determination can be very useful for distinguishing a ^2J from a ^3J coupling constant, as the latter is normally positive. The Selective Population Transfer experiment (SPT) is a simple 1D method which provides this relative sign information [1]. Furthermore, a lot can be learned about the different transitions within a spin system from this experiment. The sign information can also be obtained from a COSY-45 experiment (see Exp. 10.6)

2. Literature

[1] K. G. R. Pachler, P. L. Wessels, *J. Magn. Reson.* **1973**, *12*, 337–339.
[2] M. L. Martin, J. J. Delpuech, G. J. Martin, *Practical NMR Spectroscopy*, Heyden, London, **1980**, 222–226.

3. Pulse Scheme and Phase Cycle

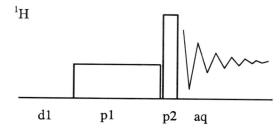

^{1}H

p1: x, x, -x, -x, y, y, -y, -y
p2: x, x, -x, -x, y, y, -y, -y
aq: x, x, -x, -x, y, y, -y, -y

d1   p1   p2   aq

4. Acquisition

Time requirement: 1 h

Sample: 5% 2,3-dibromopropionic acid in [D$_6$]benzene

Depending on the age of the spectrometer this experiment may need to be modified to the available hardware. Older spectrometers have no variable transmitter attenuation; p1 must then be taken from the decoupler and o1 = o2 phase coherence between decoupler and transmitter/receiver should be established. Another possibility is to perform the experiment completely with the decoupler (both p1 and p2) in the inverse mode of the spectrometer. On modern instruments the rectangular pulse p1 can also be replaced by a shaped pulse. In the following description we refer to instruments with transmitter attenuation. You have to set:

td: 8 k
sw: 2.5 ppm
o1: on resonance of a chosen multiplet line of the sample
p1: 180° ^{1}H transmitter pulse at chosen attenuation, here 0.8 s at 90 dB was
    used, see Exp. 2.6
p2: 30° ^{1}H transmitter pulse with normal attenuation (3 dB), *be sure not to use
    a 90° pulse*
d1: 5 s
two different transmitter attenuation levels
ns: 1

Record a normal ^{1}H NMR spectrum of the sample. Load a pulse program for the SPT
experiment and adjust the power of p1 to $\gamma B_1 \cong 1$Hz, typically in the order of 90 dB
(see Exp. 2.6). Adjust o1 to the left-most signal of the sample, record its SPT spectrum
and repeat the experiment for all signals of the AMX spin system.

5. Processing

Use standard 1D processing as described in Experiment 3.1

6. Result

In the figure on page 83 the normal ^{1}H NMR spectrum taken on an AMX-500 spectrometer is shown in **a**. In **b** line X_4 was irradiated and in **c** line X_3. Note that in **b**
lines A_2 and M_3 are attenuated, whereas A_1 and M_1 are enhanced. In **c** lines M_4 and
A_1 are attenuated, M_2 and A_2 are enhanced.

7. Comments

For the AMX spin system of 2,3-dibromopropionic acid the energy levels and transitions can be calculated using a spin simulation program assuming a negative coupling constant between the geminal protons on C-3. From this calculation the level scheme shown above can be drawn, indicating that the results of the SPT experiment are in agreement with the prediction from the simulation. Thus, irradiation of line X_4 in the spectrum inverts the populations of energy levels 5 and 8. This leads to enhancements of the M_1 and A_1 transitions and to attenuations of the M_3 and A_2 transitions.

8. Own Observations

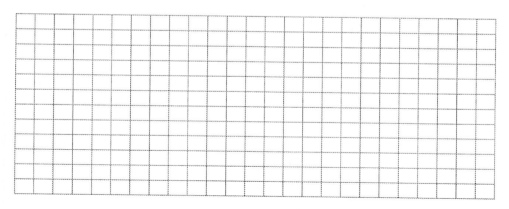

Experiment 4.6

The Heteronuclear SPT Experiment

1. Purpose

The heteronuclear SPT experiment was introduced [1] for the analysis of heteronuclear spin systems H,X with X = ^{13}C or ^{29}Si. As in the homonuclear case (see Exp. 4.5) it is especially able for determining the relative signs of long-range spin coupling constants. In addition to the sign the experiment gives information about whether a particular proton is spin-coupled to the carbon nucleus in question, and thus the experiment is very valuable in the interpretation of long-range C,H multiplets. There are many different versions [2, 3] of the experiment in addition to the basic method described here, such as difference spectroscopy and a version with proton decoupling for assignment purposes only. The theory of the experiment has been described [4, 5].

2. Literature

[1] K. G. R. Pachler, P. L. Wessels, *J. Magn. Reson.* **1973**, *12*, 337–339.
[2] S. K. Sarkar, A. Bax, *J. Magn. Reson.* **1985**, *62*, 109–112.
[3] S. A. Linde, H. J. Jakobsen, *J. Am. Chem. Soc.* **1976**, *98*, 1041–1043.
[4] R. Pachter, P. L. Wessels, *J. Magn. Reson.* **1989**, *81*, 464–473.
[5] M. L. Martin, J. J. Delpuech, G. J. Martin, *Practical NMR Spectroscopy*, Heyden, London, **1980**, 222–226.

3. Pulse Scheme and Phase Cycle

p1: x, x, -x, -x, y, y, -y, -y
p2: x, x, -x, -x, y, y, -y, -y
aq: x, x, -x, -x, y, y, -y, -y

4. Acquisition

Time requirement: 1 h

Sample: 5% 3-chloroacrylic acid in CDCl$_3$

As seen from the pulse sequence above, the experiment consists of a selective 180° proton pulse p1 with a very narrow bandwidth and low power level ($\gamma B_2 \approx$ 1Hz) centred on a particular transition of the $^{13}C,H$ spin system, followed by a hard sampling pulse p2 in the ^{13}C channel. You have to set:

td: 64 k
sw: 200 ppm
o1: middle of the ^{13}C NMR spectrum
o2: exact transition frequency of a ^{13}C satellite in the ^1H NMR spectrum
p1: 180° ^1H decoupler pulse at chosen attenuation; here 0.4 s at 90 dB
    was used, see Exp. 2.6
p2: 45° ^{13}C transmitter pulse
d1: 2s
ns =8

Measure a normal ^1H NMR spectrum and a proton-coupled ^{13}C spectrum (gated de-coupling, see Exp. 4.10) as reference spectra. Load a pulse program for the heteronu-clear SPT experiment and adjust the p1 power to $\gamma B_1 \approx 1Hz$, typically in the order of 90 db (see Exp. 2.6). Adjust o2 to a frequency 2 Hz above that of the left-most line of the proton doublet at $\delta_H = 7.5$, in order to excite the corresponding ^{13}C satellite sig-nal. Measure the SPT spectrum and repeat this for the other satellites of the spin sys-tem.

5. Processing

Use standard 1D processing as described in Experiment 3.2.

6. Result

The figure on page 85 shows at **a** the normal ^{1}H NMR spectrum taken on an AMX-500 spectrometer. In **b** the ^{1}H-coupled resonance of the carboxyl ^{13}C nucleus at δ_C = 169 is shown. In **c** o2 was set 2 Hz downfield from the left-most proton transition and in **d** 2 Hz upfield from the same transition.

7. Comments

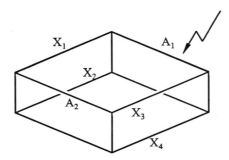

In an AMX spin system, calculated with all coupling constants positive as given in the figure, irradiation of the A_1 transition leads to population changes within the connected energy levels; thus the X_1 transition will be in emission and the X_3 transition in enhanced absorption. The reverse is true, if the A_2 transition is irradiated. Using a spin simulation program the energy levels can be calculated and the transitions are numbered; if the results of the SPT experiment agree with the predictions from the simulation, this confirms the assumed sign of the coupling constants. Note that in contrast with the homonuclear experiment (Exp. 4.5) one obtains true inversions and large enhancements due to the large difference in the γ-values for carbon and hydrogen.

8. Own Observations

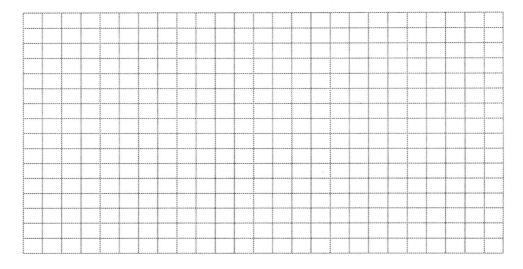

Experiment 4.7

1D Nuclear Overhauser Difference Spectroscopy

1. Purpose

Many problems of stereochemical assignment, for example differentiating between *E* and *Z* double bonds or between *exo* and *endo* groups in bicyclic compounds, cannot be solved using spin coupling constants if no suitable protons are present. In many cases, however, an NOE difference measurement provides an easy and straightforward answer. Irradiation of one group of protons causes a change in the intensities of other signals, which is related to the inverse sixth power of the distance between the spins.

2. Literature

[1] D. Neuhaus, M. Williamson, *The Nuclear Overhauser Effect*, VCH, Weinheim, **1989**.
[2] J. K. M. Sanders, B. K. Hunter, *Modern NMR Spectroscopy*, 2nd Edition, Oxford University Press, Oxford, **1993**, Ch. 6.

3. Pulsescheme and Phase Cycle

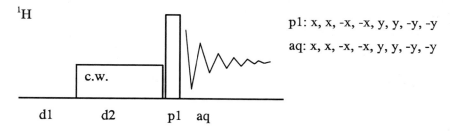

p1: x, x, -x, -x, y, y, -y, -y

aq: x, x, -x, -x, y, y, -y, -y

4. Acquisition

Time requirement: 0.5 h

Sample: 5% ethylmethacrylate in $CDCl_3$, *degassed and sealed sample*

Obtain a normal ^1H NMR spectrum and note the frequency of the methyl group signal. Depending on the instrument used, adjust the low power level for pre-irradiation by either decoupler or transmitter to $\gamma B_2 \cong 10$ Hz (see Exp 2.6). Here 70 dB attenuation was used. You should check whether the irradiated signal has disappeared from the ^1H NMR spectrum under these conditions. Record two spectra in which first the methyl group resonance and then a reference signal which does not introduce an NOE effect is irradiated. TMS or the residual proton signal of $CDCl_3$ is often used for the latter purpose. For dilute samples these two spectra are accumulated in an interleaved mode. You have to set:

td: 32 k
sw: 10 ppm
o1: middle of ^{1}H NMR spectrum
o2: on resonance for the methyl protons in the first experiment and on reso-
    nance of the residual ^{1}H signal of CHCl$_3$ in the reference spectrum
p1: 90° ^{1}H transmitter pulse
d1: 0.1 s
d2: 6 s
decoupler attenuation for selective presaturation
ds: 4
ns: 16

5. Processing

NOE difference spectra can be processed in different ways. Since one wants to observe signal intensity changes of 2 to 10%, one should use an exponential window function with lb = 2 Hz to minimize artefacts of subtraction. One can either transform the two spectra separately using a *digitally identical* phase correction and subtract the two spectra, or, more conveniently, subtract the two FIDs directly from each other. In the difference spectrum, adjust the phase of the methyl group signal to be negative and the phase of the reference signal (CHCl$_3$) to be positive. Evaluate only signals which have correct phase and have therefore not been affected by inadequate spectrometer stability.

6. Result

b

a

δ_H 6.5   6.0   5.5   5.0   4.5   4.0   3.5   3.0   2.5   2.0   1.5

The figure on page 88 shows the results obtained on an ARX-200 spectrometer. In **a** the normal ^{1}H NMR spectrum is given while in **b** the NOE difference result is shown with an expansion in the olefinic region. Integration of the methyl group signal and comparison with the integral of the *cis* olefinic proton ($\delta_H = 5.54$) gives an NOE effect of 9%, taking into account the threefold number of protons within the methyl group. Note the subtraction artefacts at $\delta_H = 4.3$.

7. Comments

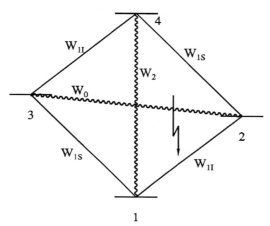

The exact theory of the NOE effect is complicated and is described in detail in the references given. In principle, saturation of one transition W_{1I} in a spin system with dipolar couplings but no indirect (scalar) couplings as given in the figure, first equalizes the populations of the two corresponding energy levels. The system reacts via the relaxation pathways W_2 or W_0, which leads to population changes of those energy levels that are connected by the W_{1S} transition. One should warn against placing too much weight on a quantitative interpretation of the results of these measurements, since the relaxation times of all neighbour protons are important, furthermore three spin effects and other complications are known to play a role. From a qualitative standpoint, however, in most cases, the experiment gives a correct answer to a stereochemical question.

8. Own Observations

Experiment 4.8

1D NOE Spectroscopy with Multiple Selective Irradiation

1. Purpose

This experiment is a technical variant of Experiment 4.7. In NOE difference spectroscopy one often encounters the problem that the large decoupler bandwidth required to irradiate a broad multiplet spills out to other nearby signals, thus making a correct NOE assignment very difficult. Instead of irradiating the center of a broad multiplet, in the experiment described here each line of the multiplet is irradiated for a short time with a bandwidth of ca. 1–2 Hz and the irradiating frequency is cycled repeatedly in a stepwise manner through the entire multiplet during the pre-irradiation time. In principle, this is a multiple SPT experiment (see Exp 4.5), but here the SPT effects are cancelled and only the NOE effects remain.

2. Literature

[1] M. Kinns, J. K. M. Sanders, *J. Magn. Reson.* **1984**, *56*, 518–520.
[2] D. Neuhaus, M. Williamson, *The Nuclear Overhauser Effect*, VCH, Weinheim, **1989**.
[3] J. K. M. Sanders, B. K. Hunter, *Modern NMR Spectroscopy*, 2nd Edition, Oxford University Press, Oxford, **1993**, Ch. 6.

3. Pulsescheme and Phase Cycle

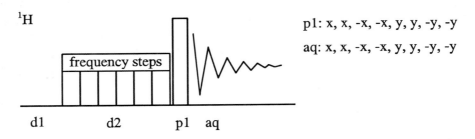

^{1}H

frequency steps

d1   d2   p1   aq

p1: x, x, -x, -x, y, y, -y, -y

aq: x, x, -x, -x, y, y, -y, -y

4. Acquisition

Time requirement: 0.5 h

Sample: 10% strychnine in CDCl$_3$, *degassed and sealed sample*

Obtain a normal ^{1}H NMR spectrum and note the single frequencies to be irradiated within the multiplets. Depending on the instrument used, adjust the low power level for pre-irradiation by either decoupler or transmitter to $\gamma B_2 \cong 1$ to 2 Hz (see Exp 2.6). Here 85 dB attenuation was used. As in Experiment 4.7 a reference signal which does not introduce an NOE effect is irradiated in a separate measurement. TMS or the residual proton signal of $CDCl_3$ is often used for this purpose. Depending on the spectrometer used, an automatic program may be loaded which organizes the stepping of the irradiation frequency through the multiplets. For dilute samples the spectra are accumulated in an interleaved mode. You have to set:

td: 32 k

sw: 10 ppm

o1: middle of spectrum

o2: lists of frequencies within the multiplets to be irradiated

p1: 90° ^{1}H transmitter pulse

d1: 0.1 s

d2: 7.2 s total pre-irradiation time; in the example multiplets with 6 lines were chosen, each line was irradiated for 400 ms, and the process was performed three times. In addition, the whole sequence for two irradiated multipletts and one reference line was repeated four times and the data averaged.

decoupler attenuation for presaturation (85 dB)

ds: 4

ns: 8

5. Processing

Use processing for NOE difference spectroscopy as described in Experiment 4.7.

6. Result

The figure on p. 92 shows the result obtained on an AMX-500 spectrometer. Spectrum **a** shows the normal spectrum in the region between $\delta_H = 6.0$ and 1.0. In spectrum **b** proton 12 at $\delta_H = 4.2$ was irradiated. Three NOE enhancements can be seen, namely for proton 13 at $\delta_H = 1.18$, one of the protons 11 at $\delta_H = 3.05$, and a slight effect at one of the protons 23 at $\delta_H = 3.98$. In spectrum **c** one of the protons 23 at $\delta_H = 4.05$ was irradiated. Note that with this technique the NOE effect of the nearby resonance of the other proton 23 at $\delta_H = 3.98$ can be observed without distortion; the olefinic proton 22 also shows an effect.

7. Comments

See Experiment 4.7 for some short remarks on the mechanism of the NOE effect. Compared with Experiment 4.7 the experiment described here requires more preparations and instruments adjustments, however is less prone to artefacts.

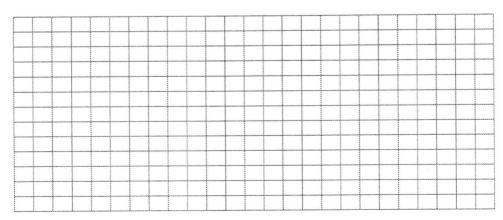

δ_H

8. Own Observations

Experiment 4.9

¹H Off-Resonance Decoupled ¹³C NMR Spectra

1. Purpose

This experiment is used to get information about the multiplicity of ¹³C NMR signals resulting from scalar coupling to the directly bound protons. In certain cases the more modern methods such as APT (see Exp. 6.4) or DEPT (see Exp. 6.9) may fail due to large differences between the C,H spin coupling constants. In these cases the old off-resonance decoupling method yields unambigous results. An additional advantage is the recognition of X-CH₂-CH₂-Y [4] and X-CH=CH-Y [5] groups which can be achieved by this technique. Here we present an ¹H-off resonance decoupled spectrum of ethyl crotonate.

2. Literature

[1] R. R. Ernst, *J. Chem. Phys.* **1966**, *45*, 3845–3861.
[2] M. L. Martin, J.-J. Delpuech, G. J. Martin, *Practical NMR Spectroscopy*, Heyden, London, **1980**, Ch. 6.2.
[3] H.-O. Kalinowski, S. Berger, S. Braun, *Carbon-13 NMR Spectroscopy*, Wiley, Chichester, **1988**, Ch. 3.3.
[4] R. A. Newmark, J. R. Hill, *J. Am. Chem. Soc.* **1973**, *95*, 4435–4437.
[5] R. Radeglia, H. Poleschner, G. Haufe, *Magn. Reson. Chem.* **1993**, *31*, 639–641.

3. Pulse Scheme and Phase Cycle

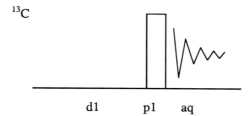

p1: x, x, -x, -x, y, y, -y, -y

aq: x, x, -x, -x, y, y, -y, -y

4. Acquisition

Time requirement: 30 min

Sample: 20% ethyl crotonate in CDCl₃

Set up the spectrometer for normal ^{13}C NMR spectroscopy with proton decoupling. Change the decoupler mode to continous wave without broad-band or CPD modulation. You have to set:

> td: 64 k
> sw: 200 ppm
> o1: middle of ^{13}C NMR spectrum
> o2: on resonance of ^{1}H TMS signal
> p1: 45° ^{13}C transmitter pulse
> d1: 0.5 s
> decoupler power for c.w. off-resonance irradiation, $\gamma B_2 \cong 3500$ Hz (see Exp. 2.6 and Exp. 4.2)
> ns: 512

5. Processing

Use standard 1D processing with lb=1 Hz as described in Experiment 3.2.

6. Result

The figure shows the result obtained for ethyl crotonate with an AM-400 spectrometer. Every signal except those of the carboxyl group and the solvent is split into a multiplet according to the number of directly attached protons (CH yields a doublet, CH$_2$ a triplet and CH$_3$ a quartet). Note that the residual splitting increases towards higher frequencies, because the decoupler offset was set on the position of the ^{1}H signal of TMS.

7. Comments

Under off-resonance conditions the $^1J(C,H)$ coupling constants are reduced according to equation (1). J_R is the residual coupling, Δv is the difference between the proton resonance frequency and the decoupler setting, and γB_2 is the strength of the decoupler

$$J_R = J \cdot \Delta v / \gamma B_2 \tag{1}$$

field. The reduced decoupler bandwidth is usually sufficient to eliminate geminal and vicinal C,H couplings. Therefore only the multiplicity which originates from the directly bonded protons is observed. In some cases additional splittings are observed e.g. in -CH_2-CH_2- or -CH=CH-groups, where the expected triplets and doublets have a fine structure due to higher-order effects.

8. Own Observations

Experiment 4.10

The Gated ¹H-Decoupling Technique

1. Purpose

This experiment is used for determining C,H spin–spin coupling constants without losing nuclear Overhauser enhancements. It yields proton-coupled ^{13}C NMR spectra which usually have to be analyzed with the help of spin simulation, since the carbon signals often form the X part of relatively complicated $A_m B_n...X$ spin systems. A knowledge of long-range C,H spin coupling constants is very helpful in structural elucidation of organic molecules.

2. Literature

[1] O. A. Gansow, W. Schittenhelm, *J. Am. Chem. Soc.* **1971**, *93*, 4294–4295.
[2] F. W. Wehrli, T. Wirthlin, *Interpretation of Carbon-13 NMR Spectra*, Heyden, London, **1978**, Ch. 3.
[3] M. L. Martin, J.-J. Delpuech, G. J. Martin, *Practical NMR Spectroscopy*, Heyden, London, **1980**, Ch. 6.2.
[4] H.-O. Kalinowski, S. Berger, S. Braun, *Carbon-13 NMR Spectroscopy*, Wiley, Chichester, **1988**, Ch. 2.3.

3. Pulse Scheme and Phase Cycle

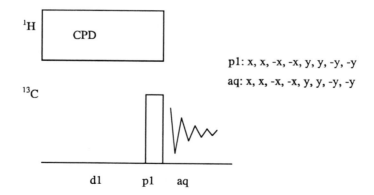

p1: x, x, -x, -x, y, y, -y, -y
aq: x, x, -x, -x, y, y, -y, -y

4. Acquisition

Time requirement: 45 min

Sample: 20% ethyl crotonate in CDCl₃

Set up the spectrometer for normal ^{13}C NMR spectroscopy. Load the pulse program for gated decoupling. Use a delay time d1 which is in the same order of magnitude as the acquisition time. You have to set:

    td: 64 k
    sw: 200 ppm
    o1: middle of ^{13}C NMR spectrum
    o2: middle of ^{1}H NMR spectrum
    p1: 45° ^{13}C transmitter pulse
    d1: 2 s
    ns: 512
    decoupler attenuation and 90° pulse for CPD

5. Processing

Use standard 1D processing with exponential multiplication (lb = 0.3 Hz); you can also use Gaussian multiplication to enhance the resolution.

6. Result

The figure shows the ^{1}H coupled ^{13}C NMR spectrum of ethyl crotonate obtained with an AM-400 spectrometer. Every signal is split into multiplets according to the underlying spin system. The inset is the expanded part of the olefinic region between δ_C = 124 and 121. This multiplet belongs to C-2 of ethyl crotonate showing a doublet of quartets of doublets due to the coupling to H-2, H-4 (CH$_3$) and H-3, with coupling constants of 161.7, 6.7 and 1.8 Hz. Note that the spectrum is field dependent owing to the fact that both the C-2 and C-3 resonances are the X parts of ABM$_3$X spin systems.

7. Comments

In this experiment composite pulse decoupling is applied during the delay d1 but not during the acquisition time. Coupling information is present immediately after switching off the decoupling field, whereas the populations of the energy levels decay with the spin–lattice relaxation times. During d1 (same order as the acquisition time) favorable ^{13}C energy level populations become established and coupled spectra with NOE can be obtained. One has to be careful about assuming a first-order interpretation of such spectra since higher order effects can occur. Make sure that the observed splittings are in fact first-order, and use spin simulation programs to analyze the spin systems.

8. Own Observations

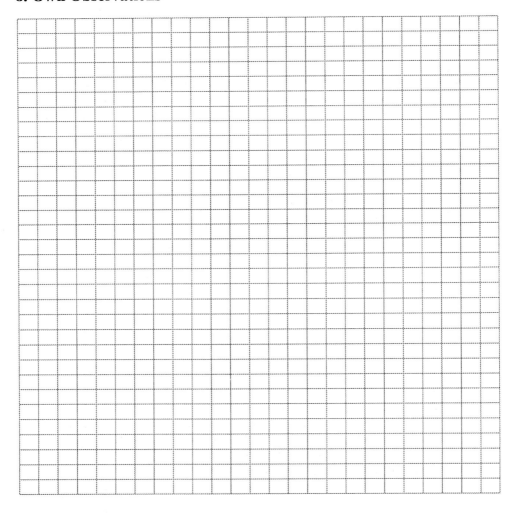

Experiment 4.11

The Inverse Gated ¹H-Decoupling Technique

1. Purpose

This experiment yields ¹H-decoupled NMR spectra of X nuclei without signal enhancement by the nuclear Overhauser effect. This is important for nuclei with a negative gyromagnetic ratio, where the Overhauser effect can completely suppress some or all signals under certain circumstances. The pulse sequence is also used for quantitative measurements of the Overhauser effect (see Exp. 4.14) and for quantitative ¹³C NMR spectroscopy (Exp. 8.7) where the Overhauser effect has to be suppressed. Here we show the basic experiment for ethyl crotonate.

2. Literature

[1] R. Freeman, H. D. W. Hill, R. Kaptein, *J. Magn. Reson.* **1972**, *7*, 327–329.
[2] M. L. Martin, J.-J. Delpuech, G. J. Martin, *Practical NMR Spectroscopy*, Heyden, London **1980**, 231–235.
[3] H.-O. Kalinowski, S. Berger, S. Braun, *Carbon-13 NMR Spectroscopy*, Wiley, Chichester, **1988**, Ch. 2.3.

3. Pulse Scheme and Phase Cycle

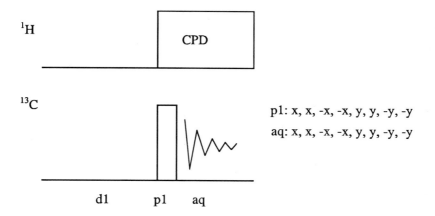

p1: x, x, -x, -x, y, y, -y, -y
aq: x, x, -x, -x, y, y, -y, -y

4. Acquisition

Time requirement: 1.5 h

Sample: 20% ethyl crotonate in CDCl₃

Set up the spectrometer for normal ^{13}C NMR spectroscopy. Load the pulse program for inverse gated decoupling. Use a delay time d1 which is about ten times the acquisition time. The latter should be rather short to avoid build up of the Overhauser effect during recording of the data. You have to set:

    td: 32 k
    sw: 200 ppm
    o1: middle of ^{13}C NMR spectrum
    o2: middle of ^{1}H NMR spectrum
    p1: 45° ^{13}C transmitter pulse
    d1: 10 s
    decoupler attenuation and 90° pulse for CPD
    ns: 512

5. Processing

Use standard 1D processing as described in Exp. 3.2. Apply zero filling to 64 k with exponential multiplication (lb = 1 Hz).

6. Result

Shown is the ^{1}H decoupled ^{13}C NMR spectrum of ethylcrotonate obtained with an AM-400 spectrometer. The signals of the protonated carbon atoms all have nearly the same height, remaining intensity differences are probably due to different spin–lattice relaxation times which affect most the signal intensity of the carboxyl atom C-1 (see exp. 6.1).

7. Comments

In this experiment composite pulse decoupling is applied only during the short acquisition time and not during the delay d1. Coupling information which is present after the delay is immediately eliminated by the decoupling field, whereas the populations of the energy levels and hence NOE enhancements require a build up time in the order of the spin–lattice relaxation times. If the delay d1 is at least 10 times the acquisition time, decoupled spectra without NOE effect can be recorded.

8. Own Observations

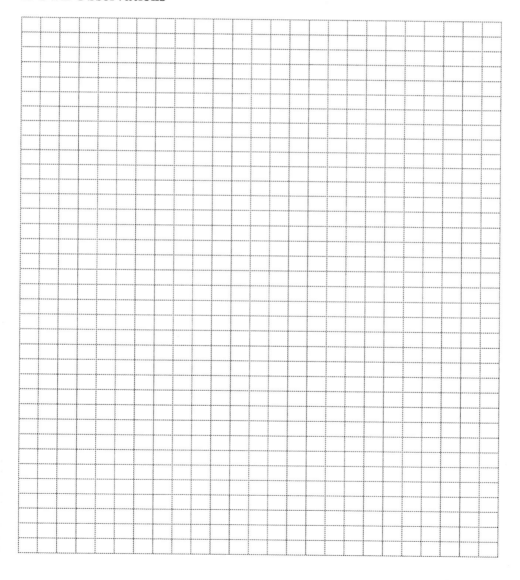

Experiment 4.12

1H Single Frequency Decoupling of ^{13}C NMR Spectra

1. Purpose

This experiment correlates a chosen ^{1}H signal with the corresponding carbon signal via $^1J(C,H)$ and is the 1D equivalent of the 2D C,H correlation (Exp 10.8). The experiment runs with ^{13}C as the observed nuclide and can therefore be performed on older instruments without difficulty. The inverse 2D H,C correlation (Exp 10.11) also has a 1D equivalent, called SELINCOR (Exp 7.6). The choice between these four techniques is dictated by the available hardware and the question whether only one specific item of information or the complete C,H correlation is needed. The experiment described here gives in a most straightforward manner the desired connectivity information, provided that the proton signals are sufficiently separated.

2. Literature

[1] M. L. Martin, J.-J. Delpuech, G. J. Martin, *Practical NMR Spectroscopy*, Heyden, London, **1980**, Ch. 6.

3. Pulse Scheme and Phase Cycle

^{1}H

c.w., single frequency

^{13}C

p1: x, x, -x, -x, y, y, -y, -y
aq: x, x, -x, -x, y, y, -y, -y

d1   p1   aq

4. Acquisition

Time requirement: 15 min

Sample: 20% ethyl crotonate in CDCl$_3$

Record a normal ^{1}H and ^{13}C NMR spectrum of ethyl crotonate and note the ^{1}H frequency of the methyl group attached to the double bond. Load a pulse program for ^{13}C detection under *continous wave* decoupling. The decoupler power γB_2 should be set to a level appropriate for the $^1J(C,H)$ coupling constant (Exp.2.6). You have to set:

td: 64 k
sw: 200 ppm
o1: middle of ^{13}C NMR spectrum
o2: center of methyl group ^{1}H resonance at $\delta_H = 1.6$
p1: 45° ^{13}C transmitter pulse
d1: 1 s
decoupler power $\gamma B_2 = 150$ Hz [45dB was used here]
ns: 8

5. Processing

Use standard ^{13}C NMR processing as described in Exp 3.2.

6. Result

In the figure **a** is the normal ^{1}H-decoupled ^{13}C NMR spectrum of ethyl crotonate and **b** is the result of the single frequency decoupling experiment obtained on an AMX-500 spectrometer. The experiment gives a singlet for C-4, whereas the other signals are multiplets according to the number of attached protons. These multiplets can display an off-resonance pattern (see Exp 4.9).

7. Comments

Single frequency decoupling only works perfectly if all transitions of the spin system are irradiated. A proton-coupled methyl carbon gives a quartet in the ^{13}C NMR spectrum, but the protons show a doublet in the ^1H NMR spectrum. The decoupler bandwidth has therefore to match the line separation of the ^{13}C satellite splitting in the ^1H NMR spectrum.

8. Own Observations

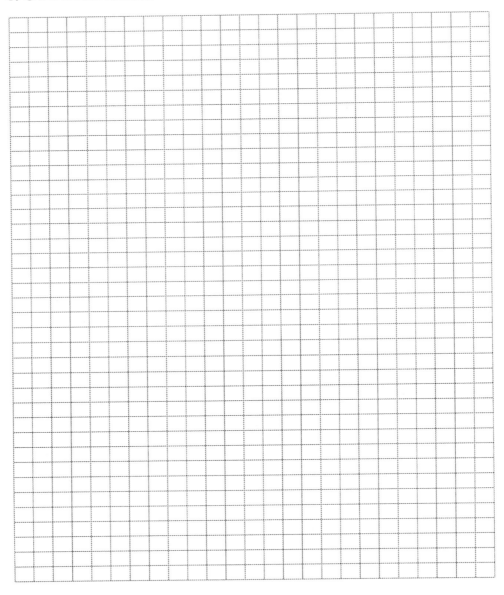

Experiment 4.13

^{1}H Low-Power Decoupling of ^{13}C NMR Spectra

1. Purpose

As in Experiment 4.12, this technique correlates an ^{1}H signal with ^{13}C signals, but in this case the nuclei concerned are separated by two, three or more bonds. As such it is a 1D equivalent of the 2D COLOC technique (Exp. 10.10). Again, this experiment can be performed in the inverse mode either as a 1D or a 2D method (gs-SELINCOR, Exp. 11.11 and HMBC, Exp. 10.13). The main purpose of the experiment described here is to simplify proton-coupled carbon spectra which can not only give assignment information but can make the analysis of the spin system much easier.

2. Literature

[1] M. L. Martin, J.-J. Delpuech, G. J. Martin, *Practical NMR Spectroscopy*, Heyden, London, **1980**, Ch. 6.

3. Pulse Scheme and Phase Cycle

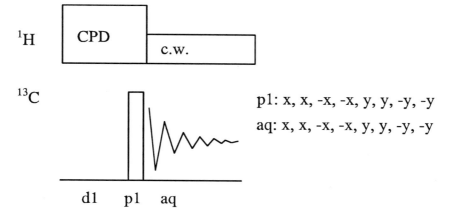

p1: x, x, -x, -x, y, y, -y, -y
aq: x, x, -x, -x, y, y, -y, -y

4. Acquisition

Time requirement: 15 min

Sample: 20% ethyl crotonate in CDCl$_3$

Record a normal ^{1}H NMR spectrum and an ^{1}H-coupled ^{13}C NMR spectrum (gated decoupling, see Exp. 4.11) of ethyl crotonate and note the ^{1}H frequency of the upfield olefinic proton. In order to avoid distortion of intensities due to SPT effects, load a pulse program for ^{13}C detection under *continous wave* decoupling during acquisition and broad-band decoupling during the delay d1. The decoupler power γB_2 during acquisition should be set to a level appropiate for the width of the ^{1}H signal, taking into account the additional splitting by the long range C,H spin coupling constant of 5–10 Hz. The decoupler power γB_2 during the pulse delay should be set to an appropriate value to maintain the NOE effect. You have to set:

td: 64 k
sw: 200 ppm
o1: middle of ^{13}C NMR spectrum
o2: center of ^{1}H signal of the upfield olefinic proton
p1: 45° ^{13}C transmitter pulse
d1: 1 s
decoupler attenuation during acquisition γB_2 = 15 Hz [70 dB were used here]
decoupler attenuation and 90° pulse for CPD
ns: 8

5. Processing

Use standard ^{13}C NMR processing as described in Experiment 3.2.

6. Result

The figure on page 106 shows spectra obtained on an AMX-500 spectrometer. **a** is the expanded methyl carbon region of the ^{1}H-coupled ^{13}C NMR spectrum; the methyl group C-4 displays two long-range spin coupling constants of 6.5 and 3.6 Hz. In **b** the olefinic proton at C-2 was irradiated, leaving only the coupling to H-3 with ^2J(C,H) = 6.5 Hz.

7. Comments

Single frequency decoupling only works perfectly if all transitions of the spin system are irradiated. A proton coupled to ^{13}C forms a doublet in the ^{1}H NMR spectrum (^{13}C satellites). These satellite lines are separated by the coupling constant ^nJ(C,H). The ^1J(C,H) couplings and remaining long-range couplings of other protons can be reduced due to off-resonance effects.

8. Own Observations

Experiment 4.14

Measurement of the Heteronuclear Overhauser Effect

1. Purpose

To evaluate spin–lattice relaxation data one often needs to know the dipolar contribution $T_{1(DD)}$. This can be obtained by measuring the overall spin–lattice relaxation time $T_{1(exp)}$ (see Exp. 6.1) and the heteronuclear Overhauser effect η as described in this experiment. Selective versions of this experiment can be used for assignment purposes in certain cases [1]. The 2D variant, called HOESY, is described in Experiment 10.18.

2. Literature

[1] K. E. Köver, G. Batta, *Prog. NMR Spectrosc.* **1987**, *19*, 223–266.
[2] D. Neuhaus, M. Williamson, *The Nuclear Overhauser Effect*, VCH, Weinheim, **1989**.
[3] S. Berger, F. R. Kreissl , J. D. Roberts, *J. Am. Chem. Soc.* **1974**, *96*, 4348.

3. Pulse Scheme and Phase Cycle

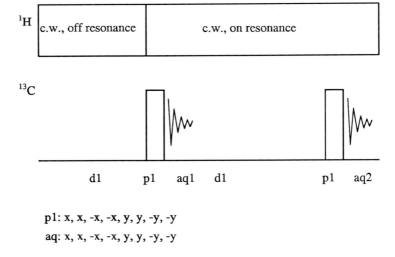

p1: x, x, -x, -x, y, y, -y, -y

aq: x, x, -x, -x, y, y, -y, -y

4. Acquisition

Time requirement: 1 h

Sample: 50% Cyclohexane in CDCl₃, *degassed and sealed*

Measure normal ^{1}H and ^{13}C NMR spectra and obtain the offsets. Load a pulse program as shown, which combines measurement with proton irradiation at two different proton offsets and which stores the two FIDs separately. This procedure ensures that the instrument performance is exactly the same in the two experiments. You have to set:

> td: 1 k (short aq, to avoid NOE buildup during acquisition)
> sw: 500 Hz
> o1: on resonance of ^{13}C signal of cyclohexane
> o2: provide a ^{1}H frequency list for the pulse program, first value 200 KHz off
> resonance, second value on resonance of ^{1}H signal of cyclohexane
> p1: 90° ^{13}C transmitter pulse
> d1: 200 s (10 times the relaxation time of cyclohexane)
> decoupler power for c.w. decoupling
> ns: 4

5. Processing

The experiment yields two FIDs which must be processed absolute identically. Use a large line-broadening value of lb = 3 Hz to obtain spectra with good signal-to-noise. Measure the two integrals and divide one by the other to obtain $\eta + 1$.

6. Result

The figure shows the spectra without (**a**) and with NOE (**b**) obtained on an AM-400 spectrometer. From integrals $\eta + 1$ is determined to be 2.84.

7. Comments

Spin–lattice relaxation involves a number of different mechanisms as indicated in Equation (1). The relative importance of these is field dependent.

$$1/T_{1(exp)} = 1/T_{1(DD)} + 1/T_{1(other)} \tag{1}$$

From the dipolar contribution to the spin–lattice relaxation one can estimate carbon–proton distances. The ratio of the integrals as measured in this experiment yields the NOE effect as defined in Equation (2), where $M_C\{H\}$ is the carbon magnetization with proton decoupling, M_C the carbon magnetization without proton decoupling, σ the cross relaxation rate, and $\rho_C = 1/T_1$.

$$M_C\{H\} / M_C = \sigma\gamma_H/\rho_C\gamma_C + 1 = \eta + 1 \tag{2}$$

In the extreme narrowing limit it can be shown that with a γ_H/γ_C ratio of approximately 4, $T_{1(DD)}$ can be calculated from Equation (3)

$$T_{1(DD)} = 2\,T_1\,/\,\eta \tag{3}$$

8. Own Observations

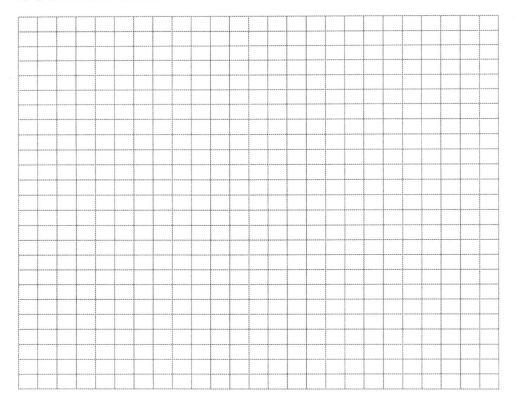

Chapter 5

Dynamic NMR Spectroscopy

In addition to its applications in the determination of static molecular structures, NMR spectroscopy can be used to detect intra- and intermolecular dynamic processes such as hindered rotations about partial double bonds, ring inversions and valence isomerizations. By measuring the temperature dependence of these processes the thermodynamic parameters $\Delta G^{\#}$, $\Delta H^{\#}$ and $\Delta S^{\#}$ can be obtained. The ability of NMR spectroscopy to determine energy barriers in the range from about 20 to 100 kJ mol^{-1} is based on the so-called NMR time-scale. Separate NMR signals are observed for nuclei at two sites A and B only when the site exchange rate constant k is much less than the difference $\Delta\omega$ between the corresponding angular resonance frequencies.

In this short chapter we first provide two basic calibration routines which enable the user to check whether the actual temperature of a sample corresponds to the setting of the temperature unit on the spectrometer. These are very important experiments which have to be performed prior to any dynamic NMR investigation. It cannot be stressed enough that depending on many instrumental factors, such as the position of the thermocouple in the probe-head, there might be quite a difference between actual and indicated temperature.

The chapter also includes a description of a basic dynamic NMR experiment using dimethylformamide as an example, and concludes with the saturation transfer experiment which can be viewed as the 1D analog of the two-dimensional EXSY technique, given in Experiment 10.20.

Literature

[1] G. Binsch, *Top. Stereochem.* **1968**, *3*, 97–192.
[2] G. Binsch, H. Kessler, *Angew. Chem. Int. Ed. Engl.* **1980**, *19*, 411–429.
[3] L. M. Jackman, F. A. Cotton (eds.) *Dynamic NMR Spectroscopy*, Academic Press, New York, **1975**.
[4] J. I. Kaplan, G. Fraenkel, *NMR of Chemically Exchanging Systems*, Academic Press, New York, **1980**.
[5] M. Oki, *Applications of Dynamic NMR Spectroscopy to Organic Chemistry*, VCH, Weinheim, **1985**.

Experiment 5.1

Low Temperature Calibration with Methanol

1. Purpose

There are many NMR experiments which are performed at different temperatures or where the emphasis lies on the measurement of a temperature-dependent effect. Hence, it is most important to know whether the temperature controller of the instrument used gives a correct reading of the actual temperature within the sample. Many different calibration samples have been proposed, working at different temperature ranges and for different nuclides. Here we restrict the description to the most common low temperature standard, methanol, where the chemical shift difference between the OH proton and those of the methyl group is used for the calibration.

2. Literature

[1] A. L. van Geet, *Anal. Chem.* **1970**, *42*, 679–680; ibid. **1968**, *40*, 2227–2229.
[2] H. Friebolin, G. Schilling, L. Pohl, *Org. Magn. Reson.* **1979**, *12*, 569–573.
[3] C. Piccinni-Leopardii, O. Fabre, J. Reisse, *Org. Magn. Reson.* **1976**, *8*, 233–236.
[4] J. Bornais, S. Brownstein, *J. Magn. Reson.* **1978**, *29*, 207–211.
[5] M. L. Martin, J.-J. Delpuech, G. J. Martin, *Practical NMR Spectroscopy*, Heyden, London, **1980**, 330–341.

3. Pulse Scheme and Phase Cycle

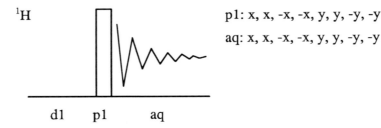

^{1}H

p1: x, x, -x, -x, y, y, -y, -y
aq: x, x, -x, -x, y, y, -y, -y

d1   p1   aq

4. Acquisition

Time requirement: 1 h

Sample: 4% MeOH in [D$_4$]Methanol containing a trace of HCl

Load standard proton parameters and connect the low temperature equipment for your instrument. Adjust for stable nitrogen flow and set the temperature controller in turn to 193, 223, and 273 K. Let each temperature equilibrate for at least 5 minutes. Measure at each temperature the chemical shift difference between the two methanol signals. Compare the values with those given in the instrument manufacturer's calibration curve or with the equations given by van Geet [1]. Outside the temperature range covered by the sample one may use a calibrated thermocouple fixed in an NMR sample. You have to set:

    td: 32 k
    sw: 8 ppm
    o1: middle of ^{1}H NMR spectrum
    p1: 45° ^{1}H transmitter pulse
    d1: 300 s
    ns: 1

5. Processing

Use standard 1D processing as described in Experiment 3.1

6. Result

CH₃—OH

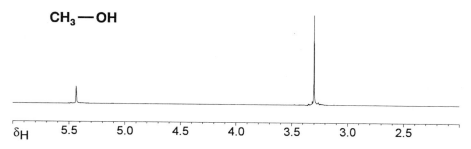

The figure shows the result obtained on an AM-400 spectrometer with the temperature unit set to 223 K. A difference of 2.136 ppm between the two signals was measured.

7. Comments

In principle, a long narrow cylinder like an NMR sample surrounded by a gas flow cannot be held at a very accurate and stable temperature compared to the performance of a large temperature bath as used in chemical kinetics. Temperature gradients in the sample are expected. Nevertheless, modern NMR instrumentation gives reasonably reproducible results if enough time is allowed for temperature equilibration. Your temperature readings should not deviate by more than 1–2 K from the calibration curve (page 114) and should be reproducible in repeated measurements.

8. Own Observations

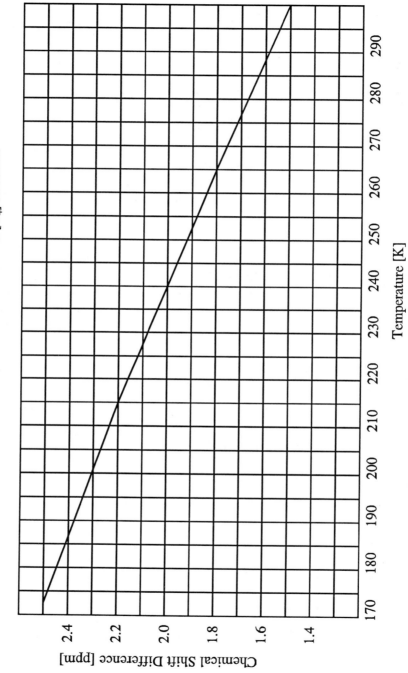

Calibration Curve for 4% Methanol in [D$_4$]Methanol

Experiment 5.2

High Temperature Calibration with 1,2-Ethanediol

1. Purpose

There are many NMR experiments which are performed at different temperatures or where the emphasis lies on the measurement of a temperature dependent effect. Hence, it is most important to know whether the temperature controller of the instrument used gives a correct reading of the actual temperature within the sample. Many different calibration samples have been proposed, working at different temperature ranges and for different nuclides. Here we restrict the description to the most common high temperature standard, 1,2-ethanediol, where the temperature-dependent chemical shift difference between the OH protons and those of the methylene groups is used for the calibration.

2. Literature

[1] A. L. van Geet, *Anal. Chem.* **1970**, *42*, 679–680; ibid. **1968**, *40*, 2227–2229.
[2] H. Friebolin, G. Schilling, L. Pohl, *Org. Magn. Reson.* **1979**, *12*, 569–573.
[3] C. Piccinni-Leopardii, O. Fabre, J. Reisse, *Org. Magn. Reson.* **1976**, *8*, 233–236.
[4] M. L. Martin, J.-J. Delpuech, G. J. Martin, *Practical NMR Spectroscopy*, Heyden, London, **1980**, 330–341.

3. Pulse Scheme and Phase Cycle

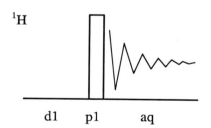

p1: x, x, -x, -x, y, y, -y, -y
aq: x, x, -x, -x, y, y, -y, -y

4. Acquisition

Time requirement: 1 h

Sample: 80% 1,2-ethanediol in [D$_6$]DMSO

Load standard proton parameters and connect the high temperature equipment for your instrument. Adjust for stable nitrogen flow and set the temperature controller in turn to 300, 330, and 400 K. Let each temperature equilibrate for at least 5 minutes. Measure at each temperature the chemical shift difference between the two 1,2-ethanediol signals. Compare the values with those given in the instrument manufacturer's calibration curve or with the equations given by van Geet [1]. You have to set:

td: 32 k
sw: 8 ppm
o1: middle of ^{1}H NMR spectrum
p1: 45° ^{1}H transmitter pulse
d1: 300 s
ns: 1

5. Processing

Use standard 1D processing as described in experiment 3.1

6. Result

The figure shows the result obtained on an AM-400 spectrometer with the temperature unit set to 330 K. A difference of 1.262 ppm between the two signals was measured.

7. Comments

In principle, a long narrow cylinder like an NMR sample surrounded by a gas flow cannot be held at a very accurate and stable temperature compared to the performance of a large temperature bath as used in chemical kinetics. Temperature gradients in the sample are expected. Nevertheless, modern NMR instrumentation gives reasonably reproducible results if enough time is allowed for temperature equilibration. Your temperature readings should not deviate by more than 1–2 K from the calibration curve (page 117) and should be reproducible in repeated measurements.

8. Own Observations

Calibration Curve for 1,2-Ethanediol in [D₆]DMSO

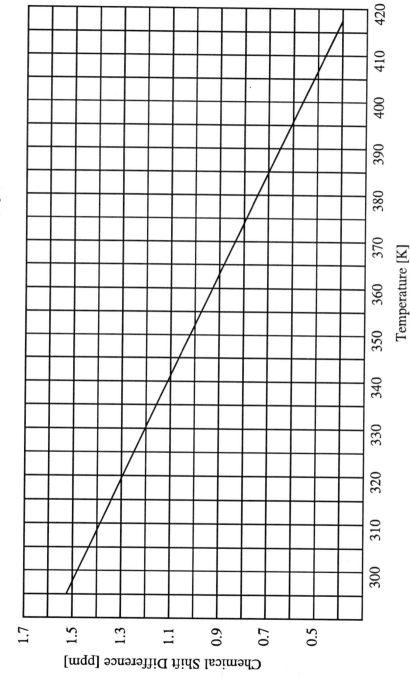

Temperature [K]

Chemical Shift Difference [ppm]

Experiment 5.3

Dynamic 1H NMR Spectroscopy on Dimethylformamide

1. Purpose

The measurement and evaluation of dynamic equilibria and the determination of activation enthalpies and entropies are important tasks which can be performed by high resolution NMR spectroscopy [1-3]. Dimethylformamide (DMF) was one of the earliest molecules investigated when the methodology of dynamic NMR measurements was beeing developed [4-6]. It still provides an easy starting point to learn the procedures involved in performing measurements at different temperatures and evaluating the results for a simple, non-coupled two-site exchange. Many different results were reported in the very early literature, whereas now an agreement seems to have been reached.

2. Literature

[1] G. Binsch, *Top. Stereochemistry*, **1968**, *3*, 97–192.
[2] G. Binsch, H. Kessler, *Angew. Chem. Int. Ed. Engl.* **1980**, *19*, 411–429.
[3] H. Günther, *NMR Spectroscopy*, 2nd Ed., Wiley, Chichester, **1995**.
[4] K. Rabinowitz, A. Pines, *J. Am. Chem. Soc.* **1969**, *91*, 1585–1589.
[5] T. Drakenburg, K. J. Dahlquist, S. Forsén, *J. Phys. Chem.* **1972**, *76*, 2178–2183.
[6] G. J. Martin, M. Berry, D. Le Botlan, B. Mechin, *J. Magn. Reson.* **1976**, *23*, 523–526.

3. Pulsescheme and Phase Cycle

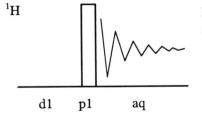

p1: x, x, -x, -x, y, y, -y, -y
aq: x, x, -x, -x, y, y, -y, -y

¹H

d1   p1   aq

4. Acquisition

Time requirement: 5 h

Sample: 5% dimethylformamide in $C_2D_2Cl_4$. **Warning: Do not overheat the sample!**

Connect your instrument for high temperature measurements, adjust a reasonable nitrogen flow, set the control to room temperature, and let the sample equilibrate for at least 5 minutes. The spectra should be recorded with homonuclear decoupling of the aldehyde proton in order to simplify the evaluation. Record a normal ^{1}H NMR spectrum, note the position of the aldehyde proton resonance, and set the decoupler offset accordingly. Run the spectrum again under decoupling conditions. The signals of the methyl groups should now have equal heights. Change the temperature in 10 K steps at first and within the actual exchange region in 5 K steps until the signals of the methyl groups coalesce, or with high field instruments to a **maximum** of 430 K. Perform the experiments in reverse order and check for reproducibility. Adjust the decoupler position for the aldehyde proton before every measurement. You have to set:

td: 32 k
sw: 12 ppm
o1: middle of ^{1}H NMR spectrum
o2: on resonance of the aldehyde proton
p1: 45° ^{1}H transmitter pulse
d1: 300 s to equilibrate temperature
decoupler attenuation corresponding to $\gamma B_2 = 10$ Hz
stable gas flow for temperature regulation
ns: 8

5. Processing

Use standard processing as described in Experiment 3.1, and for each temperature run an expanded plot of the signals of the methyl groups. For comparison with theoretically calculated line-shapes it is helpful to plot the experimental result on a transparent film with an enlargement that corresponds to a filled PC screen. Note for each temperature the line-width of the residual proton signal of the solvent.

6. Result

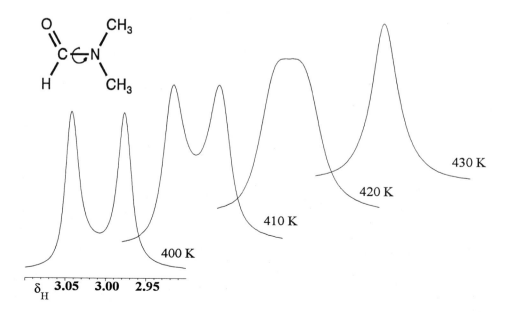

Displayed on page 119 are four typical spectra taken on an AM-400 spectrometer at 400–430 K. From the complete series the result $\Delta G^{\#}(298) = 21.4$ kcal/mol was obtained; $\Delta S^{\#}$ was essentially zero.

7. Comments

It would be beyond the scope of this book to describe the theory of line-shape investigations in NMR spectroscopy. The interested reader therefore is referred to the fundamental review articles [1–3]. For our purpose here it is sufficient to know that two exchanging sets of nuclei can only be separately observed if the rate constant of the exchange is considerably smaller than their chemical shift difference in Hz (NMR time scale). The goal of the experiment is to derive a table of rate constant vs. temperature. From such a table, using the Eyring equation, you can calculate values of $\Delta G^{\#}$. By plotting $\Delta G^{\#}$ as a function of temperature one can derive $\Delta H^{\#}$ and $\Delta S^{\#}$ for the observed exchange process.

There are many PC-based programs which are able to calculate the theoretical lineshape. These require as input the line separation in the low temperature limit Δv, the ratio of populations of the two sites, the line-width for non-exchanging protons, and the rate constant. From this they calculate a line-shape which must be compared with the experimental result at the corresponding temperature. The rate constant at the temperature of coalescence T_C is given for the simple degenerate two site exchange by Equation (1).

$$k_C = \frac{\pi \Delta v}{\sqrt{2}} \tag{1}$$

Using Equation (1) a formula (2) was derived, by which the $\Delta G^{\#}$ value at the coalescence can be obtained [3].

$$\Delta G^{\#}(T_C) = RT_C[22.96 + \ln(T_C/\Delta v)] \tag{2}$$

8. Own Observations

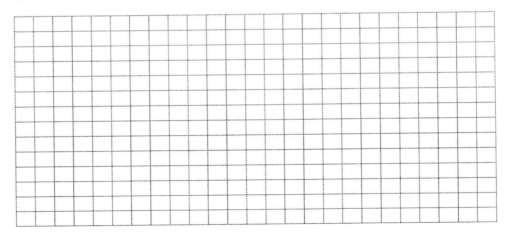

Experiment 5.4

The Saturation Transfer Experiment

1. Purpose

Dynamic NMR experiments such as that described in Experiment 5.3 can detect chemical exchange only if the exchange is fast enough to alter the NMR line-shape. However, slower chemical exchange processes can be detected by the saturation transfer experiment. One signal is irradiated and a change is observed in the intensity of another signal which is connected with the irradiated one by chemical exchange. A similar extension of the NMR time-scale is provided by the 2D EXSY experiment (Exp. 10.20). The FT modification [3] of the original Forsén–Hoffmann method shown here requires modern instruments where the transmitter power can be attenuated; on older instruments a third frequency source is necessary.

2. Literature

[1] S. Forsén, R. A. Hoffmann, *Acta Chem. Scand.* **1963**, *17*, 1787–1788.
[2] S. Forsén, R. A. Hoffmann, *Prog. NMR Spectrosc.* **1966**, *1*, 15–204.
[3] B. E. Mann, *J. Magn. Reson* **1976**, *21*, 17–23.
[4] J. J. Led, H. Gesmar, *J. Magn. Reson* **1982**, *49*, 444–463.
[4] M. L. Martin, J.-J. Delpuech, G. J. Martin, *Practical NMR Spectroscopy*, Heyden, London, **1980**, 315–321.

3. Pulse Scheme and Phase Cycle

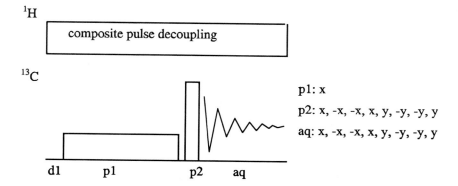

^{1}H

composite pulse decoupling

^{13}C

p1: x
p2: x, -x, -x, x, y, -y, -y, y
aq: x, -x, -x, x, y, -y, -y, y

d1   p1   p2   aq

4. Acquisition

Time requirement: 1 h

Sample: 5% dimethylformamide in $C_2D_2Cl_4$

Record a normal ^{13}C NMR spectrum of the sample and note the offsets of the signals of the methyl groups. Connect the high temperature equipment for your instrument, adjust a stable N_2 flow, and set the temperature first to 300 K. Afterwards increase the temperature to 350 K in 10 K steps. You have to set:

> td : 8 k
> sw: 25 ppm
> o1: on resonance of low frequency methyl group signal
> o2: middle of ^1H NMR spectrum
> p1: 25 s pre-irradiation pulse at high transmitter attenuation; the transmitter bandwitdh (see Exp. 2.6) must be small enough in order to saturate only the signal on resonance (70 dB)
> p2: 90° ^{13}C transmitter pulse
> d1: 0.1 s
> decoupler attenuation and 90° pulse for CPD
> ns: 8

5. Processing

Use standard 1D processing with exponential multiplication (lb = 2 Hz)

6. Result

The figure on page 122 shows a series of saturation transfer spectra obtained on an AMX-500 spectrometer. The bottom trace is the normal ^{13}C NMR spectrum of the compound at 300 K. In the other spectra the signal of the low frequency methyl group was pre-irradiated giving nearly complete saturation of the other methyl group signal at 350 K, although no line-broadening can be observed at this temperature and magnetic field strength.

7. Comments

Note that the saturation transfer is field dependent. Performing this sequence with ^{13}C rather than ^{1}H NMR has the distinct advantage that the result is not blurred by Overhauser effects since the exchanging spins are not in the same molecule. The solution consists of a mixture of isotopomers where the ^{13}C atom is located either in the cisoid or transoid methyl group. The experiment gives directly qualitative proof of chemical exchange. However, quantitative treatment is more complicated, since it requires in addition a knowledge of the T_1 relaxation times of the nuclei involved. See the cited literature for the corresponding equations.

8. Own Observations

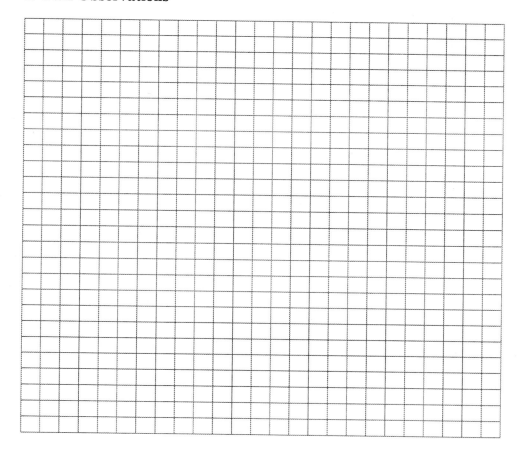

Chapter 6

1D Multipulse Sequences

In this chapter we provide several basic 1D pulse sequences where more than one r.f. pulse is applied. These pulses have to be calibrated for both the transmitter and decoupler channels. Due to error propagation these sequences are sensitive to miscalibration of the r.f. pulses and you will only succeed if these are correct.

Since a knowledge of both spin–lattice and spin–spin relaxation times is very important in multipulse NMR spectroscopy, this chapter begins with the two basic experiments for T_1 and T_2 measurements. A large part (Exp. 6.3–6.10) is then devoted to editing techniques with and without polarization transfer. There have been numerous discussions in the literature on the relative performance of these techniques. We give the basic descriptions of the most often used methods, SEFT, APT, INEPT, DEPT, and the recent PENDANT technique, and leave it to the reader to decide which editing variety best serves his or her own particular needs.

After an introduction to 1D-INADEQUATE (Exp. 6.11) three purely educational sequences are described: the use of BIRD, TANGO, and the double quantum filter is introduced. Together with the basic INEPT and reverse INEPT sequences these five experiments are shown for the simple case of the $CHCl_3$ molecule. However, we feel that a lot can be learned about modern multipulse NMR techniques from performing these experiments as shown.

Two methods for suppressing the huge solvent signal of water conclude the chapter. It should also be mentioned that another water suppression technique using pulsed field gradients is described in Chapter 11.

Literature

[1] C. L. Turner, *Prog. NMR Spectrosc.* **1984**, *16*, 311–370.

Experiment 6.1

Measurement of the Spin–Lattice Relaxation Time T_1

1. Purpose

The longitudinal or spin–lattice relaxation time T_1 is the time constant for re-establishing thermal equilibrium of the z-magnetization after an r.f. pulse and must be clearly distinguished from the transversel or spin–spin relaxation time T_2, which describes the decay of the x,y-magnetization (see Exp. 6.2). As far as structure determination is concerned, T_1 is not as important a parameter as the chemical shift or the spin–spin coupling. But even for routine work at least a qualitative knowledge of this parameter is essential, e.g. for choosing a reasonable pulse repetition time. Furthermore, T_1-values are important for setting up NOE experiments and for studying molecular motions. Here we describe the inversion recovery experiment as applied to the determination of the ^{13}C NMR T_1-values of ethyl crotonate. Other methods are based on the progressive saturation and saturation recovery experiments.

2. Literature

[1] R. L. Vold, J. S. Waugh, M. P. Klein, D. E. Phelps, *J. Chem. Phys.* **1968**, *48*, 3831–3832.
[2] J. S. Frye, *Concepts Magn. Reson.* **1989**, *1*, 27–33.
[3] D. J. Craik, G. C. Levy, *Top. Carbon-13 Spectrosc.* **1984**, *4*, 239–275.
[4] J. Kowalewski, G. C. Levy, L. F. Johnson, L. Palmer, *J. Magn. Reson.* **1977**, *26*, 533–536.

3. Pulse Scheme and Phase Cycle

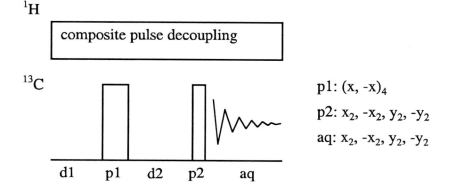

^1H

composite pulse decoupling

^{13}C

p1: $(x, -x)_4$

p2: $x_2, -x_2, y_2, -y_2$

aq: $x_2, -x_2, y_2, -y_2$

d1   p1   d2   p2   aq

4. Acquisition

Time requirement: 2 h

Sample: 80% ethyl crotonate in CDCl$_3$, *not degassed*

Set up the spectrometer for ^{13}C NMR and load a pulse program for inversion recovery with ^{1}H broad-band decoupling. Newer versions handle the data as 2D data: for example, the results of eight experiments with different delays d2 are stored as rows in a 2D matrix. So you have to create a 2D file and to set:

> td1: 8
> td2: 32 k
> sw: 200 ppm
> o1: middle of ^{13}C NMR spectrum
> o2: middle of ^{1}H NMR spectrum
> p1: 180° ^{13}C transmitter pulse
> p2: 90° ^{13}C transmitter pulse
> d1: 60 s (> 5 T_1 in order to achieve the equilibrium z-magnetization)
> d2: create a list with the follwing values [s]: 0.5, 1, 3, 6, 10, 16, 24, 50
> ds: 2
> decoupler attenuation and 90° pulse for CPD
> ns: 8

5. Processing

If a 2D file has been created, Fourier transformation has to be performed in F_2, using a line broadening factor lb = 2 Hz. In order to adjust the phase, read spectrum number 8 in which all signals have a positive phase, and transfer this phase correction to all other spectra.

6. Result

In the figure on p. 126 the results obtained on an ARX-300 spectrometer (5 mm dual probehead) are presented as a stacked plot for qualitative inspection. In the first two spectra all signals have a negative intensity, since after the first 180° pulse and the short delays of 0.5 and 1 s all spin vectors are still in the −z direction. After a delay d2 of 3 s spin–lattice relaxation has reduced the intensity of the signal of C-6 nearly to zero, whereas those of all other signals are still negative, showing that C-6 must have the shortest T_1. For a rough estimation of the T_1-values from these spectra you may use Equation (1), where t_{null} is the (interpolated) delay d2 at which the intensity of a signal is zero.

$$T_1 = 1.44\ t_{null} \tag{1}$$

For quantitative analysis apply the T_1/T_2 software which uses either the integrals or the peak heights. The basis for the evaluation is Equation (2) with M_0 = equilibrium z-magnetization and M_z = z-magnetization after delay τ (d2 above). Replacing M by I (integral or peak height) yields Equation (3) in which A and B are constants

$$M_z = M_0 \left(1 - 2e^{-\tau/T_1}\right) \tag{2}$$

$$I_t = A + B\,e^{-\tau/T_1} \tag{3}$$

The recommended procedure is an iterative exponential fitting according to Equation (3). This yields to the following T_1-values [s], based on peak heights and integrals:

	C-1	C-2	C-3	C-4	C-5	C-6
from peak height	(43.1)	8.2	7.5	7.8	7.0	5.3
from integral	(-)	7.6	7.2	8.0	6.7	4.9

It should be noted that the T_1-value for C-1 (C=O) is not reliable since the condition d1 > $5T_1$ is not fulfilled as is the case for the other carbon nuclei. A detailed discussion of the different parameters (length of d1, number and lengths of d2 etc.) is given in Ref. [3, 4]. As an exercise you may design and perform an experiment to determine T_1 for C-1 (about 50 s, not degassed).

7. Comments

The 180° pulse inverts the magnetization so that it lies along to the $-z$-direction; relaxation then takes place during the delay d2. At the end of d2 the actual magnetization is measured by the 90° read-pulse which transfers z-magnetization into measurable y-magnetization. Note that T_1-values are very dependent on concentration, temperature, oxygen content, and magnetic field strength. In this experiment the sample was not degassed, so as to give relatively short relaxation times which could be rapidly determined. In scientific applications, however, T_1 measurements should only be performed with carefully degassed samples.

8. Own Observations

Experiment 6.2

Measurement of the Spin–Spin Relaxation Time T_2

1. Purpose

The transverse or spin–spin relaxation time T_2 determines the decay of the $M_{x,y}$ magnetization and is related to the line-width. It must be clearly distinguished from the longitudinal or spin–lattice relaxation time T_1 (Exp. 6.1) and can be separately measured. Although there is hardly a direct relationship between spin–spin relaxation times and the structure of molecules, a knowledge of its value is important for planning dynamic NMR experiments, investigations on spin diffusion, and generally for devising new pulse sequences, because their evolution periods must not significantly exceed T_2. In the extreme narrowing limit the relationship $T_1 = T_2$ usually holds. The spin-echo method for measuring T_2 is described here.

2. Literature

[1] S. Meiboom, D. Gill, *Rev. Sci. Instrum.* **1958**, *29*, 688–691.
[2] M. L. Martin, J.-J. Delpuech, G. J. Martin, *Practical NMR Spectroscopy*, Heyden, London, **1980**, 280–287.
[3] R. Freeman, *A Handbook of Nuclear Magnetic Resonance*, Longman Scientific Technical, Harlow, **1987**, 262–266.
[4] S. W. Homans, *A Dictionary of Concepts in NMR*, Clarendon Press, Oxford, **1989**, 297–301.

3. Pulse Scheme and Phase Cycle

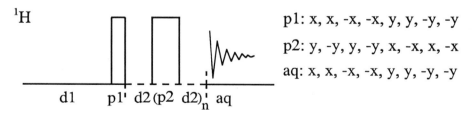

^{1}H

p1: x, x, -x, -x, y, y, -y, -y
p2: y, -y, y, -y, x, -x, x, -x
aq: x, x, -x, -x, y, y, -y, -y

d1   p1' d2 (p2 d2)$_n$ aq

4. Acquisition

Time requirement: 0.5 h

Sample: 3% $CHCl_3$ in [D_6] acetone, *degassed and sealed*

Obtain a normal ^{1}H NMR spectrum of the sample and adjust the spectral width and the offset. To avoid macroscopic motion, *turn the spinner off.* Load the CPMG (Carr–Purcell–Meiboom–Gill) pulse sequence and edit a list of ten numbers n which define the number of repeated cycles of the p2,d2 period in each of ten different experiments. On modern instruments this sequence is handled in the manner of a 2D experiment, where the ten experiments with the different repetition cycles are stored as rows in the 2D matrix. Therefore you have to create a 2D file prior to the start of the sequence. You have to set:

> td: 1 k
> sw: 500 Hz
> o1: on ^{1}H resonance
> p1: 90° ^{1}H transmitter pulse
> p2: 180° ^{1}H transmitter pulse
> d1: 150 s (5 T_1 of the $CHCl_3$ protons in the sample)
> d2: 10 ms
> preaquisition delay as short as possible
> ns: 1
> *n*-values of 2, 20, 50, 100, 200, 300, 400, 500, 750 and 1000 were used here, leading to delays between the first 90° pulse and start of the acquisition of 0.04, 0.4, 1, 2, 4, 6, 8, 10,15 and 20 s.

5. Processing

Modern software treats this experiment as a 2D file; however, transformation is only performed in the F_2 direction. Use an exponential line broadening of lb = 2 Hz and adjust the phase of the rows. After this, a normal T_1/T_2 software package detects peak integrals or heights from all rows and calculates the T_2 value from the given delays, which the user must provide in a corresponding delay list.

6. Result

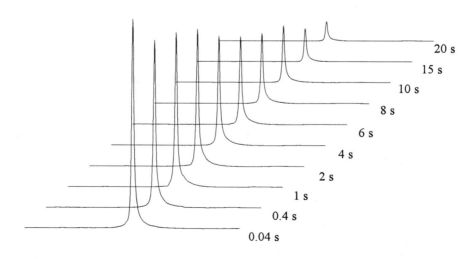

The figure on page 130 shows the ten spectra from this experiment, obtained on an AMX-500 spectrometer. From the intensities a T_2 value of 8.1 s was calculated, which corresponds to a natural linewidth of 0.04 Hz!

7. Comments

In this experiment the intrinsic value of T_2 is measured. This is related to the composite transverse relaxation time T_2^* by equation (1).

$$\frac{1}{T_2^*} = \frac{1}{T_2} + \frac{1}{T_2^{inhom}} \tag{1}$$

The second term on the right hand side describes the effect of the magnetic field inhomogeneity. T_2^* is the decay time constant of the FID and can also be approximated from the line-width using Equation (2) which is based on assuming exponential processes.

$$\Delta v_{1/2} = \frac{1}{\pi \cdot T_2^*} \tag{2}$$

For example, if the observed line-width at half height is 0.5 Hz, T_2^* can be calculated as 1.6 s; thus the inhomogeneity of the magnet is predominant for this example. As an exercise you may perform the experiment twice, first with very good resolution and then after poor shimming.

8. Own Observations

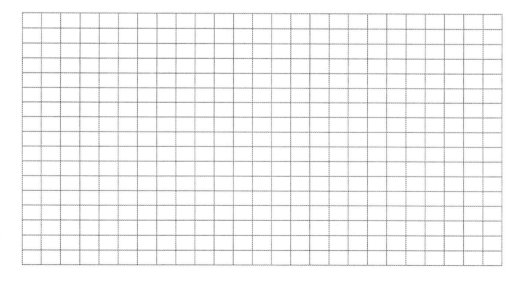

Experiment 6.3

Editing ¹³C NMR Spectra with SEFT

1. Purpose

The SEFT (Spin-Echo Fourier Transform) technique, also known as *J*-modulated spin-echo, is the simplest method of encoding the multiplicity of a ^{13}C signal into the phase of a fully decoupled ^{13}C NMR spectrum. From this method APT (Exp. 6.4) was also developed. SEFT can be performed on any instrument, because defined decoupler pulses as for DEPT (Exp. 6.10) or PENDANT (Exp. 6.11) are not needed. The method does not use polarization transfer as DEPT or INEPT, only the NOE enhancement by broad-band ^1H-decoupling is effective.

2. Literature

[1] D. W. Brown, T. T. Nakashima, D. L. Rabenstein, *J. Magn. Reson.* **1981**, *45*, 302–314.
[2] C. Le Cocq, J. Y. Lallemand, *J. Chem. Soc. Chem. Commun.* **1981**, 150–152.

3. Pulse Scheme and Phase Cycle

p1: $(x)_4$, $(y)_4$, $(-x)_4$, $(-y)_4$
p2: x, -x, y, -y, $(y, -y, -x, x)_2$, -x, x, y, -y
aq: x, x, -x, -x, y, y, -y, -y

4. Acquisition

Time requirement: 10 min

Sample: 20% ethyl crotonate in CDCl$_3$

Load standard ^{13}C NMR parameters and the pulse program. You have to set:

    td: 64 k
    sw: 200 ppm
    o1: middle of ^{13}C NMR spectrum
    o2: middle of ^1H NMR spectrum
    p1: 90° ^{13}C transmitter pulse

p2: 180° ^{13}C transmitter pulse
d1: 4 s
d2: $1/J(C,H) = 7$ ms, calculated from $^{1}J(C,H) = 140$ Hz
decoupler attenuation and 90° pulse for CPD
preacquisition delay as short as possible
ns: 16

5. Processing

Use standard 1D processing as described in Experiment 3.2. Adjust the phase for the
signals of the methyl groups to be positive and for the carboxyl nucleus negative.

6. Result

The figure shows a *J* modulated spin-echo spectrum obtained on an ARX-200 spectrometer.

7. Comments

As shown in the figure on page 134, CH$_n$ spin vectors develop differently after a 90°
pulse depending on how many hydrogens are bound to the carbon atom. If the delay d2
is set to $1/J$, CH and CH$_3$ vectors have opposite phase compared with C and CH$_2$. If
the decoupler is switched on at the end of d2 the phases are "frozen" and the corresponding signals have positive or negative sign. The second d2 delay is needed to refo-
cus phase errors caused by the chemical shift evolution. A disadvantage of this sequence is that 90° pulses are used at the start, thus requiring a relativly long relaxation
delay. This shortcoming was removed by the development of APT (Exp. 6.4).

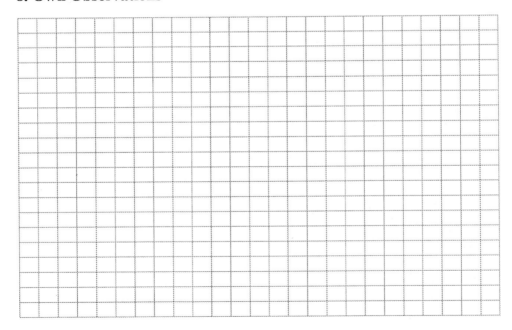

8. Own Observations

Experiment 6.4

Spectral Editing of ^{13}C NMR spectra with APT

1. Purpose

The APT (Attached Proton Test) technique is a modification of the SEFT experiment and differentiates between C, CH, CH_2 and CH_3 groups (see Exp. 6.3). The SEFT sequence suffers from the use of a 90° excitation pulse which requires long repetition times. In the APT experiment a shorter excitation pulse is used. Alternative methods which give information about the multiplicities are DEPT (see Exp. 6.9), the recently developed PENDANT (see Exp. 6.10) and the old off-resonance ^{1}H-decoupling technique (see Exp. 4.9). Unlike DEPT or INEPT, the APT method yields only NOE enhancements, but also gives information about quaternary carbon atoms. Improved modifications of APT are known [2, 3].

2. Literature

[1] S. Patt, J. N. Shoolery, *J. Magn. Reson.* **1982**, *46*, 535–539.
[2] J. C. Madsen, H. Bildsøe, H. Jakobsen, O. W. Sørensen, *J. Magn. Reson.* **1986**, *67*, 243–257.
[3] A. M. Torres, T. T. Nakashima, R. E. D. McClung, *J. Magn. Reson. Ser. A* **1993**, *101*, 285–294.

3. Pulse Scheme and Phase Cycle

p1: x, x, -x, -x, y, y, -y, -y

p2: y, y, -y, -y

p3: (y, -y)$_2$

aq: x, x, -x, -x, y, y, -y, -y

4. Acquisition

Time requirement: 30 min

Sample: 100 mg cholesteryl acetate in $CDCl_3$

Load standard ^{13}C NMR parameters and the APT pulse program. You have to set:

td: 64 k
sw: 200 ppm
o1: middle of ^{13}C NMR spectrum
o2: middle of ^{1}H NMR spectrum
p1: 45° ^{13}C transmitter pulse
p2, p3: 180° ^{13}C transmitter pulse
d1: 2s
d2: 1/ $J(C,H)$ = 7 ms, calculated from $^1J(C,H)$ = 140 Hz
d3: set d3 equal to preacquisition delay
decoupler attenuation and 90° pulse for CPD
ns = 512

5. Processing

Use standard 1D processing as described in Experiment 3.2. Adjust the phase for the TMS signal positive and for the carboxyl nucleus negative.

6. Result

The figure shows the APT spectrum of cholesteryl acetate obtained on an AM-400 spectrometer. Note that the signal of the solvent CDCl$_3$ is negative like the other signals of carbon atoms carrying no protons. Signals of CH and CH$_3$ groups are positive and signals of CH$_2$ groups are negative.

7. Comments

The APT sequence is in principle a double spin-echo experiment. By using a 45° or shorter excitation pulse a part of the initial magnetization remains in the z-direction and is inverted by the first 180° pulse. This could lead to a cancelling of signals with long spin–lattice relaxation times, but in the second spin-echo period the 180° pulse reinverts the z-magnetization, thus eliminating this problem. In comparison with all other editing techniques APT still seems to be the most simple and efficient method, since it gives in one experiment all the necessary information on *all* sorts of carbon atoms. The lower sensitivity compared with polarization transfer methods such as DEPT is in practice not important for the C,H spin pair. APT can be performed on older instruments, since no specific decoupler pulses are required.

8. Own Observations

Experiment 6.5

The Basic INEPT Technique

1. Purpose

The INEPT experiment (**I**nsensitive **N**uclei **E**nhanced by **P**olarization **T**ransfer) was developed to increase the signal strength for nuclides with a low gyromagnetic ratio and low natural abundance, such as ^{13}C, ^{29}Si, or ^{15}N. This sensitivity enhancement is usually achieved by polarization transfer from the protons via X,H spin coupling. The increase in sensitivity is γ_A/γ_X , where γ_A represents the gyromagnetic ratio of the nuclide serving as the polarization source, in most cases ^1H, although ^{19}F and ^{31}P can also be used. The polarization transfer experiment delivers larger enhancement factors than the NOE experiment (see Exps. 6.7 and 4.13). The enhancement is independent of the sign of γ. The INEPT sandwich is one of the most frequently used building blocks of modern 2D and 3D sequences. An application to ^{15}N NMR spectroscopy is given in Experiment 9.1. The basic form shown here for $CHCl_3$ is tuned to $^1J(C,H)$ and yields a coupled ^{13}C NMR spectrum.

2. Literature

[1] G. A. Morris, R. Freeman, *J. Am. Chem. Soc.* **1979**, *101*, 760–762.
[2] D. P. Burum, R. R. Ernst, *J. Magn. Reson.* **1980**, *39*, 163–168
[3] O. W. Sørensen, R. R. Ernst, *J. Magn. Reson.* **1983**, *51*, 477–489.

3. Pulse Scheme and Phase Cycle

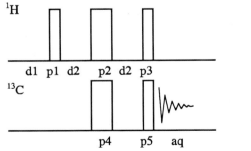

p1: $(x)_8$, $(-x)_8$

p2: x, -x

p3: $(y)_2$, $(-y)_2$

p4: x, -x

p5: $(x)_4$, $(y)_4$, $(-x)_4$, $(-y)_4$

aq: x, x, -x, -x, y, y, -y, -y

4. Acquisition

Time requirement: 10 min

Sample: 80% $CHCl_3$ in [D_6]acetone

Record normal ^{13}C and ^1H NMR spectra, note the offsets of $CHCl_3$, and load the INEPT pulse program. You have to set:

td: 4 k
sw: 500 Hz
o1: on resonance of ^{13}C NMR signal
o2: on resonance of ^{1}H NMR signal
p1, p3: 90° ^{1}H decoupler pulse
p2: 180° ^{1}H decoupler pulse
p4: 180° ^{13}C transmitter pulse
p5: 90° ^{13}C transmitter pulse
d1: 10 s
d2: 1/[4J(C,H)] = 1.18 ms, calculated from ^1J(C,H) = 212 Hz
decoupler attenuation for hard decoupler pulses
ns: 1 for the first and 4 for the second experiment

5. Processing

Use standard 1D processing as described in Experiment 3.2.

6. Result

The figure shows two INEPT spectra of CHCl$_3$ obtained on an AM-400 spectrometer. Spectrum **a** was recorded with one scan, spectrum **b** with 4 scans. Due to the phase cycle one obtains in spectrum **b** a 1 : (−1) doublet, whereas in **a** the intensities are in the ratio 5 : (−3). As an additional exercise you may perform the experiment with ethyl crotonate; see Experiment 6.6.

7. Comments

For the product operator formalism we consider a C,H spin pair. The first 90° proton pulse creates transverse magnetization of the protons which develops C,H spin coupling and ^{1}H chemical shift during both delays d2. The chemical shift, however, is refocused by the 180° ^{1}H pulse and therefore for simplicity is not included in the equations. Since a 180° ^{13}C pulse is applied simultaneously with the 180° ^{1}H pulse, the spin-echo after the second d2 delay is modulated by the C,H spin coupling. If the delay τ is set equal to 2·d2 = 1/[2J(C,H)] the cosine term becomes zero and the sine term unity, leaving pure antiphase magnetization of the proton with respect to carbon in Equation (1).

$$\gamma_H I_{Hz} \xrightarrow{I_{Hx}} -\gamma_H I_{Hy} \xrightarrow{\pi J \tau \, 2I_{Hz}I_{Cz}} -\gamma_H 2I_{Hx}I_{Cz} \tag{1}$$

This antiphase magnetization is converted into antiphase magnetization of ^{13}C with respect to ^1H by the two simultaneous 90° pulses. During acquisition C,H spin coupling develops again, forming an in-phase ^{13}C magnetization, which however is multiplied by γ_H and thus we obtain a proton-polarized ^{13}C signal. This signal appears in antiphase due to the sine term in Equation (2).

$$-\gamma_H 2I_{Hx}I_{Cz} \xrightarrow{I_{Hy}, I_{Cx}} -\gamma_H 2I_{Hz}I_{Cy} \xrightarrow{\pi J \, \text{aq} \, 2I_{Hz}I_{Cz}} \gamma_H I_{Cx} \sin\pi J \cdot \text{aq} \tag{2}$$

However, there is another contribution to the signal from the ^{13}C magnetization. I_{Cz} is first inverted by the 180° ^{13}C pulse and then converted into transverse magnetization by the 90° ^{13}C pulse. It develops C,H spin coupling during acquisition, giving an in-phase signal due to the cosine term in Equation (3).

$$\gamma_C I_{Cz} \xrightarrow{180° I_{Cx}} -\gamma_C I_{Cz} \xrightarrow{90° I_{Cx}} \gamma_C I_{Cy} \xrightarrow{\pi J \, \text{aq} \, 2I_{Hz}I_{Cz}} \gamma_C I_{Cy} \cos\pi J \cdot \text{aq} \tag{3}$$

This signal has the intensity ratio of 1 : 1, whereas the signal obtained in Equation (2) has the intensity ratio 4: (−4), superposition yields the intensity ratio 5 : (−3) as observed in spectrum **a.** The phase cycle of the INEPT sequence eliminates all signal contributions stemming from initial carbon magnetization; thus in spectrum **b** a 4 : (−4) doublet is seen. Furthermore, all signals from quaternary carbon atoms are suppressed.

In case of the polarization of ^{13}C nuclei by ^1H ($\gamma_H/\gamma_C \approx 4$) the theoretical relative intensities of the multiplets obtained in *one scan* are as follows:

CH		−3	5	
CH$_2$		−7	2	9
CH$_3$	−11	−9	15	13

This distortion of multiplets is a drawback of the INEPT sequence. Therefore the sequences INEPT+ (see Exp. 6.6) and DEPT (see Exp. 6.9) were developed.

8. Own Observations

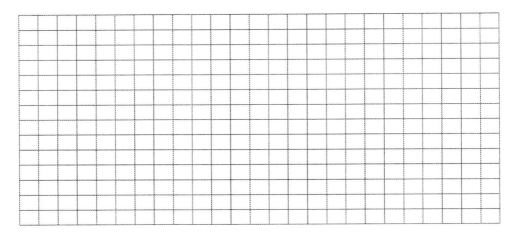

Experiment 6.6

INEPT+

1. Purpose

The disadvantage of the basic INEPT technique is the distortion of the multiplets. By adding a refocusing period with a subsequent additional purging pulse the extended version INEPT+ was developed, which yields coupled polarization-enhanced NMR spectra of X nuclei with correct intensities within the multiplets. Furthermore, the sequence can be tailored to give a different phase for CH_2 groups with respect to the signals of CH and CH_3 groups, providing editing possibilities. Here we describe the ^{13}C INEPT+ technique for ethyl crotonate.

2. Literature

[1] G. A. Morris, R. Freeman, *J. Am. Chem. Soc.* **1979**, *101*, 760–762.
[2] D. P. Burum, R. R. Ernst, *J. Magn. Reson.* **1980**, *39*, 163–168.
[3] O. W. Sørensen, R. R. Ernst, *J. Magn. Reson.* **1983**, *51*, 477–489.

3. Pulse Scheme and Phase Cycle

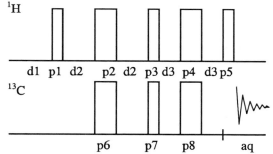

p1, p5: $(x)_8$, $(-x)_8$
p2, p4, p6: x, -x
p3: $(y)_2$, $(-y)_2$
p7: $(x)_4$, $(y)_4$, $(-x)_4$, $(-y)_4$
p8: $(x, -x)_2$, $(y, -y)_2$
aq: x, x, -x, -x, y, y, -y, -y

4. Acquisition

Time requirement: 10 min

Sample: 20% ethyl crotonate in $CDCl_3$

Load standard ^{13}C NMR parameter and the INEPT+ pulse program. You have to set:

td: 64 k
sw: 200 ppm
o1: middle of ^{13}C NMR spectrum
o2: middle of ^1H NMR spectrum
p1, p3, p5: 90° ^1H decoupler pulse
p2, p4: 180° ^1H decoupler pulse

p5, p7: 180° ^{13}C transmitter pulse
p6: 90° ^{13}C transmitter pulse
d1: 2 s
d2: 0.25/J(C,H) = 1.78 ms, calculated from ^1J(C,H) = 140 Hz
d3: 0.375/J(C,H) = 2.68 ms, calculated from ^1J(C,H) = 140 Hz
decoupler attenuation for hard decoupler pulses
ns = 128

5. Processing

Use standard 1D processing as described in Experiment 3.2

6. Result

In the figure **a** is the normal INEPT spectrum of ethyl crotonate (sequence of Exp. 6.5) and **b** (page 143) is the INEPT+ modification obtained on an AM-400 spectrometer. Compare the signal patterns of the two spectra. Note that in both spectra the signals of the quaternary carbon nuclei, i.e. those of the C=O group and CDCl$_3$, are missing.

7. Comments

In the INEPT+ sequence an additional refocusing period with two 180° pulses is added to the basic INEPT scheme. It can be shown by the product operator formalism [2] that the polarization factors obtained for CH, CH$_2$, and CH$_3$ groups are described by Equations (1).

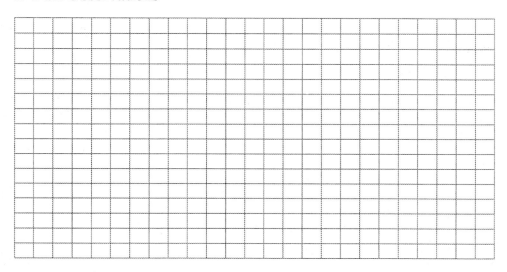

CH: $\gamma_H/\gamma_C \sin(\pi J\, d2) \sin(\pi J\, d3)$

CH$_2$: $\gamma_H/\gamma_C \sin(\pi J\, d2) \sin(2\pi J\, d3)$ (1)

CH$_3$: $3\gamma_H/4\gamma_C \sin(\pi J\, d2) [\sin(\pi J\, d3) + \sin(3\pi J\, d3)]$

Thus choosing delay d3 = 0.325/J(C,H), the CH$_2$ group gives a negative signal. The final purging pulse p5 removes intensity anomalies within the C,H multiplets.

8. Own Observations

Experiment 6.7

Refocused INEPT

1. Purpose

This variant of INEPT spectroscopy yields proton-decoupled and polarization-enhanced NMR spectra of X nuclei. It is derived from INEPT+ (see Exp. 6.6) by replacing the last proton pulse by broad-band decoupling. The experiment can be tailored to yield different phases of CH_2 groups with respect to CH and CH_3 groups and can therefore be used for editing. Another method yielding the same information is DEPT (see Exp. 6.9). Here we describe the ^{13}C experiment with ethyl crotonate.

2. Literature

[1] G. A. Morris, R. Freeman, *J. Am. Chem. Soc.* **1979**, *101*, 760–762.
[2] D. P. Burum, R. R. Ernst, *J. Magn. Reson.* **1980**, *39*, 163–168
[3] O. W. Sørensen, R. R. Ernst, *J. Magn. Reson.* **1983**, *51*, 477–489.

3. Pulse Scheme and Phase Cycle

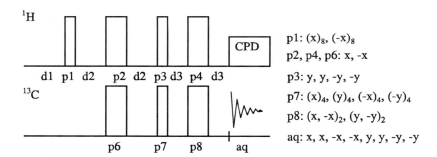

p1: $(x)_8$, $(-x)_8$

p2, p4, p6: x, -x

p3: y, y, -y, -y

p7: $(x)_4$, $(y)_4$, $(-x)_4$, $(-y)_4$

p8: $(x, -x)_2$, $(y, -y)_2$

aq: x, x, -x, -x, y, y, -y, -y

4. Acquisition

Time requirement: 10 min

Sample: 20% ethyl crotonate in $CDCl_3$

Load standard ^{13}C NMR parameter and the INEPT pulse program. You have to set:

td: 64 k
sw: 200 ppm
o1: middle of ^{13}C NMR spectrum
o2: middle of ^1H NMR spectrum
p1, p3: 90° ^1H decoupler pulse
p2, p4: 180° ^1H decoupler pulse

p6, p8: 180° ^{13}C transmitter pulse
p7: 90° ^{13}C transmitter pulse
d1: 2 s
d2: 0.25/J(C,H) = 1.78 ms, calculated from ^1J(C,H) = 140 Hz
d3: 0.375/J(C,H) = 2.68 ms, calculated from ^1J(C,H) = 140 Hz
decoupler attenuation for hard decoupler pulses
decoupler attenuation and 90° pulse for CPD
ns = 128

5. Processing

Use standard 1D processing as described in Experiment 3.2

6. Result

The figure shows the refocused INEPT spectrum of ethyl crotonate obtained on an AM-400 spectrometer. The signals of the quaternary carbon nuclei, i.e. those of the C=O group and CDCl$_3$, are missing.

7. Comments

The polarization and phase factors obtained for the refocused INEPT experiment are the same as in INEPT+ and are given there (see Exp. 6.6). Broad-band ^{1}H decoupling causes collapse of the multiplet lines, which after the refocusing period are all in-phase.

Refocused INEPT is useful for nuclides with low natural abundance and low gyro-magnetic ratio. The enhancemant factors η for different nuclides in comparison with the NOE enhancement factors are as follows:

Nuclide	^{13}C	^{15}N	^{29}Si	^{57}Fe	^{103}Rh	^{109}Ag	^{119}Sn	^{183}W
η(NOE)	2.99	−3.94	−1.52	16.48	−16.89	−9.75	−0.41	13.02
η(INEPT)	3.98	9.87	5.03	30.95	31.77	21.50	2.81	24.04

The advantage of INEPT, like all other polarization transfer methods is that the pulse repetition time of the experiment is dictated by the spin–lattice relaxation time of the protons rather than that of the nuclide under observation, here ^{13}C. The disadvantage of the INEPT sequence is its sensitivity towards both delays d2 and d3. Carbon nuclei with widely different C,H spin coupling constants can give signals with lower intensity or even the wrong sign. Therefore the DEPT sequence is more often used, since the choice of the delays is not as critical (see exp.6.9).

8. Own Observations

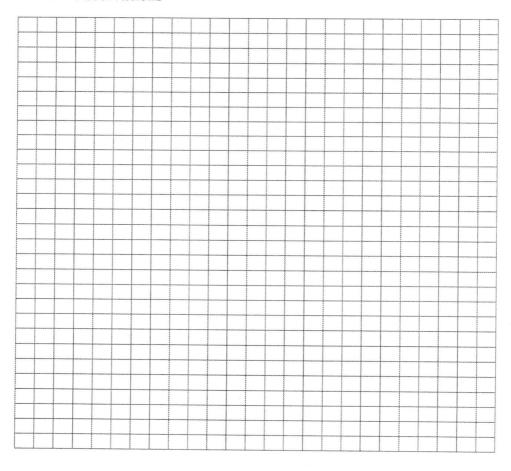

Experiment 6.8

Reverse INEPT

1. Purpose

The INEPT sandwich forms a basic building block in many modern 2D and 3D sequences, such as the HSQC technique (see Exp. 10.14). It transfers proton magnetization to an X nucleus. The reverse transfer is usually also achieved by an INEPT type sandwich, which is shown in the educational experiment given here. Starting from ^{13}C magnetization, the C,H spin coupling is observed by proton detection. Signals of protons bound to ^{12}C are suppressed.

2. Literature

[1] R. Freeman, T. H. Mareci, G. A. Morris, *J. Magn. Reson.* **1981**, *42*, 341–345.

3. Pulse Scheme and Phase Cycle

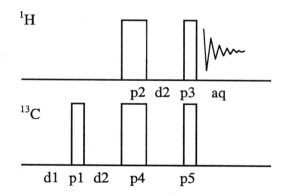

p1: $(x)_8$, $(-x)_8$

p2: x, -x

p3: $(y)_2$, $(-y)_2$

p4: x, -x

p5: $(x)_4$, $(y)_4$, $(-x)_4$, $(-y)_4$

aq: $(x)_2$, $(-x)_2$, $(y)_2$, $(-y)_2$

4. Acquisition

Time requirement: 10 min

Sample: 10% $CHCl_3$ in [D_6]acetone

Record normal ^{13}C and ^1H NMR spectra and note the offsets of $CHCl_3$. Set the instrument to ^1H observation with ^{13}C decoupling (inverse mode on older instruments) and load the reverse INEPT pulse program. You have to set:

    td: 4 k
    sw: 500 Hz
    o1: on resonance of ^1H NMR signal

o2: on resonance of ^{13}C NMR signal
p1, p5: 90° ^{13}C decoupler pulse
p2: 180° ^{1}H transmitter pulse
p3: 90° ^{1}H transmitter pulse
p4: 180° ^{13}C decoupler pulse
d1: 30 s
d2: $1/[4J(C,H)] = 1.19$ ms, calculated from $^{1}J(C,H) = 214$ Hz
decoupler attenuation for hard decoupler pulses
ns: 8

5. Processing

Use standard 1D processing with exponential multiplication (lb = 0.5 Hz) as described in Experiment 3.1

6. Result

The figure shows the result obtained on an AMX-500 spectrometer with an inverse probe-head.

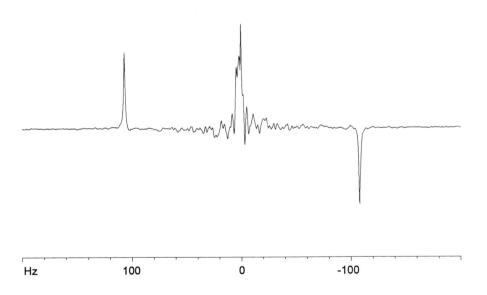

7. Comments

The product operator formalism is exactly the same as given in Experiment 6.5, except that the H and C subscripts of the operator terms have to be interchanged. Note, however, that the reverse INEPT sandwich shown in this experiment differs slightly from the one actually used in 2D experiments; see for example Experiment 10.14. In this educational experiment we have to start with in-phase carbon magnetization, created by the first pulse p1. Antiphase magnetization is developed, chemical shift effects are refocused, and the reverse transfer is achieved by the last two 90° pulses. In an actual 2D or 3D experiment, usually antiphase magnetization is already present after the t_1 evolution. Therefore, first the two 90° reverse transfer pulses are applied and the refocusing period with the two 180° pulses is used after the reverse transfer. Thus the common reverse INEPT building block in 2D or 3D sequences is a pair of 90° pulses followed by a refocusing period with a pair of 180° pulses, as seen in the HSQC sequence of Experiment 10.14. As an exercise you may add to the sequence described here an additional refocusing period with two 180° pulses, which will yield an in-phase signal. The experiment may also be performed with a normal dual probe-head.

8. Own Observations

Experiment 6.9

Editing ^{13}C NMR Spectra with DEPT

1. Purpose

The DEPT experiment (**D**istortionless **E**nhancement by **P**olarization **T**ransfer) uses, like the INEPT method (see Exps. 6.5–6.7), a polarization transfer from protons to an X nucleus to increase the signal strength. The experiment may be performed with polarization transfer over one or more bonds, with or without ^{1}H decoupling. It is therefore applied to nuclei with a low γ and a low natural abundance like ^{15}N or ^{29}Si (see Exp. 9.1–9.4) Furthermore, the sequence can also be used for distinguishing CH$_3$, CH$_2$, and CH groups (spectral editing). Alternative methods, which give information about the multiplicities, are SEFT (Exp. 6.3), APT (Exp. 6.4) and, more recently, PENDANT (Exp. 6.10). Described here is a ^{13}C DEPT experiment on cholesteryl acetate with complete editing yielding three subspectra.

2. Literature

[1] M. R. Bendall, D. M. Doddrell, D. T. Pegg, *J. Am. Chem. Soc.* **1981**, *103*, 4603–4605.
[2] D. M. Doddrell, D. T. Pegg, M. R. Bendall, *J. Magn. Reson.* **1982**, *48*, 323–327.
[3] K. V. Schenker, W. v. Philipsborn, *J. Magn. Reson.* **1986**, *66*, 219–229.

3. Pulse Scheme and Phase Cycle

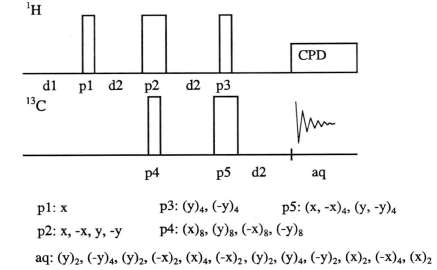

p1: x   p3: (y)$_4$, (-y)$_4$ p5: (x, -x)$_4$, (y, -y)$_4$

p2: x, -x, y, -y   p4: (x)$_8$, (y)$_8$, (-x)$_8$, (-y)$_8$

aq: (y)$_2$, (-y)$_4$, (y)$_2$, (-x)$_2$, (x)$_4$, (-x)$_2$, (y)$_2$, (y)$_4$, (-y)$_2$, (x)$_2$, (-x)$_4$, (x)$_2$

4. Acquisition

Time requirement: 1.5 h

Sample: 100 mg cholesteryl acetate in $CDCl_3$

Load standard ^{13}C NMR parameters and the DEPT pulse program. You have to set:

td: 64 k
sw: 200 ppm
o1: middle of ^{13}C NMR spectrum
o2: middle of ^1H NMR spectrum
p1: 90° ^1H decoupler pulse
p2: 180° ^1H decoupler pulse
p3: use 45°, 90°, and 135° ^1H decoupler pulses for three successive spectra a, b and c. Spectrum a will give the signals of CH, CH_2, and CH_3 groups all positive, b gives only the signals of CH groups, and the third spectrum c gives the signals of CH and CH_3 groups positive and signals of CH_2 groups negative. The second spectrum b gives a clear indication whether the decoupler pulse was determined correctly.
p4: 90° ^{13}C transmitter pulse
p5: 180° ^{13}C transmitter pulse
d1: 2 s
d2: $1/[2J(C,H)] = 3.5$ ms, calculated from $^1J(C,H) = 140$ Hz
decoupler attenuation for hard decoupler pulses
decoupler attenuation and 90° pulse for CPD
ns = 512

5. Processing

Use standard 1D processing as described in Experiment 3.2. For editing purposes the three spectra have to be further manipulated. Subtraction of 0.8·b from a yields spectrum d, where the signals of CH_2 and CH_3 groups both remain positive. Subtraction of 0.6·b from c yields spectrum e, where the signals of CH_2 are negative and those of the CH_3 groups remain positive. Subtraction of 1.2·e from d yields spectrum f with only signals of CH_2 groups, whereas addition of 1.2·e to d yields spectrum g with only signals of the CH_3 groups. The factors of 0.8, 0.6, and 1.2 may be finely adjusted according to the exact duration of pulse p3.

6. Result

The figure on page 152 shows the three edited DEPT subspectra b (CH groups), f (CH_2 groups), and g (CH_3 groups), obtained from the three different measurements a–c on an AM-400 spectrometer and calculated as described. Note that there is no information about quaternary carbon atoms. This is a disadvantage in comparison with the APT or PENDANT sequences. Compare the signal-to-noise ratio with that of Experiment 6.4 which was obtained under otherwise identical conditions.

7. Comments

For the product operator formalism we consider a C,H spin pair and neglect the effects of chemical shifts, since these are refocused by the 180° pulses. The first 90° proton pulse creates transverse magnetization of the protons which develops C,H spin coupling during the delay d2. If the delay τ is set equal to d2 = $1/[2J(C,H)]$ the cosine term becomes zero and the sine term unity, leaving pure antiphase magnetization of the proton with respect to carbon in the equation. This antiphase magnetization is converted into double quantum magnetization of carbon and proton by the first 90° ^{13}C pulse; see Equation (1).

$$\gamma_H I_{Hz} \xrightarrow{I_{Hx}} -\gamma_H I_{Hy} \xrightarrow{\pi J \tau 2 I_{Hz} I_{Cz}} \gamma_H 2 I_{Hx} I_{Cz} \xrightarrow{I_{Cx}} -\gamma_H 2 I_{Hx} I_{Cy} \qquad (1)$$

This double quantum term does not further develop spin coupling during the second d2 period. The transfer pulse p3 creates antiphase magnetization of carbon with respect to proton which during the third d2 delay develops in-phase carbon magnetization I_{Cx}. This is a polarized signal since I_{Cx} is multiplied by γ_H; see Equation (2). C,H coupling which would develop during acquisition is removed by the decoupling of the protons.

$$-\gamma_H 2^I H_x^I C_y \xrightarrow{I_{Hy}} \gamma_H 2^I H_z^I C_y \xrightarrow{\pi J \tau 2^I H_z^I C_z} \gamma_H ^I C_x \qquad (2)$$

Another signal contribution stemming from carbon magnetization I_{Cz}, which is converted into tranverse carbon magnetization by the first 90° carbon pulse, is removed by the phase cycle.

The adjustment of d2 = $1/2J$ is less crucial compared with INEPT, while the multiplicity selection is performed by the angle of the transfer pulse p3. However, signals of carbon atoms with very widely differing spin coupling constants such as sp-hybridized carbon atoms may display the wrong sign. Often the DEPT sequence is only performed once with p3 = 135°, yielding positive signals for CH and CH_3 groups and negative signals for CH_2 groups.

8. Own Observations

Experiment 6.10

Editing ^{13}C NMR Spectra with PENDANT

1. Purpose

There are several methods for distinguishing CH, CH_2, and CH_3 groups in fully ^1H decoupled carbon NMR spectra. Those most often used are INEPT (Exps. 6.5–6.8), DEPT (Exp. 6.9) or APT (Exp. 6.4), although all these methods have disadvantages. INEPT and DEPT give no chemical shift information on quaternary carbon atoms, and thus a normal ^{13}C NMR spectrum has to be measured in addition. APT is said to be less sensitive than DEPT, since only the NOE enhancement is operative. The very recently introduced PENDANT method (Polarization ENhancement During Attached Nucleus Testing) [1,2] described here is claimed to have the full sensitivity of DEPT and gives signals of quaternary carbon atoms within the same measurement.

2. Literature

[1] J. Homer, M. C. Perry, *J. Chem. Soc. Chem. Commun.* **1994**, 373–374.
[2] J. Homer, M. C. Perry, *J. Chem. Soc. Perkin Trans. 2* **1995**, 533–536.

3. Pulse Scheme with Phasecycle

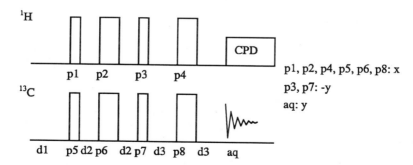

p1, p2, p4, p5, p6, p8: x
p3, p7: -y
aq: y

4. Acquisition

Time requirement: 10 min

Sample: 20% ethyl crotonate in $CDCl_3$

Load standard ^{13}C NMR parameters and the pulse program. You have to set:

    td: 64 k
    sw: 250 ppm
    o1: middle of ^{13}C NMR spectrum
    o2: middle of ^1H NMR spectrum

p1, p3: 90° ^{1}H decoupler pulse
p3, p4: 180° ^{1}H decoupler pulse
p5, p7: 90° ^{13}C transmitter pulse
p6, p8: 180° ^{13}C transmitter pulse
d1: 2 s
d2: $1/[4J(C,H)] = 1.72$ ms, calculated from $^1J(C,H) = 145$ Hz
d3: $5/[8J(C,H)] = 4.31$ ms, calculated from $^1J(C,H) = 145$ Hz
decoupler attenuation for hard decoupler pulses
decoupler attenuation and 90° pulse for CPD
de: preaquisition delay as short as possible
ns: 16

5. Processing

Use standard 1D processing as described in Experiment 3.2. Adjust the phase for the signal of the methyl groups to be positive and for the carboxyl nucleus negative.

6. Result

The figure shows a PENDANT spectrum of ethyl crotonate obtained on an ARX-200 spectrometer.

7. Comments

The authors do not provide an explanation in terms of the product operator formalism. One can, however, first consider a quaternary carbon spin I_C, which has no interaction with protons, giving Equation (1).

$$I_{Cz} \xrightarrow{90°I_{Cx}} -I_{Cy} \xrightarrow{180°I_{Cx}} I_{Cy} \xrightarrow{90°I_{C-y}} I_{Cy} \xrightarrow{180°I_{Cx}} -I_{Cy} \quad (1)$$

The first 90° pulse aligns the z-magnetization vector along the $-y$ direction. Chemical shift evolution before acquisition can be neglected as the two 180° carbon pulses only change the sign of the operator, and the 90° pulse in the $-y$ direction has no effect on the y-magnetization, thus the receiver detects a negative signal.

For a CH group we start with $\gamma_H I_{Hz}$, which is transformed into transverse proton magnetization by the first 90° proton pulse, giving Equation (2). During the following two delays d2 C,H spin coupling evolves, which is not refocused due to the simultaneous 180° proton and carbon pulses. Since we set τ equal to d2 = $1/4J$ and use two d2 periods in this sequence, the cosine term becomes zero and the sine term unity. Chemical shift evolution of the protons is refocused by the 180° pulse. Thus at the end of the second delay τ we find antiphase magnetization of the ^1H with respect to the ^{13}C.

$$\gamma_H I_{Hz} \xrightarrow{90°I_{Hx}} -\gamma_H I_{Hy} \xrightarrow{\pi J \tau \, 2I_{Hz}I_{Cz}} -\gamma_H I_{Hy}\cos(\pi J\tau) + 2\gamma_H I_{Hx}I_{Cz}\sin(\pi J\tau)$$

$$\xrightarrow{180°I_{Hx}, \, 180°I_{Cx}} -2\gamma_H I_{Hx}I_{Cz} \xrightarrow{90°I_{H-y}, \, 90°I_{Cy}} 2\gamma_H I_{Hz}I_{Cx} \quad (2)$$

The two simultaneous 90° proton and carbon pulses perform the polarization transfer by transforming $-2\gamma_H I_{Hx}I_{Cz}$ into antiphase magnetization of the carbon with respect to the proton. In the final part of the sequence an observable in-phase ^{13}C magnetization is generated. Note that this magnetization bears the factor γ_H, and is thus four times stronger than a normal carbon signal. To choose a suitable d3 value, one has to compromise for CH, CH$_2$, and CH$_3$. For a CH group we find that with d3 close to $1/2J$ the sine term disappears, leaving a positive ^{13}C signal at the receiver, giving Equation (3).

$$2\gamma_H I_{Hz}I_{Cx} \xrightarrow{\pi J \, d3 \, 2I_{Hz}I_{Cz}} -\gamma_H I_{Cy}\cos(\pi J d3) + 2\gamma_H I_{Hz}I_{Cx}\sin(\pi J d3) \quad (3)$$

In summary, the sequence can be viewed as a refocused INEPT with an additional ^{13}C pulse at the beginning.

8. Own Observations

Experiment 6.11

1D-INADEQUATE

1. Purpose

$^{13}C,^{13}C$ spin coupling constants are valuable parameters for the structure elucidation of organic molecules, but are difficult to determine at natural abundance since only every 10 000th molecule contains the necessary two ^{13}C nuclei. Their signals appear as doublets with an intensity 0.5% of that of the singlets from the mono-^{13}C isotopomers, so that only the large $^1J(C,C)$ couplings are accessible under normal conditions. However, the strong singlets can be suppressed by the INADEQUATE (Incredible Natural Abundance Double Quantum Transfer Experiment) pulse sequence, so that, at least in principle, even small $^{13}C,^{13}C$ couplings over two or three bonds may be observed. The version given here is the basic experiment tuned to $^1J(C,C)$, leading to antiphase signals [1]. Other variants described elsewhere are SELINQUATE (Exp. 7.7) and 2D-INADEQUATE (Exp. 10.19). 1D variants are refocused INADEQUATE, INEPT-INADEQUATE and DEPT-INADEQUATE [2], as well as a method which uses cross-polarization for signal enhancement [3]. Currently the difficult problem of suppressing the central signal is investigated using pulsed field gradients (see Experiment 11.12).

2. Literature

[1] A. Bax, R. Freeman, S. P. Kempsell, *J. Am. Chem. Soc.* **1980**, *102*, 4849–4851.
[2] J. Buddrus, H. Bauer, *Angew. Chem. Int. Ed. Engl.* **1987**, *26*, 625–643.
[3] C. Dalvit, G. Bovermann, *J. Magn. Reson. Ser. A* **1994**, *109*, 113–116.

3. Pulse Scheme and Phase Cycle

p1: $(x)_4$, $(y)_4$, $(-x)_4$, $(-y)_4$, $(-x)_4$, $(-y)_4$, $(x)_4$, $(y)_4$

p2: $[(x)_4$, $(y)_4$, $(-x)_4$, $(-y)_4]_2$, $[(-x)_4$, $(-y)_4$, $(x)_4$, $(y)_4]_2$

p3: $(x)_4$, $(y)_4$, $(-x)_4$, $(-y)_4$

p4: x, -y, -x, y   aq: $(x, y, -x, -y, -x, -y, x, y)_2 (-x, -y, x, y, x, y, -x, -y)_2$

4. Acquisition

Time requirement: 1 h

Sample: 90% 1-hexanol in [D$_6$]acetone

Tune the probe-head to the actual sample and record a normal ^{13}C NMR spectrum with ^{1}H-broad-band decoupling. Optimize the spectral width and determine the 90° and 180° pulse lengths (see Exp. 2.2) for *this* sample. Load the pulse program and set the following parameters:

> td: 32 k
> sw: 60 ppm (spectral range for C$_6$H$_{13}$OH)
> o1: 40 ppm downfield from TMS (middle of that range)
> o2: middle of ^{1}H NMR spectrum
> p1, p3, p4: 90° ^{13}C transmitter pulse
> p2: 180° ^{13}C transmitter pulse
> d1: 3 s
> d2: 1/[4 J(C,C)] = 7.6 ms, calculated from ^1J(C,C) = 33 Hz
> d3: 3 μs
> decoupler attenuation and 90° pulse for CPD
> ds: 4
> ns: 512

5. Processing

Use standard 1D processing as described in Exp. 3.2; apply zero filling to 64 k, use exponential multiplication with lb = 0.5 Hz.

6. Result

The figure on p. 158 shows the ^{13}C-1D-INADEQUATE spectrum of 1-hexanol obtained on an ARX-300 spectrometer using a 5 mm ^{1}H/^{13}C dual probe-head. Note the remarkable suppression of the singlets of the mono-^{13}C isotopomers. Closer inspection of the observed splittings (see expansion) shows that some couplings are obviously equal. For instance, the signal at δ_C = 32.4 (C-4) is just one doublet so that an unequivocal assignment based solely on the ^1J(C,C) values is not possible. Furthermore, doublets may show a "roof effect", characteristic of AB systems (see signal at δ_C = 33.2). The problem of assignment may be overcome by using the 2D version (see Exp. 10.19) in which the various AB spectra are spread out into the second dimension of double quantum frequencies or by using SELINQUATE (Exp. 7.7). As an exercise you may measure the 1D-INADEQUATE spectrum of 2-cyclohexene-1-one, where all C,C couplings are different and clearly resolved. Compare the results with Experiment 7.7.

7. Comments

Using the product operator formalism we consider a C,C spin pair. The first pulse p1 creates transverse magnetization, which develops C,C spin coupling during both delays d2. The 180° pulse refocuses the chemical shifts and is for simplicity not shown in the equations. Thus at the end of the spin-echo period we have in-phase and antiphase carbon magnetization multiplied by the respective cosine and sine terms as seen in Equation(1).

$$I_{Cz} \xrightarrow{\ I_{Cx}\ } -I_{Cy} \xrightarrow{\ \pi J \tau 2 I_{Cz} I_{Cz}\ } -I_{Cy}\cos\pi J\tau \ +2I_{Cx}I_{Cz}\sin\pi J\tau \tag{1}$$

If the delay τ is set equal to $2 \cdot d2 = 1/[2J(C,C)]$ the cosine term becomes zero and the sine term unity. The pulse p3 transfers the antiphase magnetization into double quantum magnetization, which is immediately transformed back into antiphase magnetization by pulse p4. During acquisition, C,C spin coupling develops again, forming an observable in-phase ^{13}C magnetization which is multiplied by a sine term containing the spin coupling as in Equation (2). Therefore the doublets appear in antiphase.

$$2I_{Cx}I_{Cz} \xrightarrow{I_{Cx}} -2I_{Cx}I_{Cy} \xrightarrow{I_{Cx}} 2I_{Cx}I_{Cz} \xrightarrow{\pi J \text{ aq } 2I_{Cz}I_{Cz}} I_{Cy}\sin\pi J\text{aq} \quad (2)$$

The mechanism for suppressing the central signal is based on the fact that the desired observable coherences must have passed the double quantum filter. This gives them a phase response different from that of ^{13}C signals from molecules which contain only one ^{13}C atom, and thus cannot develop spin–spin coupling. The sequence can therefore be viewed as a spin-echo method with a subsequent homonuclear double quantum filter. For a heteronuclear double quantum filter see Experiment 6.14. It is possible to set the delays d2 according to Equation (3); in cases where the ^{13}C signals have only a small chemical shift difference it is advisable to use n = 1 or 2.

$$d2 = (2n + 1)/[4J(C,C)] , n = 0, 1, 2... \quad (3)$$

8. Own Observations

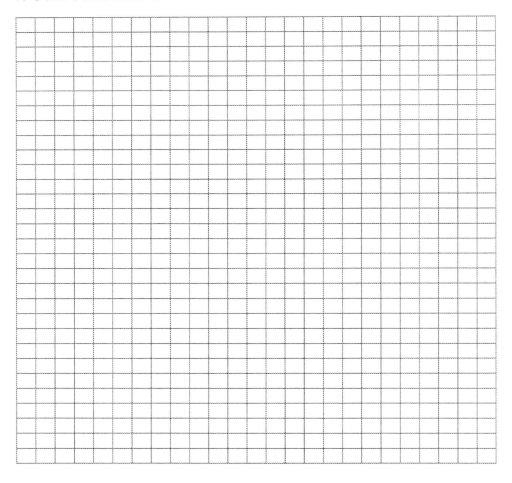

Experiment 6.12

The BIRD Filter

1. Purpose

In many experiments one wants to selectively observe protons that are attached to ^{13}C or ^{15}N. The strong signals of those protons attached to ^{12}C or ^{14}N need to be suppressed prior to the actual pulse sequence in order to be able to adjust the receiver gain for the desired signals only. One method of discriminating between these two kinds of signals is to insert the BIRD (**BI**linear **R**otation **D**ecoupling) sandwich, which rotates the magnetization of the protons attached to ^{12}C into the $-z$-direction of the rotating frame, but leaves the magnetization of the ^{13}C-bound protons unchanged. If one waits a suitable time after the BIRD sandwich, the signals of the former are at the null point and therefore not excited during the following pulse sequence. In this educational experiment the use of the BIRD sandwich is shown for chloroform.

2. Literature

[1] J. R. Garbow, D. P. Weitekamp, A. Pines, *Chem. Phys. Lett.* **1982**, *93*, 504–508.

3. Pulse Scheme and Phase Cycle

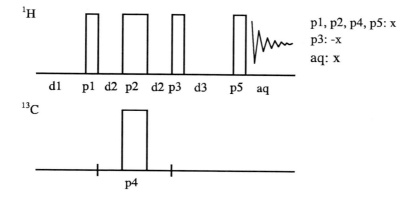

Note that the actual BIRD sandwich consists of the pulses p1 to p4, whereas p5 is only used for detection.

4. Acquisition

Time requirement: 10 min

Sample: 10% $CHCl_3$ in [D_6]acetone

Record normal ^{13}C and ^1H NMR spectra and note the offsets of $CHCl_3$. Set the instrument to ^1H observation with ^{13}C decoupling (inverse mode on older instruments) and load the BIRD pulse program. You have to set:

td: 4 k
sw: 500 Hz
o1: on ^1H resonance
o2: on ^{13}C resonance
p1, p3, p5: 90° ^1H transmitter pulse
p2: 180° ^1H transmitter pulse
p4: 180° ^{13}C decoupler pulse
d1: 60 s
d2: 1/[2J/C,H)] = 2.38 ms, calculated from ^1J (C,H) = 214 Hz
d3: 20 s, to be varied
ns: 1

Observe the incoming FID and adjust d3 until you find a minimum intensity, adjust the receiver gain accordingly.

5. Processing

Use standard ^1H processing as described in Experiment 3.1 with an exponential multiplication of lb = 1 Hz.

6. Result

The figure shows the result obtained on an ARX-200 spectrometer with a normal forward dual probe-head. Note that the BIRD filter has suppressed the central line roughly to the height of the ^{13}C satellites. The actual d3 value was 90 s (degassed and sealed sample); it depends greatly on the oxygen content of the sample.

7. Comments

The BIRD sandwich can be understood both either from usual vector diagrams or with the product operator formalism. With the latter we find for a proton bound to ^{12}C:

$$I_{Hz} \xrightarrow{90°I_{Hx}} -I_{Hy} \xrightarrow{180°I_{Hx}} I_{Hy} \xrightarrow{90°I_{H-x}} -I_{Hz} \qquad (1)$$

Since this proton develops no spin coupling its magnetization vector reaches the $-z$-direction after the BIRD sandwich as seen in Equation (1). Proton chemical shifts are refocused by the 180° ^{1}H pulse. In contrast, protons bound to ^{13}C develop spin coupling, and due to the two simultaneous 180° pulses this is also refocused. By setting the delay τ equal to d2 = 1/[2J(C,H)] the cosine terms become zero and the sine terms unity:

$$I_{Hz} \xrightarrow{90°I_{Hx}} -I_{Hy} \xrightarrow{\pi J\tau I_{Hz}I_{Cz}} -I_{Hy}\cos(\pi J\tau) + 2I_{Hx}I_{Cz}\sin(\pi J\tau) =$$

$$2I_{Hx}I_{Cz} \xrightarrow{180°I_{Hx}} \xrightarrow{180°I_{Cx}} -2I_{Hx}I_{Cz} \xrightarrow{\pi J\tau I_{Hz}I_{Cz}}$$

$$-2I_{Hx}I_{Cz}\cos(\pi J\tau) - I_{Hy}\sin(\pi J\tau) = -I_{Hy} \xrightarrow{90°I_{H-x}} I_{Hz} \qquad (2)$$

As can be seen from Equation (2), the magnetization vector of these protons is returned into the $+z$-direction.

Note that for typical organic or bioorganic applications the BIRD delay d3 is much shorter than for the degassed example used here; typically one finds d3 values in the order of 0.5 s.

8. Own Observations

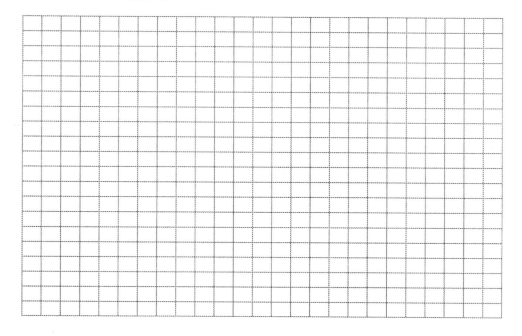

Experiment 6.13

TANGO

1. Purpose

The TANGO sequence (**T**esting for **A**djacent **N**uclei with a **G**yration **O**perator) acts as a 90° pulse for protons bound to ^{13}C, whereas the magnetization vector of protons bound to ^{12}C, which have no or only long-range couplings to ^{13}C remain in the positive z-direction. In contrast the BIRD sandwich (see Exp. 6.12) separates protons bound to ^{13}C and protons bound to ^{12}C so that their magnetization vectors are in the positive and negative z-direction. Thus, the TANGO sandwich introduces an 90° phase angle between these two sorts of proton spins whereas the BIRD sandwich an angle of 180°. The sequence is used, like BIRD, as a basic building block in many pulse techniques. In this educational experiment we demonstrate the use of the sequence on $CHCl_3$.

2. Literature

[1] S. Wimperis, R. Freeman, *J. Magn. Reson.* **1984**, *58*, 348–353.
[2] T. Parella, F. Sanchez-Ferrando, A. Virgili, *J. Magn. Reson. Ser. A* **1995**, *112*, 241–245.

3. Pulse Scheme with Phasecycle

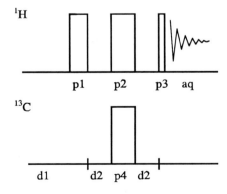

p1, p2, p3: $(x)_2$, $(-x)_2$, $(y)_2$, $(-y)_2$

p4: x, -x, -x, x, y, -y, -y, y

aq: $(x)_2$, $(-x)_2$, $(y)_2$, $(-y)_2$

4. Acquisition

Time requirement: 10 min

Sample: 10% $CHCl_3$ in [D_6]acetone

Obtain first ^1H and ^{13}C spectra of the sample and note the offsets of the $CHCl_3$ signals. The instrument must be in the inverse mode, using the proton channel as transmitter and the ^{13}C channel as decoupler. You have to set:

> td: 4 k
> o1: on ^1H resonance
> o2: on ^{13}C resonance
> sw: 500 Hz
> p1: 135° ^1H transmitter pulse
> p2: 180° ^1H transmitter pulse
> p3: 45° ^1H transmitter pulse
> p4: 180° ^{13}C decoupler pulse
> d1: 20 s
> d2: $1/[2J(C,H)] = 2.38$ ms, calculated from $^1J(C,H) = 214$ Hz
> ns: 8

5. Processing

Use standard ^1H processing as described in Experiment 3.1 with exponential multiplication of lb = 1 Hz.

6. Result

The figure shows the result obtained on an AMX-500 spectrometer with an inverse probe-head. Note that the suppression of the central signal is less efficient compared to the BIRD sequence of Experiment 6.12, since only a slight misadjustment of the pulse-length causes a central signal.

7. Comments

For analysis with the product operator formalism we consider first a proton bound to ^{12}C and thus not being able to develop C,H spin coupling. The effects of chemical shifts are neglected since they are removed by the 180° pulses. The first 135° proton pulse creates transverse magnetization and leaves part of the z-magnetization. The 180° proton pulse changes the signs of the terms, then the final 45° proton pulse creates four magnetizations, which simplify due to the different sine and cosine terms to give I_{Hz} unchanged. Thus, for protons without or small C,H spin coupling the TANGO sandwich acts as a 360° pulse, as indicated in Equation (1).

$$I_{Hz} \xrightarrow{\ 135°I_{Hx}\ } -I_{Hy}\sin(135) + I_{Hz}\cos(135) \xrightarrow{\ 180°I_{Hx}\ } I_{Hy}\sin(135)$$

$$-I_{Hz}\cos(135) \xrightarrow{\ 45°I_{Hx}\ } I_{Hy}\sin(135)\cos(45) + I_{Hy}\cos(135)\sin(45)$$

$$-I_{Hz}\cos(135)\cos(45) + I_{Hz}\sin(135)\sin(45) = I_{Hz} \qquad (1)$$

In contrast, a proton bound to ^{13}C develops C,H spin coupling after the first 45° pulse. Since both ^{1}H and ^{13}C 180° pulses are applied the spin coupling is not refocused but develops further in the second d2 period. If the delay τ is set equal to $2 \cdot d2 = 1/J$ the corresponding sine terms become zero and the cosine terms -1. Thus, compared with Equation (1), we observe a sign change before the last proton pulse as indicated in Equation (2). This again creates four magnetizations which simplify to $-I_{Hy}$, and therefore the TANGO sandwich acts like a 90° pulse for these protons.

$$I_{Hz} \xrightarrow{\ 135°I_{Hx}\ } -I_{Hy}\sin(135) + I_{Hz}\cos(135) \xrightarrow{\ \pi J \tau\, 2I_{Hz}I_{Cz}\ } -I_{Hy}\sin(135)$$

$$+ I_{Hz}\cos(135) \xrightarrow{\ 45°I_{Hx}\ } -I_{Hy}\sin(135)\cos(45) + I_{Hy}\cos(135)\sin(45)$$

$$-I_{Hz}\cos(135)\cos(45) - I_{Hz}\sin(135)\sin(45) = -I_{Hy} \qquad (2)$$

Note that both the BIRD and TANGO sandwiches can be used in a reversed sense by changing the appropriate pulse phases. Then TANGO would act as a 90° pulse for protons bound to ^{12}C and BIRD as a 180° pulse for protons bound to ^{13}C.

8. Own Observations

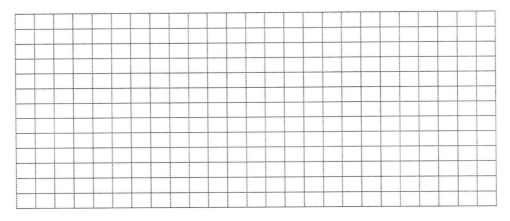

Experiment 6.14

The Heteronuclear Double Quantum Filter

1. Purpose

In many experiments one wants to selectively observe protons that are attached to ^{13}C or ^{15}N. The strong signals of protons attached to ^{12}C or ^{14}N need to be suppressed prior to the actual pulse sequence in order to be able to adjust the receiver gain for the desired signals only. One method of discriminating between these two kinds of signals is to use the double quantum filter. It is applied in many pulse sequences and consists essentially of two 90° pulses. Double quantum magnetization passes through this filter, whereas single quantum magnetization is filtered out by the phase cycle. In this educational experiment the use of a heteronuclear double quantum filter is shown for chloroform, an experiment which, in addition, reveals any instability of the spectrometer. In the homonuclear case one type of application is the suppression of a strong solvent signal, e. g. that of water (see Exp 10.7), or of the central signal in INADEQUATE (see Exp. 6.11).

2. Literature

[1] R. Freeman, *A Handbook of Nuclear Magnetic Resonance*, Longman Scientific Technical, Harlow, **1987**, p. 128–133.
[2] S. W. Homans, *A Dictionary of Concepts in NMR*, Clarendon Press, Oxford, **1989**, 93–106.

3. Pulse Scheme and Phase Cycle

p1: (x)$_4$, (-x)$_4$
p2: x, -x
p3: (x)$_2$, (-x)$_2$
aq: x, x, -x, -x, y, y, -y, -y

4. Acquisition

Time requirement: 0.5 h

Sample: 10% CHCl$_3$ in [D$_6$]acetone

The instrument must be in the inverse mode, using the proton channel as transmitter and the ^{13}C channel as decoupler. First obtain ^1H and ^{13}C spectra of the sample and note the offsets of the CHCl$_3$ signals. You have to set:

td: 4 k
sw: 500 Hz
o1: on ^1H resonance
o2: on ^{13}C resonance
p1: 90° ^1H transmitter pulse
p2, p3: 90° ^{13}C decoupler pulse
d1: 200 s
d2: $1/[2J(C,H)] = 2.38$ ms, calculated from $^1J(C,H) = 214$ Hz
d3: 10 μs
ns: 8

5. Processing

Use standard ^1H processing as described in Experiment 3.1.

6. Result

The figure shows the result obtained on an ARX-200 spectrometer with a normal forward dual probe-head. Note that the double quantum filter has suppressed the central line roughly to the height of the ^{13}C satellites.

7. Comments

The double quantum filter can be only understood with the product operator formalism or the density matrix approach. With the former we find for a proton bound to ^{13}C:

$$I_{Hz} \xrightarrow{\ 90° I_{Hx}\ } -I_{Hy} \xrightarrow{\ \pi J \tau\, 2I_{Hz}I_{Cz}\ } -I_{Hy}\cos(\pi J\tau) + 2I_{Hx}I_{Cz}\sin(\pi J\tau) \ =$$

$$2I_{Hx}I_{Cz} \xrightarrow{\;90°I_{Cx}\;} -2I_{Hx}I_{Cy} \xrightarrow{\;90°I_{Cx}\;} -2I_{Hx}I_{Cz} \xrightarrow{\;\pi J \tau \, 2I_{Hz}I_{Cz}\;}$$

$$-2I_{Hx}I_{Cz}\cos(\pi J\tau) - I_{Hy}\sin(\pi J\tau) = -I_{Hy} \tag{1}$$

By setting the delay τ equal to d2 $= 1/[2J(C,H)]$ the cosine terms become zero and the sine terms unity. As can be seen from Equation (1), the double quantum magnetization $-2I_{Hx}I_{Cy}$ is generated by the first ^{13}C pulse, whereas the second ^{13}C pulse converts this back into antiphase magnetization $-2I_{Hx}I_{Cz}$. Spin coupling evolution within the second d2 period reverts this to an observable single quantum magnetization $-I_{Hy}$. In comparison, a proton bound to ^{12}C does not develop spin coupling, and hence remains after the first proton pulse also as $-I_{Hy}$. However, if in the second scan the phase of the first ^{13}C pulse is changed along with the receiver phase, all signals of protons bound to ^{12}C are cancelled, whereas signals which developed via double quantum magnetization are accumulated.

Note that for typical organic or bioorganic applications the relaxation delay d1 is much shorter than for the sample used here. As an additional exercise you may combine the BIRD filter (Exp 6.12) with the double quantum filter, which should improve the signal suppression further.

8. Own Observations

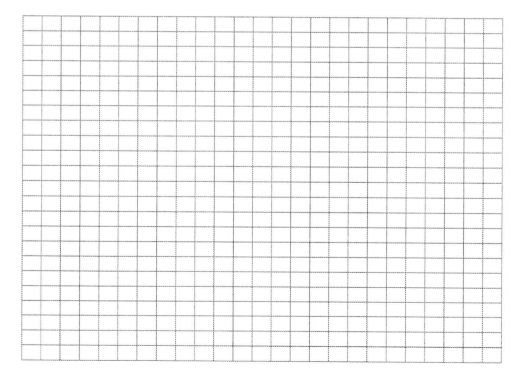

Experiment 6.15

Water Suppression by Presaturation

1. Purpose

For biological and biochemical applications ^{1}H NMR spectra usually have to be recorded in normal water, with the addition of only 10% D_2O to provide the necessary lock signal. Higher D_2O content would cause the exchangeable NH protons to dissapear. Thus, there is a need to suppress the huge solvent signal. For this purpose a multitude of techniques have been proposed. However, all techniques require that the magnet is well shimmed and a probe-head yielding a reasonable line-shape (see Exp. 3.3) must be available. In this experiment the presaturation method is described. It provides a check on whether the spectrometer set-up is capable of effective water suppression. For other methods see Experiments 6.16 and 11.13.

2. Literature

[1] M. Guéron, P. Plateu, M. Decorps, *Prog. NMR Spectrosc.* **1991**, *23*, 135–209.

3. Pulse Scheme and Phase Cycle

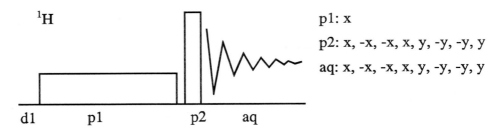

p1: x

p2: x, -x, -x, x, y, -y, -y, y

aq: x, -x, -x, x, y, -y, -y, y

4. Acquisition

Time requirement: 15 min

Sample: 2 mmol sucrose in 90% H_2O / 10% D_2O + 0.5 mmol DSS (2,2-dimethyl-2-silapentane-5-sulfonate, sodium salt) + trace of NaN_3 against bacteria growth

The magnet is well shimmed on the water sample. A normal ^{1}H NMR spectrum is recorded and the offset of the transmitter adjusted on the water resonance. The program for presaturation is loaded, where a weak transmitter pulse p1 of 2 s duration is used for irradiation of the water signal.

   On older instruments power switching of the transmitter is often not possible, and therefore the decoupler has to be used as the pre-irradiation source, which may give inferior results. If possible, the decoupler channel should be set to phase coherence with the transmitter. You have to set:

td: 32 k
sw: 10 ppm
o1: on resonance of water signal
p1: 2 s, presaturation pulse at transmitter power level corresponding to $\gamma B_1 \approx$
     25 Hz (90° pulse of $\approx$10ms, about 65 dB, see exp 2.6)
p2: 90° ^{1}H transmitter pulse
d1: 100 ms
rg: receiver gain for correct ADC input
for inverse probeheads: spinner off
ds: 2
ns: 8

5. Processing

Use standard 1D processing as described in Experiment 3.1, no window multiplication should be used.

6. Result

The figure on page 171 shows the result of the above procedure using an inverse probe-head on an AMX-500 spectrometer. The quality of the result is checked by two observations, first the line-width of the residual water signal at half height of the DSS signal and second the signal-to-noise ratio and resolution of the doublet of the anomeric proton under these conditions. The residual water line-width should be below 100 Hz and the splitting of the anomeric signal at $\delta_H = 5.41$ should be visible at least down to 40% of the signal height. Note that even better supression of the water could be obtained, although at the cost of the nearby anomeric signal.

7. Comments

The water suppression method shown here has the drawback that exchanging NH protons are also saturated and can therefore disappear from the spectrum. There are many other water suppression techniques in the literature; one, the jump and return sequence, is demonstrated in Experiment 6.16. More recent techniques work with coherence selection by pulsed field gradients, see the WATERGATE Experiment 11.13.

8. Own Observations

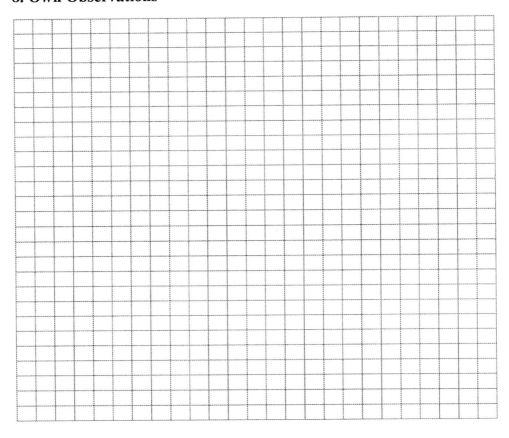

Experiment 6.16

Water Suppression by the Jump and Return Method

1. Purpose

For biological and biochemical applications ^{1}H NMR spectra usually have to be recorded in normal water with the addition of only 10% D_2O to provide the necessary lock signal. Higher D_2O content would cause the exchangeable NH protons to disappear. Thus, there is a need to suppress the huge solvent signal. For this purpose a multitude of techniques have been proposed [1]. The presaturation method (Exp. 6.15) does also affect exchangeable protons, but this is not true for the jump and return technique [2] described here. A method using pulsed field gradients is described in Experiment 11.13.

2. Literature

[1] Guéron, P. Plateu, M. Decorps, *Prog. NMR Spectrosc.* **1991**, *23*, 135–209.
[2] Guéron, P. Plateu, *J. Am. Chem. Soc.* **1982**, *104*, 7310–7311.

3. Pulse Scheme and Phase Cycle

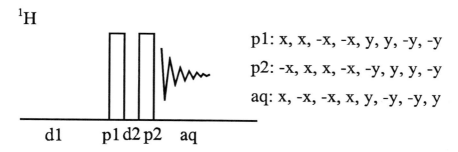

[1]H

p1: x, x, -x, -x, y, y, -y, -y

p2: -x, x, x, -x, -y, y, y, -y

aq: x, -x, -x, x, y, -y, -y, y

d1   p1 d2 p2   aq

4. Acquisition

Time requirement: 15 min

Sample: 2 mmol sucrose in 90% H_2O / 10% D_2O + 0.5 mmol DSS (2,2-dimethyl-2-silapentane-5-sulfonate, sodium salt) + a trace of NaN_3 (against bacteria growth).

The magnet is well shimmed on the water sample. A normal ^{1}H NMR spectrum is recorded and the offset of the transmitter adjusted on the water resonance. You have to set:

td: 32 k
sw: 10 ppm
o1: on resonance of water signal
p1: 90° ^{1}H transmitter pulse
p2: 90° ^{1}H transmitter pulse
d1: 2 s
d2: 125 µs
rg: receiver gain for correct ADC input
ds: 2
ns: 8

5. Processing

Use standard 1D processing as described in experiment 3.1

6. Result

The figure shows the result of the above procedure using an inverse probe-head on an AMX-500 spectrometer. Note that with the jump and return method there is a phase change of 180° at the water resonance position. Compared with the performance of the presaturation method the result is less convincing.

7. Comments

The sequence can be easily understood using the classical vector picture. The first pulse aligns all magnetization vectors in the $-y$-direction, where they start to fan out corresponding to their chemical shifts. Only the water signal has no chemical shift with respect to the rotating frame, and thus the second pulse brings it back to the z-direction, yielding in theory no signal during acquisition.

Compare the performance of this sequence with the result of the presaturation method described in Experiment 6.15 and the WATERGATE technique described in Experiment 11.13

8. Own Observations

Chapter 7

NMR Spectroscopy with Selective Pulses

The traditional method of continous wave NMR spectroscopy was in principle based on selective excitation. In the field- or frequency-swept instruments of the early days of NMR spectroscopy, each signal of a spectrum was selectively excited in turn when its resonance condition was met. With the advent of pulse Fourier transform spectroscopy these techniques were largely replaced so that all signals of a spectrum are excited non-selectively at the same time by a radiofrequency pulse. According to the Fellgett principle this leads to a much higher sensitivity than could be reached with continous wave-instruments.

However, for some applications it would be extremely useful to be able to excite a particular signal and transfer selected coherences to other spins. Therefore, in the early eighties the use of selective "shaped" or "soft" r.f. pulses of low power and relatively long duration was introduced. Their use in combination with the non-selective "hard" pulses (short rectangular high-power pulses) lead to entirely new possibilities in NMR spectroscopy.

There are some hardware requirements which have to be met before one is able to apply shaped pulses, such as waveform memories, special amplifiers, and the corresponding routers which feed these pulses into the transmitter or decoupler channel. On recent instruments this equipment is already, or will soon become, a standard feature.

Working with selective pulses does, however, require the skills of an experienced spectroscopist. These experiments cannot be performed in the manner of the routine 1D or 2D standard pulse sequences, where meaningful results can be achieved even by robots. The shape of the selective pulses has to be chosen from a large menu of possibilities to obtain the desired action and selectivity. The r.f. power and phase has to be calibrated. Thus, prior to an experiment which uses selective pulses a certain amount of preparation has to be performed. The achievable results, as shown in this chapter, should be worth the greater effort required.

After some calibration methods we show first the DANTE experiment, which can be performed without a pulse shaping unit. Homonuclear experiments such as selective COSY or TOCSY and SELINQUATE follow, and we demonstrate also some heteronuclear applications such as INAPT and SELINCOR. The chapter ends with three procedures in which selective pulses are applied within a 2D sequence, thus reducing a problem which is in principle three-dimensional in a two-dimensional one.

Literature

[1] W. S. Warren, M. S. Silver, *Adv. Magn. Reson.* **1988**, *12*, 247–384.
[2] H. Kessler, S. Mronga, G. Gemmecker, *Magn. Reson. Chem.* **1991**, *29*, 527–557.
[3] R. Freeman, *Chem. Rev.* **1991**, *91*,1397–1412.

Experiment 7.1

Determination of a Shaped 90° ^{1}H Pulse

1. Purpose

Many advanced experiments such as SELCOSY (Exp. 7.5) or selective TOCSY (Exp. 7.8) use "soft" or shaped ^{1}H pulses in the transmitter channel. Prior to these experiments the pulse shapes have to be chosen and their pulse-lengths must be selected in accordance with the desired selectivity. Thus, the 90° shaped pulse must be determined by varying the attenuation of the transmitter and not the pulse-length. After having determined the 90° pulse the relative phase of this pulse with respect to a hard 90° pulse has to be adjusted, since their signal pathways might be quite different. This experiment describes the complete calibration procedure.

2. Literature

[1] H. Kessler, S. Mronga, G. Gemmecker, *Magn. Reson. Chem.* **1991**, *29*, 527–557.

3. Pulse Scheme and Phase Cycle

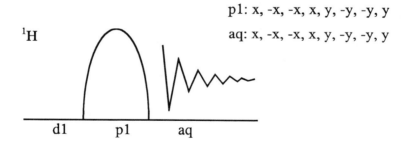

p1: x, -x, -x, x, y, -y, -y, y

aq: x, -x, -x, x, y, -y, -y, y

^{1}H

d1   p1   aq

4. Acquisition

Time requirement: 30 min

Sample: 10% CHCl$_3$ in [D$_6$]acetone; *do not use a degassed and sealed sample*, since that would make the relaxation time of the CHCl$_3$ protons exceedingly long.

The spectrometer should be in normal operation for protons. First the shape and length of the soft pulse has to be selected. For this experiment a Gaussian shape on 1024 data points of 50 ms length was chosen. As a rule of thumb the selectivity in Hz of a shaped pulse corresponds the reciprocal of its length. You have to set:

    td: 4 k
    sw: 500 Hz
    o1: on ^{1}H resonance

p1: shaped ^{1}H transmitter pulse, 50 ms
d1: 20 s
transmitter attenuation, to be varied in steps of 2 dB, initial value 90 dB
rg: receiver gain for correct ADC input
ns: 1

Since it is not allowed to change the pulse length in this experiment you have to determine the signal strength as a function of the transmitter attenuation. This is best done by recording the integrals. Having determined the optimum transmitter attenuation, a spectrum with a hard 90° pulse is obtained and the necessary phase correction noted. This phase correction value is subsequently used to adjust the phase of the spectrum which was obtained with the soft pulse. Most likely, it will be out of phase. The difference of the phases obtained in these two experiments is then put into the pulse program as the excitation phase of the shaped pulse. Recent software also allows this to be treated as an adjustable parameter of the data set. Both experiments should then give identical results with the same phase correction in the processing routine.

5. Processing

Use standard 1D processing as described in Experiment 3.1

6. Result

The figure shows a typical plot of integral values versus transmitter attenuation obtained on a AMX-500 spectrometer, an attenuator setting of ca. 67 dB corresponds to the 90° pulse. Note that the dB scale is logarithmic resulting in a compression of the expected sine curve. In addition, there is often some deviation from the ideal curve.

7. Comments

The determination of the relative phase is only necessary if, in the actual pulse sequence used, both hard and soft pulses are applied on the same channel. Recent software allows an offset modulation of the shaped pulse. Thus one can excite signals distant from the offset of the transmitter. Note, however, that the phase of these shaped pulses is dependent on the offset modulation and has to be adjusted for each different offset.

8. Own Observations

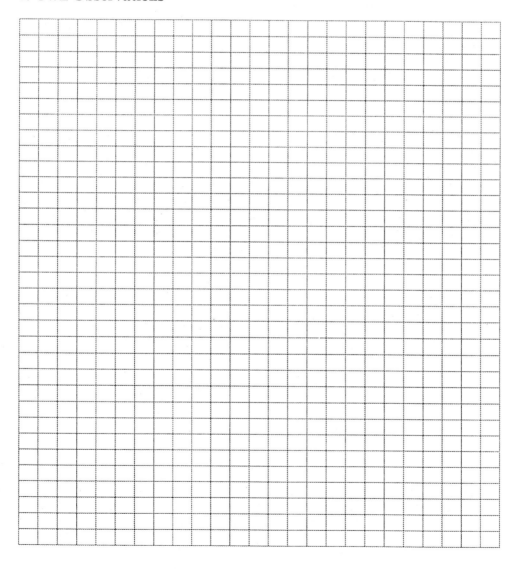

Experiment 7.2

Determination of a Shaped 90° ^{1}H Decoupler Pulse

1. Purpose

Some heteronuclear experiments use shaped pulses in the decoupler channel (see Exp. 7.10). Prior to these experiments the pulse shapes have to be chosen and their pulse-lengths must be selected in accordance with the desired selectivity. Thus, the 90° shaped ^{1}H decoupler pulse must be determined by varying the attenuation of the de-coupler and not the pulse-length. After having determined the 90° shaped decoupler pulse the relative phase of this pulse with respect to a hard 90° decoupler pulse has to be adjusted if in the actual experiment both hard and soft pulses are applied in the de-coupler channel, since their signal pathways might be quite different. Note that in Ex-periment 7.3 the inverse form of this procedure with proton detection and a shaped decoupler pulse on the ^{13}C channel is described.

2. Literature

[1] H. Kessler, S. Mronga, G. Gemmecker, *Magn. Reson. Chem.* **1991**, *29*, 527–557.
[2] J.-M. Bernassau, J.-M. Nuzillard, *J. Magn. Reson. Ser. A* **1993**, *104*, 212–221.

3. Pulse Scheme and Phase Cycle

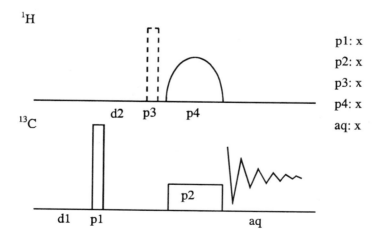

p1: x
p2: x
p3: x
p4: x
aq: x

4. Acquisition

Time requirement: 30 min

Sample: 80% CHCl$_3$ in [D$_6$]acetone; *do not use a degassed and sealed sample*, since that would make the relaxation time of the CHCl$_3$ nuclei exceedingly long.

Obtain normal ^{1}H and ^{13}C spectra of the sample and note the offsets. The spectrometer is set to ^{13}C operation. First the desired pulse shape of the decoupler soft pulse and its length must be selected. For this experiment a Gaussian shape on 1024 data points of 30 ms length was chosen. You have to set:

td: 4 k
sw: 500 Hz
o1: on ^{13}C resonance
o2: on ^{1}H resonance
p1: 90° ^{13}C transmitter pulse
p2: ^{13}C spin-lock pulse at 15 dB transmitter attenuation, length = p4
p3: leave at zero for the determination of the correct attenuation of the shaped
     pulse. For phase determination set to hard 90° ^{1}H decoupler pulse.
p4: shaped ^{1}H decoupler pulse, 30 ms
d1: 10 s
d2: $1/[2J(C,H)] = 2.36$ ms, calculated from $^1J(C,H) = 212$ Hz
decoupler attenuation for soft pulse, initial value 80 dB, to be varied
rg: receiver gain for correct ADC input
ns: 1

Since it is not allowed to change the pulse length in this experiment you have to determine the signal-to-noise ratio of the signal as a function of the decoupler attenuation. With a very high decoupler attenuation (about 80 dB) adjust the phase of the C,H doublet to an antiphase pattern. Then repeat the experiment with different decoupler attenuations until you get a spectrum with zero intensity of the doublet which corresponds to the soft 90° decoupler pulse. To obtain the correct phase of the soft decoupler pulse one introduces another hard 90° decoupler pulse p3 before the soft pulse in the pulse program. If both have the same phase, they are additive and yield an antiphase pattern with opposite phases to those adjusted before.

5. Processing

Use standard 1D processing as described in Experiment 3.2.

6. Result

The figure on page 182 shows spectra obtained on an AMX-500 spectrometer. **a** is the initial spectrum with high decoupler attenuation; **b** is the spectrum obtained with a shaped 90° decoupler pulse where both signals disappear, and **c** was obtained with an additional hard 90° decoupler pulse p3, where both hard and soft pulses have the same effective phase.

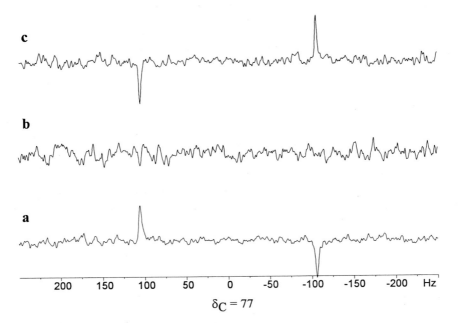

c

b

a

200   150   100   50   0   -50   -100   -150   -200   Hz

$\delta_C = 77$

7. Comments

The product operator formalism of the basic mechanism of this experiment has been outlined in Experiment 2.3. This calibration experiment follows the description given in a very recent publication [2]. In earlier work it was found difficult to obtain a correct calibration because of phasing problems. This problem is removed by using the ^{13}C spin-lock pulse p2, which decouples the ^{13}C spins during the application of the shaped ^1H decoupler pulse, reducing the ^{13}C satellites of $CHCl_3$ to one singlet. Therefore the shaped pulse can be applied at the center of the proton resonance.

8. Own Observations

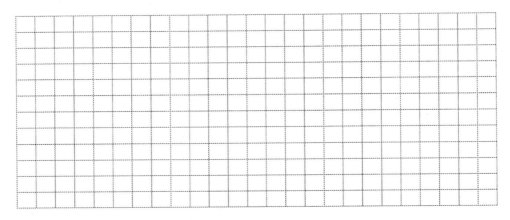

Experiment 7.3

Determination of a Shaped 90° 13C Decoupler Pulse

1. Purpose

Some inverse experiments use shaped pulses in the ^{13}C decoupler channel (Exps. 7.6, 7.11). Prior to these experiments the pulse shapes have to be chosen and their pulse-length selected in accordance with the desired selectivity (reciprocal of pulse-length). Thus, the 90° pulse must be determined by varying the attenuation of the decoupler and not the pulse-length. After having determined the attenuation of the shaped 90° pulse, the relative phase of this pulse with respect to a hard 90° decoupler pulse has to be adjusted. This is necessary if in the actual application both hard and soft pulses are used, since their signal pathways might be different.

2. Literature

[1] J.-M. Bernassau, J.-M. Nuzillard, *J. Magn. Reson. Ser. A* **1993**, *104*, 212–221.

3. Pulse Scheme and Phase Cycle

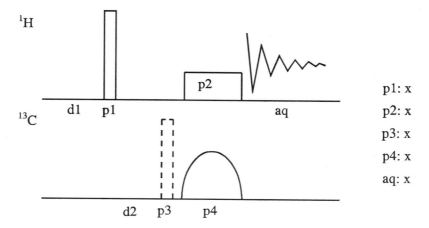

p1: x
p2: x
p3: x
p4: x
aq: x

4. Acquisition

Time requirement: 30 min

Sample: 10% $CHCl_3$ in [D_6]acetone; *do not use a degassed and sealed sample*, since that would make the relaxation time of the $CHCl_3$ nuclei exceedingly long.

First the ^1H and ^{13}C offsets of the sample have to be determined. The spectrometer is set up for ^1H obervation with ^{13}C decoupling (inverse mode on older instruments).

td: 4 k
sw: 500 Hz
o1: on ^{1}H resonance
o2: on ^{13}C resonance
p1: 90° ^{1}H transmitter pulse
p2: ^{1}H spin lock pulse, same length as p4, typical attenuation 12 dB
p3: leave at zero for the determination of the correct attenuation of the shaped
    pulse. For phase determination set to hard 90° ^{13}C decoupler pulse.
p4: shaped ^{13}C decoupler pulse, 10 ms
decoupler attenuation for soft pulse, initial value 80 dB, to be varied
d1: 10 s
d2: 1/[2J(C,H)] = 2.33 ms, calculated from ^{1}J(C,H) = 215 Hz
rg = receiver gain for correct ADC input
ns = 1

In order not to change the selectivity you have to determine the effect of the shaped pulse as a function of the decoupler attenuation. With a very high decoupler attenuation (ca. 80 dB) adjust the phase of the C,H doublet to an antiphase pattern. Then repeat the experiment with different decoupler attenuations until the satellites disappear, which corresponds to the soft 90° decoupler pulse. To obtain the correct phase of the soft decoupler pulse one introduces another hard 90° decoupler pulse before the soft pulse in the pulse program. If both have the same phase, they are additive and yield an antiphase pattern with opposite phases as adjusted before.

5. Processing

Use standard 1D processing as described in Experiment 3.1.

6. Result

The figure on page 185 shows spectra obtained on an AMX-500 spectrometer. **a** is the initial spectrum with high decoupler attenuation and in **b** the effect of a shaped 90° decoupler pulse is shown. In **c** p3 was set to 90° and the phase of the shaped pulse was adjusted correctly in order to form, in combination with p3, a 180° pulse.

7. Comments

This calibration experiment follows the description given in a very recent publication [1]. In earlier work, due to phase problems, it was found very difficult to obtain a correct calibration. With the spin lock pulse p2 these problems are removed. It serves two purposes. First, it decouples the protons during the application of the shaped pulse, leaving the ^{13}C resonance as a singlet. Therefore the shaped pulse can be applied at the center of the ^{13}C resonance. Secondly, it purges the signals of all protons bound to ^{12}C, allowing a far easier detection of the ^{13}C satellites. The product operator formalism for this experiment is the same as described in Experiment 2.3 with exchanging the notation for C and H.

c

b

a

| Hz | 200 | 150 | 100 | 50 | 0 | -50 | -100 | -150 | -200 |

$\delta_H = 7.25$

8. Own Observations

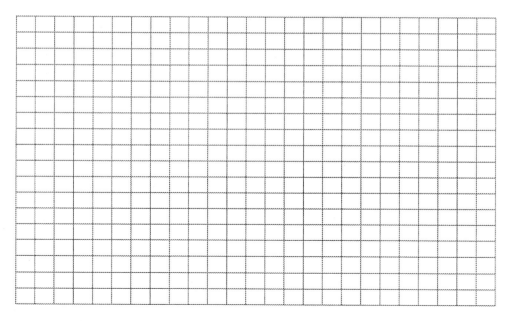

Experiment 7.4

Selective Excitation with DANTE

1. Purpose

One often wants to excite a single resonance selectively. On modern instruments this selective excitation is usually performed with shaped r.f. pulses which require additional hardware. With the DANTE (**D**elays **A**lternating with **N**utation for **T**ailored **E**xcitation) sequence [1] this can be performed on any older instrument. Care must be taken to ensure that the sidebands produced by the DANTE sequence do not excite additional signals. In the experiment presented here selective DANTE excitation is combined with a gated ^{1}H decoupling ^{13}C experiment (Exp. 4.10), demonstrating that overlapping multiplets can be individually analyzed with this technique [2].

2. Literature

[1] G. A. Morris, R. Freeman, *J. Magn. Reson.* **1978**, *29*, 433–462.
[2] G. Bodenhausen, R. Freeman, G. A. Morris, *J. Magn. Reson.* **1976**, *23*, 171–175.
[3] R. Freeman, *A Handbook of Nuclear Magnetic Resonance*, Longman, Harlow, **1987**, 207–215.

3. Pulse Scheme and Phase Cycle

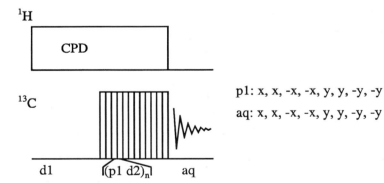

p1: x, x, -x, -x, y, y, -y, -y

aq: x, x, -x, -x, y, y, -y, -y

4. Acquisition

Time requirement: 0.5 h

Sample: 20% ethyl crotonate in CDCl$_3$

First obtain a normal ^{13}C NMR spectrum in order to get the exact resonance positions of the two methyl C-atoms. Then measure a proton coupled ^{13}C NMR spectrum using the gated decoupling method (Exp. 4.10), with the sweep width and offset adjusted to cover the area of the two methyl groups. To record the DANTE spectra you have to attenuate the transmitter power (see Exp. 2.6) until the 90° pulse is about 90 µs, so that a 1° pulse corresponds to about 1 µs. On older instruments, where software control of the transmitter attenuation is not possible, you simply introduce an attenuator box of about 20 dB into the ^{13}C transmitter line. You have to set:

td: 4 k
sw: 10 ppm
o1: on ^{13}C resonance of the selected methyl group
o2: middle of ^{1}H NMR spectrum
p1: 1° ^{13}C transmitter pulse
d1: 2 s
d2: 0.5 ms, yielding a total length of the DANTE excitation of 25.05 ms
n: number of p1 pulses, 50
decoupler attenuation and 90° pulse for CPD
ns: 128

5. Processing

Use standard ^{13}C NMR processing as described in Experiment 3.2 with exponential multiplication (lb = 0.5 Hz).

6. Result

In the figure **a** is the normal ^{1}H coupled ^{13}C NMR spectrum of ethyl crotonate in the area of the two overlapping methyl group quadruplets, obtained on an ARX-200 spectrometer. In **b** and **c** the DANTE spectra of the two selected methyl groups are shown.

7. Comments

The flip angle θ caused by an r.f. pulse of duration p and field strength B_1 is given by Equation (1).

$$\theta = \gamma B_1 p \tag{1}$$

If n very short pulses exactly on resonance are applied in a pulse train, their net effect is given by (2)

$$\theta = n\gamma B_1 p \tag{2}$$

However, if the frequency is offset from resonance by an amount Δv, then during each pulse cycle the nuclei precess in the rotating frame through an angle $2k\pi + \lambda$ given by Equation (3), where k is an integer, τ is the repetition time of the pulses, and λ is a phase angle less than 2π.

$$2k\pi + \lambda = 2\pi\Delta v \, \tau \tag{3}$$

Thus the DANTE sequence produces signal responses at the sidebands k. In quadrature detection it is most convenient to set $k = 0$ with the transmitter directly on the resonance of the desired signal. However, excitation also occurs at $k = 1$ and 2.

Very roughly, one can estimate the selectivity of a selective pulse as the reciprocal of its length; thus the DANTE excitation pulse train of 25 ms length used here corresponds to a selectivity of about 40 Hz. Attenuation of the transmitter is necessary, since the normal pulse programmers are not able to produce very short pulses; therefore the 90° pulse should be in the order of 90 μs to give a 1° pulse angle for a pulse duration of 1 μs.

8. Own Observations

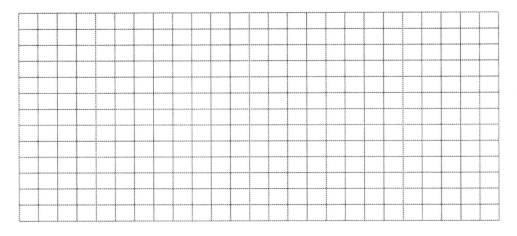

Experiment 7.5

Selective COSY

1. Purpose

This is the 1D variant of the most common 2D experiment. Instead of recording the full 2D matrix, one can simply measure one "row" by replacing the first 90° pulse of the COSY experiment (see Exp. 10.3) with a soft pulse, thus looking only for spin couplings that affect the particular proton excited. The selective COSY method yields the same connectivity information as the homonuclear decoupling technique (Exp. 4.4). In contrast to the latter, however, the multiplets of the coupling partners remain to be seen and can easily be evaluated. Because this is a 1D experiment, it can be performed at high resolution. The most recent extended version of this experiment uses gradient selection [4].

2. Literature

[1] C. J. Bauer, R. Freeman, T. Frenkiel, J. Keeler, A. J. Shaka, *J. Magn. Reson.* **1984**, *58*, 442–457.
[2] H. Kessler, H. Oschkinat, C. Griesinger, W. Bermel, *J. Magn. Reson.* **1986**, *70*, 106–133.
[3] H. Kessler, S. Mronga, G. Gemmecker, *Magn. Reson. Chem.* **1991**, *29*, 527–557.
[4] M. A. Bernstein, L. A. Trimble, *Magn. Reson. Chem.* **1994**, *32*, 107–110.

3. Pulse Scheme and Phase Cycle

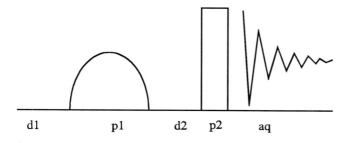

p1: y, -y, -y, y, x, -x, -x, x
p2: x, -x, x, -x, y, -y, y, -y
aq: x, -x, -x, x, y, -y, -y, y

d1   p1   d2   p2   aq

4. Acquisition

Time requirement: 15 min

Sample: 10% strychnine in CDCl$_3$

Record a normal ^{1}H NMR spectrum of the sample. Determine the 90° pulse width for the hard ^{1}H transmitter pulse, select a Gaussian pulse shape for the soft pulse and determine the correct attenuation corresponding to a 90° pulse at 50 ms duration (see

Exp. 7.1). Determine the phase difference between the hard and the soft pulse and take this into account for the actual phases used in the pulse program. You have to set:

td: 32 k

sw: 10 ppm

o1: on resonance of selected signal. If the software allows offsets for selective pulses, one can also put o1 in the middle of the ^{1}H NMR spectrum. However, the different phases of the selective pulses at different offsets must be determined.

p1: Gaussian shape, 50 ms length, transmitter attenuation corresponding to 90° excitation

p2: 90° ^{1}H transmitter pulse

d1: 2s

$$d2 = \frac{1}{2J(H,H)} - \frac{p1}{2}, \text{ typically 37 ms, calculated from } J(H,H) = 8 \text{ Hz}$$

ds: 4

ns: 16

5. Processing

Use standard ^{1}H processing as described in Experiment 3.1. Note that the selective COSY produces antiphase signals of the active coupling partners.

6. Result

The figure on page 191 shows the result obtained on an AMX-500 spectrometer. In **a** an expanded portion of the normal ^{1}H NMR spectrum is shown, in **b** H-12 was selected, giving the responses of both H-11 and (weakly) of H-13, and in **c** (d2 = 50 ms) H-15β was selected, giving the responses of H-15α, H-14, and H-16. Note that the coupling constant between H-15β and H-16 (4 Hz) can be measured selectively.

7. Comments

For the COSY part of the sequence exactly the same theory applies as given in Experiment 10.3. Note that the delay d2 determines the intensity of the "cross peak". It may be necessary to perform the experiment twice, for example in order to identify spin coupling partners with both small and large spin–spin coupling constants. In the spectrum **c** d2 was set to 50 ms.

The 90° Gaussian soft pulse used here can be replaced by many other types. You may try a 270° Gaussian, a half Gaussian with or without an additional purge pulse [3], or DANTE excitation (Exp. 7.4).

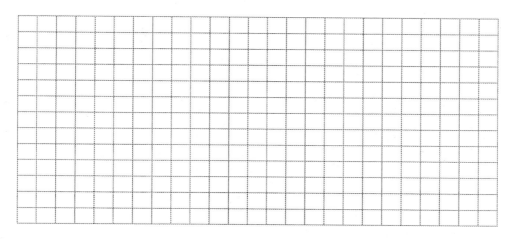

8. Own Observations

Experiment 7.6

SELINCOR: Selective Inverse H,C Correlation via ^1J(C,H)

1. Purpose

This experiment is the selective 1D version [1] of the two-dimensional inverse H,C correlation (HMQC, see Exp. 10.11). It can also be regarded as the inverse of the single-frequency decoupled ^{13}C NMR spectrum (see Exp. 4.11). The experiment correlates a selected carbon atom with the attached proton via one bond C,H coupling, using proton sensitivity for observation. In the current literature [2–5], there are many modifications and improvements of the basic experiment shown here. With a gradient selected modification, the sequence can also be used as an initial stage in various advanced ^{13}C-resolved proton experiments [6].

2. Literature

[1] S. Berger, *J. Magn. Reson.* **1989**, *81*, 561–564.
[2] R. C. Crouch, J. P. Shockar, G. E. Martin, *Tetrahedron Letters* **1990**, *31*, 5273–5276.
[3] P. Berthault, B. Perly, M. Petitou, *Magn. Reson. Chem.* **1990**, *28*, 696–670.
[4] J.-M. Bernassau, J.-M. Nuzillard, *J. Magn. Reson. Ser. A* **1993**, *104*, 212–221.
[5] W. Willker, J. Stelten, D. Leibfritz, *J. Magn. Reson. Ser. A* **1994**, *107*, 94–98.
[6] T. Fäcke, S. Berger, *Magn. Reson. Chem.* **1995**, *33*, 144–148.

3. Pulse Scheme and Phase Cycle

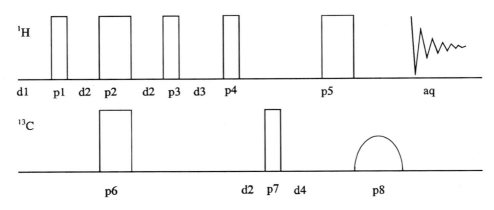

p1, p2, p6: x

p3: -x

p4: $(x)_8$, $(-x)_8$

p5: $(x)_8$, $(-x)_{16}$, $(x)_8$

p7: $(x, y, -x, -y)_2$, $(-x, -y, x, y)_2$

p8: $(x)_4$, $(-x)_8$, $(x)_4$

aq: x, -y, -x, y, $(-x, y, x, -y)_2$, x, -y, -x, y

4. Acquisition

Time requirement: 0.5 h

Sample: 20% ethyl crotonate in $CDCl_3$

Prior to the experiment you have to choose a Gaussian pulse shape and to determine the attenuation and the relative phase of a selective ^{13}C pulse in the inverse mode of the spectrometer (see Exp. 7.3). Record normal ^1H and ^{13}C NMR spectra and note the offsets of the desired carbon signals. The sequence given above consists of the BIRD filter (see Exp. 6.12) and the actual SELINCOR sequence. You have to set:

td: 32 k
sw: 8 ppm
o1: middle of ^1H NMR spectrum
o2: on resonance of selected ^{13}C nucleus
p1, p3, p4: 90° ^1H transmitter pulse
p2, p5: 180° ^1H transmitter pulse
p6: 180° ^{13}C decoupler pulse
p7: 90° ^{13}C decoupler pulse
p8: Gaussian shaped ^{13}C decoupler pulse, 5 ms length, attenuation corresponding to 90° or 270° excitation.
d1: 3s
d2: $1/[2J(C,H)] = 3.57$ ms, calculated from $^1J(C,H) = 140$ Hz
d3: BIRD relaxation delay, optimized for minimum FID intensity, typically 1 s
d4: same length as selective pulse p8, 5 ms was used here
ds: 4
ns: 64

5. Processing

Use standard ^1H processing as given in Experiment 3.1. Since the phase of the satellites is not very pure process the spectrum in magnitude mode.

6. Result

The figure on page 194 shows spectra obtained on an AMX-500 spectrometer. **a** is the normal ^1H NMR spectrum and **b** to **e** are the SELINCOR spectra, all processed in magnitude mode. In **b** C-2, in **c** C-5, in **d** C-4, and in **e** C-6 was selected. Note that the selective ^{13}C pulse of 5 ms length is just able to distinguish between C-4 and C-6, which are separated by 450 Hz at the field strength used, but is broad enough to cover the width of a typical C,H doublet.

7. Comments

The theory is the same as for the HMQC experiment (Exp.10.11) and is given there. Instead of the evolution of the carbon chemical shifts in t_1 only the double quantum magnetization of the selected carbon nucleus is transformed back into an observable magnetization; all other coherences are suppressed by the phase cycle.

8. Own Observations

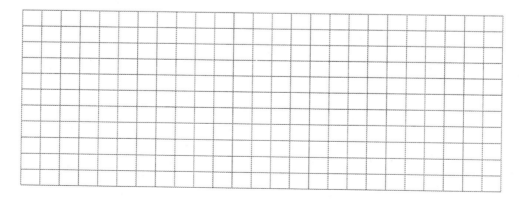

Experiment 7.7

SELINQUATE

1. Purpose

The SELINQUATE method [1] is the selective version of the INADEQUATE [2] sequence. Whereas with 1D-INADEQUATE (see Exp. 6.11) the $^{13}C, ^{13}C$ spin coupling constants can yield partially overlapping signals, the 2D version (see Exp 10.19) is very time-consuming and has limited digital resolution [3]. With SELINQUATE it is possible to measure specific $^{13}C, ^{13}C$ coupling constants over one or more bonds selectively with the high digital resolution of a 1D method. Thus, the experiment yields connectivity information for the irradiated carbon nucleus and $^{13}C, ^{13}C$ spin coupling constants with high accuracy.

2. Literature

[1] S. Berger, *Angew. Chem. Int. Ed. Engl.* **1988**, *27*, 1196–1197.
[2] A. Bax, R. Freeman, S. P. Kempsell, *J. Am. Chem. Soc.* **1980**, *102*, 4849–4851.
[3] A. Bax, R. Freeman, T. A. Frenkiel, M. H. Levitt, *J. Magn. Reson.* **1981**, *43*, 478–483.
[4] J. Buddrus, H. Bauer, *Angew. Chem. Int. Ed. Engl.* **1987**, *26*, 625–643.

3. Pulse Scheme and Phase Cycle

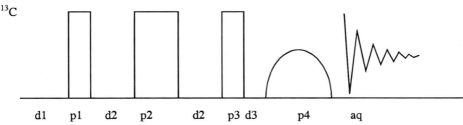

p1: (x)$_4$, (y)$_4$, [(-x)$_4$, (-y)$_4$]$_2$, (x)$_4$, (y)$_4$
p2: [(x)$_4$, (y)$_4$, (-x)$_4$, (-y)$_4$]$_2$, [(-x)$_4$, (-y)$_4$, (x)$_4$, (y)$_4$]$_2$
p3: (x)$_4$, (y)$_4$, (-x)$_4$, (-y)$_4$
p4: y, x, -y, -x
aq: (x, y, (-x, -y)$_2$, x, y)$_2$, (-x, -y, (x, y)$_2$, -x, -y)$_2$

4. Acquisition

Time requirement: 2 h

Sample: 90% 2-cyclohexen-1-one in [D$_6$]acetone

Prior to the experiment you have to determine the r.f. attenuation and phase for a selective ^{13}C pulse on carbon as described in Experiment 7.1. Record a normal ^{13}C NMR spectrum of the sample and adjust the spectral width to the aliphatic region. Note the offsets for the three signals of the aliphatic carbon nuclei and adjust the frequency of the selective pulse to one of them. You have to set:

> td: 16 k
> sw: 23 ppm
> o1: on resonance of selected signal. If the software allows offsets for selective pulses, one can also set o1 in the middle of the ^{13}C NMR spectrum. However, the different phases of the selective pulses at different offsets must be determined.
> o2: middle of ^{1}H NMR spectrum
> p1, p3: 90° ^{13}C transmitter pulse
> p2: 180° ^{13}C transmitter pulse
> p4: Gaussian shaped ^{13}C transmitter pulse, 10 ms length, attenuation corresponding to 270° excitation, which gives better phase behavior of the satellites than with a 90° pulse.
> d1: 4s
> d2: 1/[2*J*(C,C)] = 7 ms calculated from ^{1}*J*(C,C) = 33 Hz; for long-range couplings use *J*(C,C) = 4 Hz, d2 = 62.5 ms
> d3: 10 µs
> decoupler attenuation and 90° pulse for CPD
> ds: 4
> ns: 256

5. Processing

Use standard ^{13}C NMR processing as described in Experiment 3.2. Note that the experiment yields ^{13}C satellites in antiphase. The residual signal of the molecules containing only one ^{13}C atom should not be used for phasing.

6. Result

In the figure on page 197 **a** is the normal ^{13}C NMR spectrum of the aliphatic region. In **b** C-4 was irradiated, giving a response of C-5 with *J*(C,C) = 33.4 Hz. In **c** C-5 was irradiated, giving a response of both C-4 and C-6 with *J*(C,C) values of 33.4 Hz and 31.7 Hz respectively, and in **d** C-6 was irradiated giving a response of C-5 with *J*(C,C) = 31.7 Hz. In **e** the selective pulse was adjusted to the carbon nucleus of the C=O group, and d2 was adjusted to long-range interaction; the figure shows the signal of C-

4 with $^3J(C,C)$ = 4.8 Hz. In **f** C-6 was irradiated; the figure shows the signal of C-4 with $^2J(C,C)$ = 2.5 Hz.

7. Comments

The theory of the experiment is the same as for the 1D-INADEQUATE experiment and is outlined there (see Exp. 6.11). In SELINQUATE only the double quantum coherence of the selectively irradiated carbon atom is transformed back into an observable magnetization. Note that the excitation bandwidth of the selective pulse used must be broad enough to excite both satellites of the carbon signal.

8. Own Observations

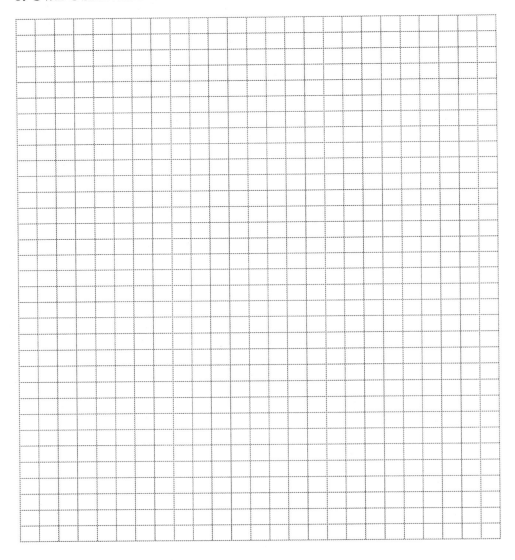

Experiment 7.8

Selective TOCSY

1. Purpose

This experiment is the selective 1D version of the 2D TOCSY (**TO**tal **C**orrelation **S**pectroscop**Y**) method (Exp. 10.15), also known as HOHAHA (**HO**monuclear **HA**rt-mann–**HA**hn). One proton is excited by a shaped pulse and this produces a response from all protons that are connected by spin coupling within a chain. Thus it is possible, for example, to trace all protons in a sugar moiety by starting from the anomeric proton or in one amino acid side-chain by starting from the α proton. Since the publication of the original experiment [1,2] given here, there have been several attempts to improve the performance and to eliminate some shortcomings [3–6].

2. Literature

[1] D. G. Davis, A. Bax, *J. Am. Chem. Soc.* **1985**, *107*, 7197–7198; A. Bax, D. G. Davis, *J. Magn. Reson.* **1985**, *65*, 355–360.

[2] H. Kessler, H. Oschkinat, C. Griesinger, W. Bermel, *J. Magn. Reson.* **1986**, *70*, 106–133.

[3] V. Sklenár, J. Feigon, *J. Am. Chem. Soc.* **1990**, *112*, 5644–5645.

[4] J. P. Shockcor, R. C. Crouch, G. E. Martin, A. Cherif, J.-K. Luo, R. N. Castle, *J. Heterocycl. Chem.* **1990**, *27*, 455–458.

[5] L. Poppe, H. van Halbeek, *J. Magn. Reson.* **1992**, *96*, 185–190.

[6] T. Fäcke, S. Berger, *J. Magn. Reson. Ser. A* **1995**, *113*, 257-259.

3. Pulse Scheme and Phase Cycle

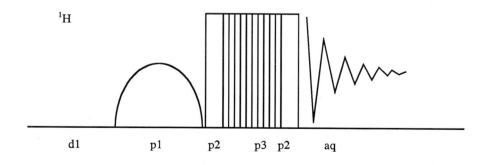

p1: y, (−y)$_2$, y, x, (−x)$_2$, x   aq: y, (−y)$_2$, y, x, (−x)$_2$, x
p2: (x, −x)$_2$, (y, −y)$_2$ (trim pulses)

p3: MLEV-17 spin-lock out of composite 180° pulses (90°, 180°, 90°); sequence:

90 (ph1), 180 (ph2), 90 (ph1)
[90 (ph3), 180 (ph4), 90 (ph3)]₂
90 (ph1), 180 (ph2), 90 (ph1)
[90 (ph3), 180 (ph4), 90 (ph3)]₂
[90 (ph1), 180 (ph2), 90 (ph1)]₂
90 (ph3), 180 (ph4), 90 (ph3)
[90 (ph1), 180 (ph2), 90 (ph1)]₂
90 (ph3), 180 (ph4), 90 (ph3)
[90 (ph1), 180 (ph2), 90 (ph1)]₂
[90 (ph3), 180 (ph4), 90 (ph3)]₂
60 (ph2)

ph1: (−y, y)₂, (x, −x)₂
ph2: (x, −x)₂, (y, −y)₂
ph3: (y, −y)₂, (−x, x)₂
ph4: (−x, x)₂, (−y, y)₂

4. Acquisition

Time requirement: 30 min

Sample: 10% strychnine in $CDCl_3$

Prior to the experiment the attenuator setting needed to give a 90° shaped pulse of a chosen duration has to be determined (see Exp 7.1). Its phase relative to the phase of the spin-lock pulses must be known, and the 90° pulse duration and the attenuation of the spin-lock pulses must also be calibrated (see Exp. 2.6). Run a normal ^1H NMR spectrum of the sample and note the offsets of the protons to be irradiated. You have to set:

    td: 32 k
    sw: 10 ppm
    o1: on resonance of selected signal. If the software allows offsets for selective pulses, one can also put o1 in the middle of the ^1H NMR spectrum. However, the different phases of the selective pulses at different offsets must be determined.
    p1: Gaussian shaped ^1H transmitter pulse, 50 ms length, transmitter attenuation corresponding to 90° excitation
    p2: trim pulse 2.5 ms at power level of spin-lock
    p3: series of composite 180° pulses (90°, 180°, 90°) at power level of spin-lock, typically 90° pulse width of 40 μs at 12 dB transmitter attenuation corresponding to an effective spin-lock field of ca. 7000 Hz. Total length of spin-lock set to 200 ms by loop parameter of spin-lock sequence.
    d1: 2s
    ns: 8
    ds: 4

5. Processing

Use standard ^1H processing as described in Experiment 3.1

6. Result

In the figure **a** is an expanded region of the normal ¹H NMR spectrum of strychnine obtained on an AMX-500 spectrometer. In **b** H-12 was irradiated, giving responses from H-13, both H-11 protons, H-8, and H-14. In **c** H-16 was irradiated, giving responses from both H-15 protons, H-14, H-13, and H-8.

7. Comments

As for the 2D TOCSY experiment there exists a simple picture which explains the result of a spin-lock. The various protons "see" as the effective field only the weak r.f. field of the spin-lock, therefore chemical shift differences vanish and the spin systems are all of higher order leading to a mixing of all spin states. Exciting one proton at the end of a chain connected by spin coupling produces a response from all spins affected by the spin-lock. However, the phase of the response signals is not pure, but a mix of in-phase and antiphase components, thus it is difficult to extract correct spin coupling constants.

8. Own Observations

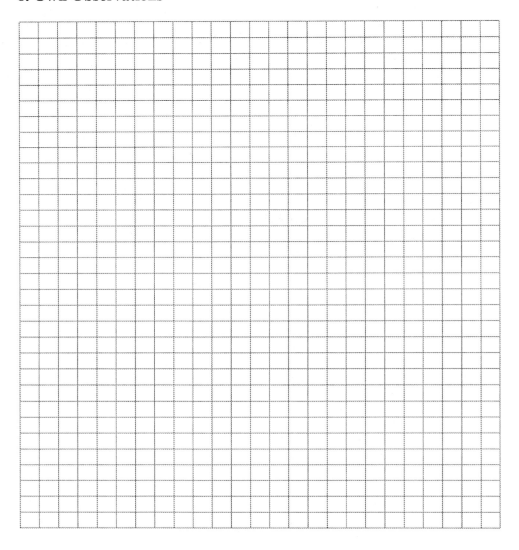

Experiment 7.9

INAPT

1. Purpose

This experiment is the selective version of INEPT (see Exp. 6.7). Here only a particular proton is excited and used for polarization transfer, in order to identify ^{13}C nuclei that are connected to this proton via spin–spin coupling. The experiment is mainly used for detecting long-range interactions and provides a good method for assigning quaternary carbon nuclei. The relative popularity of this experiment in the literature is probably due to the fact that only soft rectangular pulses are used in the proton channel [1,2], and thus it can be implemented on any instrument. Many applications of the INAPT technique have been reported [2–5] and a J resolved 2D version is also known [6].

2. Literature

[1] A. Bax, *J. Magn. Reson.* **1984**, *57*, 314–318.
[2] A. Bax, J. A. Ferretti, N. Nahsed, D. M. Jerina, *J. Org. Chem.* **1985**, *50*, 3029–3038.
[3] A. N. Abdel Sayed, L. Bauer, *Tetrahedron* **1988**, *44*, 1883–1892
[4] M. A. Bernstein, *Magn. Reson. Chem.* **1989**, *27*, 659–662.
[5] W. H. Gmeiner, J. W. Lown, *Magn. Reson. Chem.* **1992**, *30*, 101–106.
[6] C. A. Drake, N. Rabjohn, M. S. Tempesta, R. B. Taylor, *J. Org. Chem.* **1988**, *53*, 4555–4562.

3. Pulse Scheme and Phase Cycle

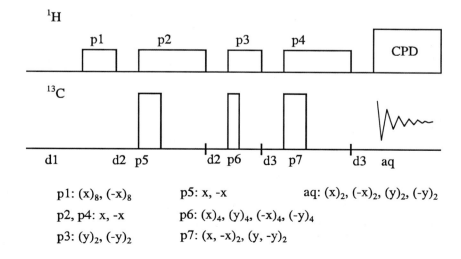

p1: $(x)_8$, $(-x)_8$ p5: x, -x   aq: $(x)_2$, $(-x)_2$, $(y)_2$, $(-y)_2$

p2, p4: x, -x   p6: $(x)_4$, $(y)_4$, $(-x)_4$, $(-y)_4$

p3: $(y)_2$, $(-y)_2$ p7: $(x, -x)_2$, $(y, -y)_2$

4. Acquisition

Time requirement: 0.5 h

Sample: 2-hydroxynaphthalene, saturated solution in $CDCl_3$

Prior to this experiment the decoupler attenuation for a rectangular soft pulse must be known (see Exp 7.2). Record an ^1H NMR spectrum and note the offsets of the different proton signals. Switch the instrument to ^{13}C operation, record as a reference a normal ^{13}C NMR spectrum, and load the INAPT pulse program. You have to set:

> td: 32 k
> sw: 55 ppm
> o1: center of aromatic region of the ^{13}C NMR spectrum
> o2: on resonance of selected ^1H NMR signal
> p1, p3: 20 ms rectangular shaped ^1H decoupler pulse at 67 db attenuation
> p2, p4: 40 ms rectangular shaped ^1H decoupler pulse at 67 db attenuation
> p5, p7: 180° ^{13}C transmitter pulse
> p6: 90° ^{13}C transmitter pulse
> decoupler attenuation and 90° pulse for CPD
> d1: 3 s
> d2: 10 ms
> d3: 20 ms
> ns: 64

5. Processing

Use standard ^{13}C NMR processing as described in Experiment 3.2.

6. Result

In the figure on p. 203 **a** is the normal ^1H NMR spectrum recorded on an AMX-500 spectrometer with the assignments obtained by inspection of a NOESY experiment. **b** is the normal ^{13}C NMR spectrum. In **c** the selective proton pulse was adjusted to H-8, giving responses from carbon nuclei C-6, C-10 and C-1, all of which are connected to H-8 via $^3J(C,H)$. Note that the sign of the signals may be positive or negative. In **d** proton H-1 was irradiated, giving responses from C-10, C-8, C-2 and C-3.

7. Comments

The product operator formalism description is identical with that for the normal refocused INEPT experiment (Exp 6.7) which is given there. Here especially the signals of
quaternary carbon nuclei are enhanced by polarization transfer and thus appear with
high intensity. Since the experiment can easily be implemented on older instruments it
is highly attractive.

8. Own Observations

Experiment 7.10

Determination of Long-Range C,H Coupling Constants

1. Purpose

The NMR spectroscopist is often interested in one specific long-range C,H spin coupling constant [1]. There are several methods for simplifying complicated C,H multiplets, such as selective decoupling (see Exp. 4.13), though these methods usually yield residual multiplets which still have to be analyzed by spin simulation. The experiment presented here demonstrates a 2D method related to 2D *J*-resolved spectroscopy and employing a selective pulse. It yields directly the desired spin coupling constant of a chosen C,H pair free of other passive spin couplings. Unlike the original method [2] the pulse sequence given here uses a shaped RE-BURP pulse [3,4].

2. Literature

[1] M. Eberstadt, G. Gemmecker, D. F. Mierke, H. Kessler, *Angew. Chem. Int. Ed. Engl.* **1995**, *34*, 1671-1695.
[2] A. Bax, R. Freeman, *J. Am. Chem. Soc.* **1982**, *104*, 1099–1100.
[3] H. Geen, R. Freeman, *J. Magn. Reson.* **1991**, *93*, 93–141.
[4] T. Fäcke, S. Berger, unpublished results.

3. Pulse Scheme and Phase Cycle

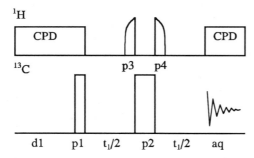

p1: (x)$_4$, (y)$_4$, (-x)$_4$, (-y)$_4$

p2: x, -x, y, -y, (y, -y, -x, x)$_2$, -x, x, -y, y

p3, p4: x, -x, y, -y, (y, -y, -x, x)$_2$, -x, x, -y, y

aq: (x)$_2$, (-x)$_2$, (y)$_2$, (-y)$_2$

4. Acquisition

Time requirement: 1.5 h

Sample: 20% ethyl crotonate in CDCl$_3$

Record a normal ^{1}H NMR spectrum and note the ^{1}H frequency offset of the methyl group attached to the double bond at δ_H = 1.8. Define and calibrate RE-BURP pulses for p3 and p4 in the ^{1}H channel, so that p3 forms the first half and p4 the second half of the shaped pulse (see Exp. 7.2). Change to the 2D mode of the spectrometer software. You have to set:

td2: 1 k data points in F_2
td1: 128 data points in F_1
sw2: 200 ppm
sw1: 50 Hz
o1: middle of ^{13}C NMR spectrum
o2: on resonance of the methyl group at $\delta_H = 1.8$
p1: 90° ^{13}C transmitter pulse
p2: 180° ^{13}C transmitter pulse
p3: selective 180° ^1H decoupler pulse, first half of RE-BURP shape (20 ms
 length at 46 dB)
p4: selective 180° ^1H decoupler pulse, second half of RE-BURP shape (20 ms
 length at 46 dB)
d1: 2 s
initial value for t_1 evolution: 3 µs
increment for t_1 evolution = 1/[2·sw1]
ds: 2
preacquisition delay: as small as possible
ns: 8

5. Processing

Apply zero filling in F_1 to 256 real data points. Use $\pi/2$ shifted sinusoidal windows in both dimensions. Apply complex Fourier transformation corresponding to the N type signal selection using the quadrature off mode in F_1. Phase correction is not necessary, since the data are processed in the magnitude mode.

6. Result

The figure on page 208 shows the result obtained on an AMX-500 spectrometer for the signals of C-2 and C-3. The coupling of these carbon nuclei and the protons of the methyl group C-4 can be seen in F_1 from the splitting of the quartets. Note that in this case the geminal coupling constant ^2J(C-3,H-4) of 7.1 Hz is slightly larger than the vicinal coupling constant ^3J(C-2,H-4) of 6.7 Hz. A reliable assignment of these spin couplings by any other means would be very difficult. Compare the signal patterns with the result obtained in Exp. 10.2.

7. Comments

This method can be thought of as the selective version of the heteronuclear 2D *J*-resolved technique. The selective 180° pulse consisting of p3 and p4 acts only on the chosen protons. At the end of the t_1 period the spin-echo is modulated only by this selected spin coupling. The spin coupling to all other protons is not refocused and is therefore not observable in the final spectrum.

This method provides a unique means of analyzing C,H multiplets without assignment ambiguities, although it is rather insensitive since it is based on a 2D method with ^{13}C detection. The corresponding inverse experiment is described in Experiment 7.11.

8. Own Observations

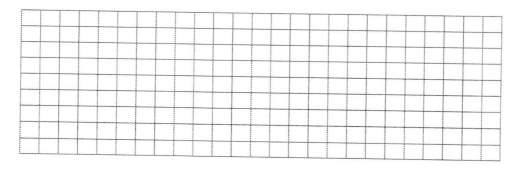

Experiment 7.11

SELRESOLV

1. Purpose

The NMR spectroscopist is often interested in one specific long-range C,H spin coupling constant [1]. There are several methods for simplifying complicated C,H multiplets, such as selective decoupling (see Exp. 4.13), though these methods usually yield residual multiplets which still have to be analyzed by spin simulation. The experiment presented here demonstrates a 2D method related to 2D *J*-resolved spectroscopy and employing a selective pulse [2]. It yields directly the desired spin coupling constant of a chosen C,H pair independent of other passive spin couplings. In contrast to Experiment 7.10, however, the SELRESOLV method is a proton detected experiment and hence more sensitive.

2. Literature

[1] M. Eberstadt, G. Gemmecker, D. F. Mierke, H. Kessler, *Angew. Chem. Int. Ed. Engl.* **1995**, *34*, 1671-1695.
[2] M. Ochs, S. Berger, *Magn. Reson. Chem.* **1990**, *28*, 994–997.

3. Pulse Scheme and Phase Cycle

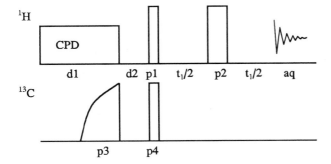

p1: -x, x, x, -x, -y, y, y, -y

p2: (x)$_2$, (-x)$_2$, (y)$_2$, (-y)$_2$

p3: x, -x, -x, x, y, -y, -y, y

p4: (y)$_2$, (-y)$_2$, (-x)$_2$, (x)$_2$

aq: (x)$_2$, (-x)$_2$, (y)$_2$, (-y)$_2$

4. Acquisition

Time requirement: 1.2 h

Sample: 20% ethyl crotonate in CDCl$_3$

Record a normal ^{13}C NMR spectrum and note the offset of the olefinic carbon nucleus C-2 at δ_C = 123.6. Change to ^{1}H observation with ^{13}C decoupling (inverse mode on older instruments) and calibrate a 10 ms soft pulse p3 with half-Gaussian shape as decoupler pulse in the ^{13}C channel. Change to the 2D mode of the spectrometer software. You have to set:

td2: 2 k data points in F_2
td1: 32 data points in F_1
sw2: 1 ppm
sw1: 45 Hz
o1: center of methyl group region in ^{1}H NMR spectrum
o2: on resonance of the olefinic carbon atom C-2 at $\delta_C = 123.6$
p1: 90° ^{1}H transmitter pulse
p2: 180° ^{1}H transmitter pulse
p3: selective 90° ^{13}C decoupler pulse, half-Gaussian shape (10 ms length at 66 dB)
d1: 6 s
d2: $1/[2J(C,H)] = 50$ ms, calculated from $^nJ(C,H) = 10$ Hz
^{1}H transmitter attenuation and 90° pulse width for broad-band presaturation (16 dB, 18 µs)
initial value for t_1 evolution: 3 µs
increment for t_1 evolution $= 1/[2 \cdot sw1]$
preacquisition delay: as small as possible
ds: 4
ns: 16

5. Processing

Apply zero filling in F_2 and in F_1 to 2 k and 128 real data points respectively. Use unshifted sinusoidal windows in both dimensions. Apply complex Fourier transformation corresponding to the N type signal selection using the quadrature off mode in F_1. Phase correction is not necessary, since the data are processed in the magnitude mode.

6. Result

The figure on page 211 shows the result obtained on an AMX-500 spectrometer, with the region of the methyl group attached to the olefinic carbon expanded. The ^3J(C-2,H-4) spin coupling of 6.6 Hz can be seen in F_2, whereas the homonuclear couplings to the two olefinic protons are observed in F_1. This long range C,H coupling constant can also be obtained by Experiment 7.10, using ^{13}C rather than proton detection, and is then observed in the F_1 dimension. Note that some axial peak breakthrough at 0 Hz in F_1 is unavoidable; residual signals from protons bound to ^{12}C may also appear, but are outside the region of interest. Along the F_1 axis the normal signal of H-4 is shown.

7. Comments

The method consists of a selective reverse INEPT transfer from ^{13}C to protons followed by a subsequent 2D J-resolved sequence. In this 2D part only the proton selected by the ^{13}C selective pulse is active. The homonuclear spin couplings of this proton are observed in the F_1 dimension, leaving only the heteronuclear spin coupling to the chosen carbon nucleus in F_2. The signals of protons bound to ^{12}C are suppressed by the phase cycle and the presaturation period.

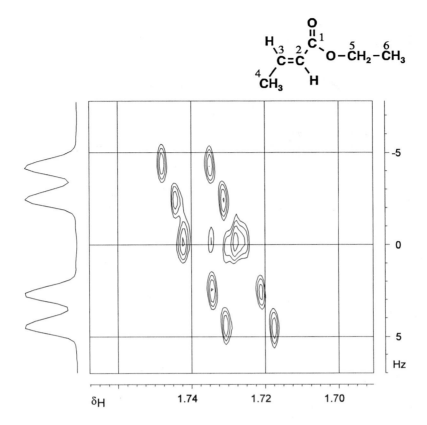

This is a considerable drawback of the method; thus the sensitivity gain obtained through inverse detection is somewhat diminished due to the necessary suppression of unwanted coherences. More effective approaches use pulsed field gradients (Chapter 11).

8. Own Observations

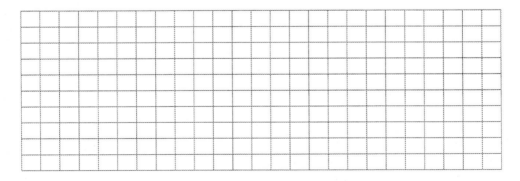

Experiment 7.12

SERF

1. Purpose

The NMR spectroscopist is often interested in determining a specific H,H spin coupling constant [1]. There are several methods for simplifying complicated multiplets, such as homonuclear decoupling (see Exp. 4.4) or selective COSY (see Exp. 7.5); however, these methods usually yield residual multiplets which still have to be analyzed by spin simulation. The SERF (**SE**lective **ReF**ocussing) experiment [2] presented here is a 2D method employing two selective pulses. It directly yields the desired coupling constant of a chosen spin pair without other passive spin couplings.

2. Literature

[1] M. Eberstadt, G. Gemmecker, D. F. Mierke, H. Kessler, *Angew. Chem. Int. Ed. Engl.* **1995**, *34*, 1671-1695.
[2] T. Fäcke, S. Berger, *J. Magn. Reson. Ser. A* **1995**, *113*, 114–116.

3. Pulse Scheme and Phase Cycle

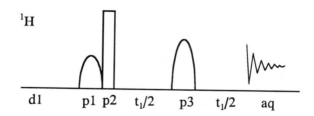

p1: x, -x, -x, x   p3: x

p2: y, y, -y, -y   aq: x, -x, -x, x

4. Acquisition

Time requirement: 20 min

Sample: 5% ethyl crotonate in CDCl$_3$

Record a normal ^{1}H NMR spectrum and note the offsets of the olefinic protons and of the methyl group attached to the double bond. Define and calibrate for p1 an E-BURP pulse shape and check its phase relative to the purging pulse p2. Define and calibrate for p3 a double selective RE-BURP pulse shape, so that this pulse acts simultaneously on the olefinic proton at $\delta_H = 6.9$ (H-3) and the methyl group at $\delta_H = 1.8$. For a second spectrum set this pulse to act on both olefinic protons. Change to the 2D mode of the spectrometer software. You have to set:

td2: 1 k data points in F_2
td1: 64 data points in F_1
sw2: 8 ppm
sw1: 50 Hz
o1: middle of ^{1}H NMR spectrum
p1: selective 90° ^{1}H transmitter pulse, E-BURP shape; 50 ms length at 55 dB
     was used here
p2: 5 ms ^{1}H purging pulse
p3: double selective 180° ^{1}H transmitter pulse, RE-BURP shape; 50 ms length
     at 45 dB was used here
d1: 2 s
initial value for t_1 evolution: 3 μs
increment for t_1 evolution = 1/[2·sw1]
preacquisition delay: as small as possible
ds: 2
ns: 4

5. Processing

Apply zero filling in F_1 to 128 real data points. Use unshifted sinusoidal windows in both dimensions. Apply complex Fourier transformation corresponding to the N type signal selection using the quadrature off mode in F_1. Phase correction is not necessary, since the data are processed in magnitude mode.

6. Result

The figures show the result obtained on an AMX-500 spectrometer. In spectrum **a** the double selective pulse was set to act on the olefinic proton at δ_H = 6.9 (H-3) and on the methyl protons at $\delta_H = 1.8$. Only J(H-3,CH$_3$) is observed in F_1, whereas J(H-2, CH$_3$) appears in F_2. In spectrum **b** the double selective pulse was set to act on both olefinic protons, so that only the large olefinic spin coupling constant can be seen in F_1. Compare the signal patterns with the result of Experiment 10.1.

7. Comments

This method can be thought of as the double selective version of the 2D J-resolved technique. After excitation by the selective pulse p1 the selected proton develops spin–spin coupling to all other protons that are coupled to it. The purging pulse p2 suppresses unwanted coherences. The double selective pulse p3 acts only on the chosen spin pair so that at the end of the t1 period the spin echo is only modulated by this selected spin coupling.

8. Own Observations

Chapter 8

Auxiliary Reagents, Quantitative Determinations, and Reaction Mechanism

This chapter describes typical applications of routine NMR spectroscopy in organic, inorganic and physical organic chemistry. The emphasis is therefore not on how to perform a special pulse sequence, to set up a certain 2D file, or to tune the spectrometer to a seldom used heteronucleus; instead the NMR experiments shown here mainly use the simple "zero/go" acquisition sequence given in Experiment 3.1, and additionally introduce special reagents such as lanthanide shift reagents or Pirkle's reagent to illustrate how one can obtain meaningful information with these auxiliaries. The analytical application of NMR for quantitative determinations is also demonstrated. Finally, an important experiment in physical organic chemistry, the CIDNP effect, is described.

Literature

[1] M. L. Martin, J. J. Delpuech, G. J. Martin, *Practical NMR Spectroscopy*, Heyden, London, **1980**, Chs. 9 and 10.
[2] D. Wendisch, *Appl. Spectrosc. Rev.* **1993**, *28*, 165–229.

Experiment 8.1

Signal Separation Using a Lanthanide Shift Reagent

1. Purpose

Lanthanide shift reagents are used for simplifying complex NMR spectra. Chiral lanthanide shift reagents can also be used to determine enantiomeric purity (see Exp. 8.2). In the experiment described here tris[1,1,1,2,2,3,3-heptafluoro-7,7-dimethyloctane-4,6-dionato]-europium, Eu(fod)$_3$, is used to separate multiplets of an alkyl chain.

2. Literature

[1] M. L. Martin, J. J. Delpuech, G. J. Martin, *Practical NMR Spectroscopy,* Heyden, London, **1980**, Ch. 5.4.
[2] O. Hofer, *Top. Stereochem.* **1976**, *9*, 111–197.
[3] J. Reuben, *Prog. Nucl. Magn. Reson. Spectrosc.* **1975**, *9*, 1–70.
[4] T. C. Morrill (ed.): *Lanthanide Shift Reagents in Stereochemical Analysis,* in *Methods in Stereochemical Analysis,* VCH, Weinheim, **1985**.
[5] G. R. Sullivan, *Top. Stereochem.* **1978**, *10*, 288–329.

3. Pulse Scheme and Phase Cycle

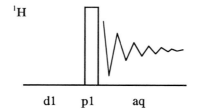

^{1}H

p1: x, x, -x, -x, y, y, -y, -y
aq: x, x, -x, -x, y, y, -y, -y

d1   p1   aq

4. Acquisition

Time requirement: 30 min

Sample: 10 mg 1-octanol in 0.7 ml CDCl$_3$

Load standard ^{1}H NMR acquisition parameters (see Exp. 3.1), set the spectral width to 15 ppm, and record a spectrum of 1-octanol. Add a *very* small portion (about 1 mg) of tris[1,1,1,2,2,3,3-heptafluoro-7,7-dimethyloctane-4,6-dionato]-europium,   Eu(fod)$_3$, allow sufficient time to reach equilibrium, and record the spectrum again. Increase the amount of the shift reagent until all the seven CH$_2$ signals are separated.

   For quantitative work it is advisable to prepare substrate and reagent stock solutions. Fill six NMR tubes with 0.1 ml substrate stock solution and varying amounts of reagent solution. Add solvent to each NMR tube to give the same total amount of liquid, so that the substrate concentration remains constant. For experiments with constant susceptibility the reagent concentration is kept constant and the substrate concentration is varied.

solvent

reagent

substrate

5. Processing

Use standard 1D processing for ^{1}H NMR spectra (see Exp. 3.1).

6. Result

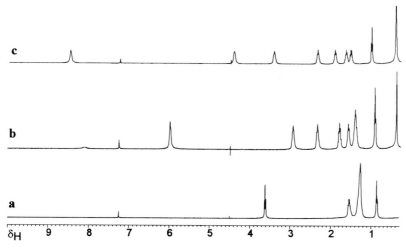

The figure shows in **a** the ^{1}H NMR spectra of 1-octanol without Eu(fod)$_3$ and in **b** and **c** with varying amounts of Eu(fod)$_3$, obtained on an AM-400 spectrometer. The signals which are shifted most are also severely broadened. The signal of the OH group at δ_H = 8.2 in **b** is no longer visible in **c**. Note that in spectrum **c** the CH$_2$O group now has a chemical shift of δ_H = 8.5 and all CH$_2$ groups of the octyl chain are separated. The signal at δ_H = 0.5 comes from the *t*-butyl group of the shift reagent Eu(fod)$_3$.

7. Comments

Lanthanide shift reagents act like an additional magnetic field in the sample and dramatically change the chemical shifts of the signals, especially for nuclei in the vicinity of the complexation site ("the poor man's 1 GHz NMR spectrometer"). Thus, they make it possible to separate signals or to simplify an NMR spin system. The use of lanthanide shift reagents usually gives an unambigious answer to problems such as *cis*/*trans*, *E*/*Z*, *endo*/*exo* or *syn*/*anti* assignments. The change in chemical shift resulting from the addition of a shift reagent can be expressed as the sum of three components, as given by Equation (1).

$$\Delta = \Delta_{DIA} + \Delta_{CON} + \Delta_{DIP} \tag{1}$$

The diamagnetic contribution Δ_{DIA} is caused by the complexation of the substrate, whereas the contact contribution Δ_{CON} has its origin in the delocalization of electron spin density from the lanthanide ion to the substrate. Usually both are small and can be neglected. The dipolar contribution Δ_{DIP} depends on the distance r between the lanthanide ion and the nuclear spin being observed, and the angle θ between the principal magnetic dipolar axis of the complex and the distance vector. The complex usually has axial symmetry in solution and the McConnell–Robertson Equation (2) holds:

$$\Delta_{DIP} = K\,(3\cos^2\theta - 1)\,r^{-3} \tag{2}$$

This equation can be used to give quantitative information about the structure or conformation of a compound, if the bound shifts are known [3]. Lanthanide shift experiments are only successful when the substrate acts as a Lewis base to which complexing can occur. The degree of Lewis basicity decreases in the following order:

$$RNH_2 > ROH > RCOR > RCOOR > RCN$$

The commercially available lanthanide shift reagents are 1,3 diketone complexes. In contrast to europium, praseodymium complexes shift the signals to lower frequency, while the ytterbium reagents are best used in ^{13}C NMR spectroscopy. Binuclear shift reagents such as $Ag(fod)/Eu(fod)_3$ can be used for unsaturated hydrocarbons.

8. Own Observations

Experiment 8.2

Signal Separation of Enantiomers Using a Chiral Shift Reagent

1. Purpose

Chiral lanthanide shift reagents are used for the determination of enantiomeric purity (for other techniques see Exp. 8.3 and 8.4). In this experiment the chiral tris[3-(hepta-fluoropropylhydroxymethylene)-*d*-camphorato]-praseodymium complex, Pr(hfc)$_3$, is used, which (unlike europium, Exp. 8.1) results in low frequency rather than high frequency shifts.

2. Literature

[1] G. R. Sullivan, *Top. Stereochem.* **1978**, *10*, 288–329.
[2] W. H. Pirkle, D. J. Hoover, *Top. Stereochem.* **1982**, *13*, 263–331.
[3] D. Parker, *Chem. Rev.* **1991**, *91*, 1441–1457.
[4] O. Hofer, *Top. Stereochem.* **1976**, *9*, 111–197.
[5] J. Reuben, *Prog. Nucl. Magn. Reson. Spectrosc.* **1975**, *9*, 1–70.
[6] T. C. Morrill (ed.): *Lanthanide Shift Reagents in Stereochemical Analysis*, in *Methods in Stereochemical Analysis*, VCH, Weinheim, **1985**.

3. Pulse Scheme and Phase Cycle

p1: x, x, -x, -x, y, y, -y, -y
aq: x, x, -x, -x, y, y, -y, -y

4. Acquisition

Time requirement: 1 h

Sample: 10 mg rac 1-phenylethanol in 0.7 ml CDCl$_3$

Load standard ^{1}H NMR acquisition parameters, set the spectral width to 15 ppm and adjust the offset so that signals up to $\delta_H = -3$ are covered. Record a spectrum of 1-phenylethanol, add a very small portion (about 1 mg) of tris[3-(heptafluoropropyl-hydroxy-methylene)-*d*-camphorato]-praseodymium, Pr(hfc)$_3$, allow sufficient time to reach equilibrium, and record the spectrum again. Increase the amount of the chiral shift reagent until the separation of the two quartets of the methine group (initially at $\delta_H = 4.9$) is sufficient for reasonable integration.

5. Processing

Use standard 1D processing for ^1H NMR spectra (see Exp. 3.1).

6. Result

The figure shows the ^1H NMR spectrum of rac 1-phenylethanol (**a**) in the absence of and (**b**) in the presence of Pr(hfc)$_3$. The signals originally at $\delta_H = 1.5$ (CH$_3$) and $\delta_H = 4.9$ (CH) are shifted to $\delta_H = -0.3$ and $\delta_H = 1.7$ and 1.9 in spectrum **b**. The methine signals of the two enantiomers are completely separated, but are also significantly broadened. The signals of the methyl group are not yet separated. They begin to separate when the concentration of the added shift reagent is such that the signal is shifted to $\delta_H = -2$ ppm.

7. Comments

Chiral shift reagents (L$_S$) form diastereomeric complexes with the substrate molecules S$_S$ and S$_R$ which are in a rapid equilibrium with the uncomplexed species:

$$L_S + S_S \rightleftharpoons [L_S S_S]$$

$$L_S + S_R \rightleftharpoons [L_S S_R]$$

With increasing concentration of the reagent the equilibrium is shifted to the right and the lanthanide-induced shifts increase. Since the shift reagent is paramagnetic one observes significant line broadening at higher concentrations of the shift reagent, especially for nuclei (in this case protons) which are near to the complexation site. Instead of performing several weighing procedures for quantitative work it is better to start with the highest concentration of the lanthanide shift reagent and to dilute by means of a substrate stock solution. Another method is to prepare stock solutions of the reagent and the substrate and to increase the ratio of reagent solution to substrate solution, while always keeping the same total volume of solution by adding solvent (see figure in Exp. 8.1).

Normally the enantiomeric excess *ee* is calculated using to the following equation:

$$ee = (I_1 - I_2) / (I_1 + I_2)$$

where I_1 and I_2 are the integrals of the corresponding signals. The *ee* value is zero for the example shown, because the racemate was investigated. Although it is no problem to separate and integrate the signals of racemates, this method has its limitations if the ratio of the integrals of the enantiomers is about 9:1 or greater. The choice of a reagent shifting the signals to lower frequencies, as shown here, compared with one shifting to higher frequencies (see Exp. 8.1) must be carefully considered for each substrate.

8. Own Observations

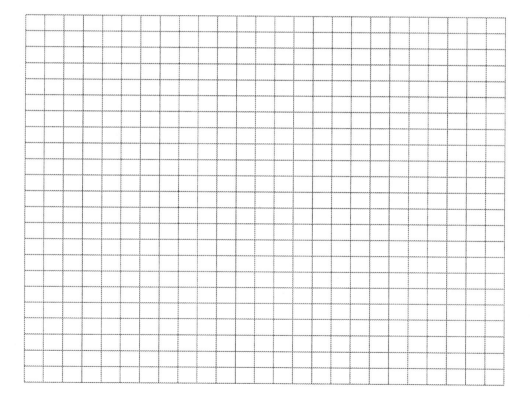

Experiment 8.3

Signal Separation of Enantiomers Using a Chiral Solvating Agent

1. Purpose

This ^{1}H NMR experiment is used to prove the presence of enantiomers or to determine the enantiomeric purity of a compound. A chiral solvating agent, R-(–)-α-acetoxy-phenylacetic acid (R-(–)-O-acetyl-mandelic acid), which is commercially available in pure enantiomeric form is employed [1-3]. A similar application is described in Experiment 8.4.

2. Literature

[1] G. R. Sullivan, *Top. Stereochem.* **1978**, *10*, 288–329.
[2] W. H. Pirkle, D. J. Hoover, *Top. Stereochem.* **1982**, *13*, 263–331.
[3] D. Parker, *Chem. Rev.* **1991**, *91*, 1441–1457.

3. Pulse Scheme and Phase Cycle

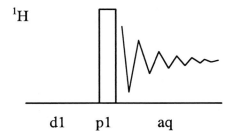

¹H

p1: x, x, -x, -x, y, y, -y, -y
aq: x, x, -x, -x, y, y, -y, -y

d1   p1   aq

4. Acquisition

Time requirement: 20 min

Sample: 10 mg rac 1-phenylethylamine in 0.7 ml CDCl$_3$

Load standard ^{1}H NMR acquisition parameters (see Exp. 3.1) and record a spectrum of 1-phenylethylamine. Add about 10 mg of R-(–)-O-acetyl-mandelic acid and record the spectrum again. Increase the amount of the chiral solvating agent until the separation of the two doublets of the methyl group at $\delta_H = 1.2$ is sufficient for integration.

5. Processing

Use standard 1D processing for ^{1}H NMR spectra (Exp. 3.1).

6. Result

The figure shows the ^{1}H-NMR spectrum of rac 1-phenylethylamine obtained on an AM-400 spectrometer (**a**) without and (**b**) in the presence of the chiral solvating agent R-(−)-O-acetyl-mandelic acid. The signals at δ_H = 1.2 (CH$_3$) and at δ_H = 4.05 (CH) are doubled and the CH$_3$ signals are suitably separated for integration. The phenyl-ethylamine signals in (**b**) are slightly upfield from those in (**a**).

7. Comments

Chiral solvating agents form diastereomeric solvation complexes which are in rapid equilibrium with the uncomplexed species. Solvents with low solvating ability should therefore be used, such as CDCl$_3$, CCl$_4$ or C$_6$D$_6$. Other common commercially available agents are 2,2,2-trifluoro-1-phenylethanol and 1-(9-anthryl)-2,2,2-trifluoro-ethanol (Pirkle's reagent, see Exp. 8.4). In the example presented here the chiral auxiliary forms a salt with the basic phenylethylamine. The salt is still in rapid equilibrium with the base and the acid, so this is not a derivatizing agent like, for example, Mosher esters.

For quantitative determinations use stock solutions of the substrate and the chiral solvating agent to make up a series of solutions of constant volume containing a fixed amount of substrate solution and varying amounts of the chiral agent solution (see figure in Exp. 8.1).

The enantiomeric excess *ee* can be calculated from the following equation:

$$ee = (I_1 - I_2) / (I_1 + I_2)$$

where I_1 and I_2 are the integrals of the corresponding signals. The *ee*-value is zero for the example given, as the racemic form was investigated.

8. Own Observations

Experiment 8.4

Determination of Enantiomeric Purity with Pirkle's Reagent

1. Purpose

This ^{1}H NMR experiment is used to prove the presence of enantiomers or to determine the enantiomeric purity of a compound, and employs a chiral solvating agent, 1-(9-anthryl)-2,2,2-trifluoroethanol (Pirkle's reagent), which is commercially available in both pure enantiomeric forms [1–3]. A similar application is described in Experiment 8.3.

2. Literature

[1] G. R. Sullivan, *Top. Stereochem.* **1978**, *10*, 288–329.
[2] W. H. Pirkle, D. J. Hoover, *Top. Stereochem.* **1982**, *13*, 263–331.
[3] D. Parker, *Chem. Rev.* **1991**, *91*, 1441–1457.

3. Pulse Scheme and Phase Cycle

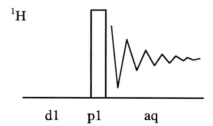

^{1}H

p1: x, x, -x, -x, y, y, -y, -y
aq: x, x, -x, -x, y, y, -y, -y

d1   p1   aq

4. Acquisition

Time requirement: 30 min

Sample: 10 mg rac 1-phenylethanol in 0.7 ml CDCl$_3$

Load standard ^{1}H NMR acquisition parameters (see Exp. 3.1) and record a spectrum of 1-phenylethanol. Add about 40 mg of S-(+)-1-(9-anthryl)-2,2,2-trifluoroethanol and record another ^{1}H NMR spectrum. Increase the amount of the chiral solvating agent until the separation of the two doublets of the methyl group at $\delta_H = 1.2$ is sufficient.

5. Processing

Use standard 1D processing for ¹H NMR spectra (see Experiment 3.1). A Gaussian window (gb = 0.2, lb = −0.5 Hz) was used to process spectrum **b**.

6. Result

The figure shows the ¹H NMR spectrum of rac 1-phenylethanol obtained on an AM-400 spectrometer (**a**) without and (**b**) in the presence of the chiral solvating agent S-(+)-1-(9-anthryl)-2,2,2-trifluoroethanol. The signals at δ_H = 1.2 (CH$_3$) and at δ_H = 4.9 (CH) are doubled. Note, however, that the separation of the two CH$_3$ doublets is not sufficient for an integation. This is due to a weaker interaction of the the chiral solvating agent with the 1-phenylethanol, which is less basic than 1-phenylethylamine (see Exp. 8.3). On the other hand the chiral auxiliary used here is not acidic enough to form strong solvation complexes. Better results were achieved for 1-phenylethanol with a chiral shift reagent (see Exp. 8.2).

7. Comments

Chiral solvating agents form diastereomeric solvation complexes, which are in rapid equilibrium with the uncomplexed species. Solvents with low solvating ability should therefore be used, such as CDCl$_3$, CCl$_4$ or C$_6$D$_6$. Frequently used commercially available agents are 2,2,2-trifluoro-1-phenylethanol, or R-(−)-O-acetyl-mandelic acid (see Exp. 8.3). It is difficult to predict which chiral solvating agent is the best for a certain compound. The enantiomeric excess *ee* can be calculated from the following relationship:

$$ee = (I_1 - I_2) / (I_1 + I_2)$$

where I_1 and I_2 are the integrals of the corresponding signals. For the example shown here the *ee* value is zero, because the racemate was used.

8. Own Observations

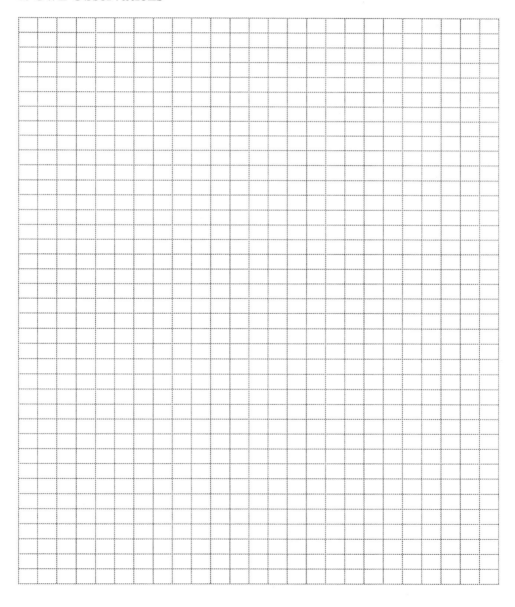

Experiment 8.5

The Relaxation Reagent Cr(acac)$_3$

1. Purpose

The paramagnetic relaxation reagent Cr(acac)$_3$ is used to increase the intensity of the signals of quaternary ^{13}C nuclei which suffer from long relaxation times T_1. The addition of increasing amounts of the reagent results in a shortening of the relaxation times T_1 and an increase in line-width. The chemical shift is usually unaffected. The relaxation reagent is important for quantitative ^{13}C NMR investigations (see Exp. 8.7). Cr(dpm)$_3$ was reported to be more soluble, however is not commercially available.

2. Literature

[1] M. L. Martin, G. J. Martin, J. J. Delpuech, *Practical NMR Spectroscopy,* Heyden London, **1980**, Ch. 10.3.
[2] G. C. Levy, U. Edlund, *J. Am. Chem. Soc.* **1986**, *97*, 4482–4485.

3. Pulse Scheme and Phase Cycle

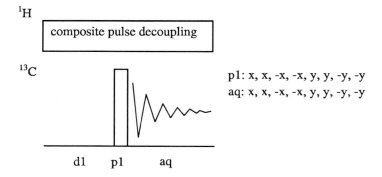

p1: x, x, -x, -x, y, y, -y, -y
aq: x, x, -x, -x, y, y, -y, -y

4. Acquisition

Time requirement: 15 min

Sample: 20% ethyl crotonate in CDCl$_3$.

Load standard ^{13}C NMR acquisition parameters (see Exp. 3.2) and record a ^{13}C NMR spectrum. Then add about 20 mg of chromium acetylacetonate, Cr(acac)$_3$. The solution should become slightly purple. A concentration of 0.1 M is ideal for quantitative work. The highest concentration which is reported in the literature to give reasonable results is 0.4 M. At higher concentrations one gets severe line broadening and it is difficult to lock on the solvent signal. You have to set:

td: 64 k
sw: 250 ppm
o1: middle of ^{13}C NMR spectrum
o2: middle of ^{1}H NMR spectrum
d1: 0.5 s
p1: 45° ^{13}C transmitter pulse
decoupler attenuation and 90° pulse for CPD
ns: 64

5. Processing

Use standard 1D processing for ^{13}C NMR (see Experiment 3.2).

6. Result

The figure shows the result obtained on an ARX-200 spectrometer. Note that after the addition of Cr(acac)₃ in (**b**) the intensities of all signals of ethyl crotonate are almost the same and the signal of CDCl₃ dominates, whereas the spectrum (**a**) without the relaxation reagent shows small intensities for the signal of the carboxyl group of ethyl crotonate and for the solvent signal. However, addition of Cr(acac)₃ also causes a reduction in the signal-to-noise ratio due to line broadening.

7. Comments

Routine ^{13}C NMR spectra are recorded under conditions which maximize sensitivity, such as using the Ernst angle and ^{1}H broad-band decoupling. This results in reduced intensities for signals of quaternary carbon nuclei, which usually have long relaxation times T_1 and smaller NOE values. The NOEs are dependent on the dipole–dipole interaction between ^{1}H and ^{13}C. The addition of paramagnetic compounds such as Cr(acac)$_3$, Mn(acac)$_2$, Cu(acac)$_2$ or Gd(acac)$_3$ reduces T_1 to less than 1 s for all types of carbon atoms. Because of the large gyromagnetic ratio of the unpaired electrons the mechanism of the relaxation is now an (electron dipole)–(^{13}C dipole) interaction. For excitation one can use 90° pulses and higher pulse repetition rates. Therefore relaxation reagents can also be used for advanced experiments like INADEQUATE (see Exps. 6.10 and 10.19).

8. Own Observations

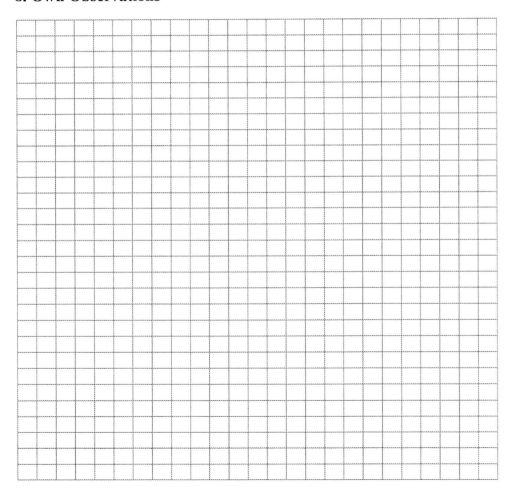

Experiment 8.6

Quantitative ^{1}H-NMR Spectroscopy: Determination of the Alcohol Content of Polish Vodka

1. Purpose

In ^{1}H NMR spectroscopy the signal area is normally proportional to the number of nuclei contributing to the signal, provided that saturation is avoided. It is therefore possible to use ^{1}H NMR for quantitative determinations in chemistry. The integrals are usually used; they are proportional to molar ratios.

2. Literature

[1] M. L. Martin, G. J. Martin, J. J. Delpuech, *Practical NMR Spectroscopy*, Heyden, London, **1984**, Ch. 9, 350–376.
[2] E. D. Becker, *High Resolution NMR*, Academic Press, New York, **1980**, Ch. 12.
[3] D. D. Traficante, *Concepts Magn. Reson.* **1992**, *4*, 145–160.
[4] D. D. Traficante, L. R. Steward, *Concepts Magn. Reson.* **1994**, *6*, 131–135.
[5] J. Peterson, *J. Chem. Educ.* **1992**, *69*, 843–845.

3. Pulse Scheme and Phase Cycle

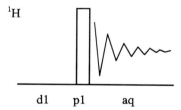

p1: x, x, -x, -x, y, y, -y, -y
aq: x, x, -x, -x, y, y, -y, -y

d1   p1   aq

4. Acquisition

Time requirement: 5 min

Sample: 0.7 ml Polish vodka containing a few drops of dry [D$_6$]acetone

Record a standard ^{1}H NMR spectrum with a large data set (10 points/Hz digital resolution). The spectral width should be large enough that the signals at both ends are not affected by the analog audio filter of the spectrometer. Be sure to obtain a good signal-to-noise ratio, at least 35:1. The pulse repetition time must be long enough for complete relaxation ($5T_1$, where T_1 is the longest spin–lattice relaxation time). It is advisable to repeat the experiment with different spectrometer settings and calculate an average of the results. You have to set:

td: 32 k
sw: 10 ppm
o1: middle of ^{1}H NMR spectrum
p1: 45° ^{1}H transmitter pulse (for optimization see literature [3])
d1: 5 s
ns: 16

5. Processing

Use standard 1D processing with additional zero-filling to 64 k. Perform a baseline correction on the FID before the Fourier transformation. Phase-adjust the spectrum accurately and perform a baseline correction on the spectrum, then integrate the signals. Ensure the integral limits are far enough apart to give a complete integration. Adjust slope and bias of the individual integrals. This is especially important for the integration of broad signals. In the present case there are three signals (H_2O + OH, CH_2 and CH_3 of ethanol).

6. Result

The figure shows the ^{1}H NMR spectrum of vodka obtained with an AM-400WB spectrometer. The water/alcohol ratio by weight is calculated using the following equation:

$$\frac{Ga}{Gb} = \frac{Fa}{Fb} \cdot \frac{Nb}{Na} \cdot \frac{Ma}{Mb}$$

where G_a and G_b are the parts by weight of the components a and b, in this example water and alcohol respectively and F_a and F_b the areas of the signals of H_2O and CH_2. N_a and N_b are the numbers of nuclei which cause the signals, in this case 2 and 2 respectively, and M_a and M_b are the molecular masses of the two components, 18 and 46 respectively. Using the measured integrals (1152, 202.6) the water/alcohol ratio by weight is calculated to be 2.029/1; in other words the vodka contains 33.0% alcohol by weight or, taking into account the density of the actual ethanol-water mixture, 39.6% by volume. This is in good agreement with the alcohol content given on the label (Bison Brand Vodka 40° by volume). Because the OH signal contains both water and ethanol OH protons, one has to subtract the intensity of one proton from the value of the integral of water before calculating this ratio.

7. Comments

The integrals of NMR signals are relative measures of the numbers of resonating nuclei. If one component is present at much lower concentration than another, the percentage error in measurement of the quantity of this minor component could by quite high (see Exp. 3.10). For quantitative determinations deconvolution and curve-fitting methods have been proposed in the literature, especially for cases where peaks are not fully resolved. Curve-fitting procedures are often included in the commercially available software packages.

8. Own Observations

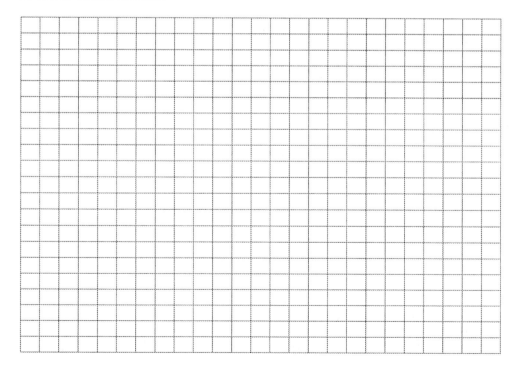

Experiment 8.7

Quantitative ^{13}C NMR Spectroscopy with Inverse Gated ^{1}H-Decoupling

1. Purpose

Quantitative ^{13}C NMR spectroscopy is not as straightforward as quantitative ^{1}H NMR spectroscopy (see Exp. 8.6) as both NOE effects (see Exp. 4.14) and widely varying relaxation times affect the intensity of the signals. For quantitative ^{13}C NMR determinations a relaxation reagent (see Exp. 8.5) should be added and the Overhauser effect suppressed (see Exp. 4.11).

2. Literature

[1] M. L. Martin, G. J. Martin, J. J. Delpuech, *Practical NMR Spectroscopy*, Heyden, London, **1984**, Ch. 9, 350–376.
[2] E. D. Becker, *High Resolution NMR*, Academic Press, New York, **1980**, Ch. 12.
[3] C. H. Sotak, C. L. Dumoulin, G. C. Levy, *Top. Carbon-13 NMR Spectrosc.* **1984**, *4*, 91–121.
[4] L. D. Field, S. Sternhell, *Analytical NMR*, Wiley, Chichester, **1989**, Ch. 3, 41–63.

3. Pulse Scheme and Phase Cycle

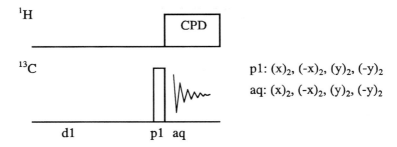

p1: $(x)_2$, $(-x)_2$, $(y)_2$, $(-y)_2$
aq: $(x)_2$, $(-x)_2$, $(y)_2$, $(-y)_2$

4. Acquisition

Time requirement: 30 min

Sample: 156.4 mg naphthalene and 70.0 mg phenanthrene in 1 ml CDCl$_3$. Add 35 mg Cr(acac)$_3$, which corresponds to a 0.1 M solution.

Record a ^{13}C NMR spectrum with the inverse gated decoupling sequence. The spectral width should be large enough that the signals at both ends are not affected by the analog audio filter of the spectrometer. Be sure to obtain a good signal-to-noise ratio, at least 35:1. You have to set:

td: 2 k (short aq to avoid NOE build-up during acquisition)
sw: 20 ppm
o1: middle of aromatic region of the ^{13}C NMR spectrum
o2: middle of aromatic region of the ^{1}H NMR spectrum
p1: 90° ^{13}C transmitter pulse
d1: 10 s
decoupler attenuation and 90° pulse for CPD
ns: 160

5. Processing

Use standard 1D processing as described in Experiment 3.2. Zero-filling to 8 k yields an adequate digital resolution. Perform a baseline correction on the FID before the Fourier transformation. Phase-adjust the spectrum accurately and perform a baseline correction on the spectrum, then integrate the signals. Ensure the integral limits are far enough from both sides of the signal to give a complete integration. In general use as many signal pairs for integration as possible and calculate an average. It is advisable to repeat the experiment with different spectrometer settings and calculate an average of the results.

6. Result

| Integral | 291.0 | | 87.6 | | 84.1 | | 84.9 563.9 266.5 570.3 | | | 86.1 |
| δC | | 132 | | 130 | | 128 | | 126 | 124 | | 122 |

The figure shows the aromatic region of the ^{13}C NMR spectrum obtained on an AM-400WB spectrometer. The ratio of the components by weight is calculated using the following equation:

$$\frac{Ga}{Gb} = \frac{Fa}{Fb} \cdot \frac{Nb}{Na} \cdot \frac{Ma}{Mb}$$

where G_a and G_b are the parts by weight of the components a (naphthalene) and b (phenanthrene) and N_a and N_b the numbers of nuclei, which cause the signals. M_a and M_b are the molecular masses of the two components, 128.16 and 178.23 respectively. Using the measured averaged integrals F_a for naphthalene (signals at δ_C = 132.8, 127.3, 125.2, relative intensity ratio 2:4:4) and F_b for phenanthrene (signals at δ_C = 131.4, 129.6, 127.9, 126.3. 125.9, 122.1, relative intensity ratio 2:2:2:2:4:2) the naphthalene/phenanthrene ratio by weight is calculated to be 2.27/1, which corresponds to 69.5/30.5 percentage weight. This is in very good agreement with the percentage ratio of 69.1/30.9 corresponding to the weighed amounts used.

7. Comments

The integrals of NMR signals are relative measures of the numbers of nuclei producing that signal. If one component is present at much lower concentration than another, the percentage error in measurement of the quantity of this minor component could by quite high (see Exp. 3.10). It is only when the line shapes and line widths are identical that the relative peak heights are a measure of the relative concentration.

The inverse gated [1]H-decoupling experiment is described in Experiment 4.11. Small NOE enhancement build up during the acquisition time, but are dissipated during the relaxation delay which should be at least 10 times longer than the acquisition time. In addition, the paramagnetic relaxation reagent Cr(acac)$_3$ shortens the ^{13}C spin–lattice relaxation times.

8. Own Observations

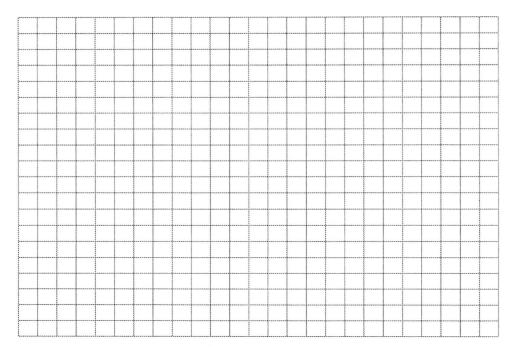

Experiment 8.8

Determination of Paramagnetic Susceptibility by NMR

1. Purpose

Magnetic susceptibilities are traditionally measured using a Gouy balance. This experiment demonstrates how the same information can be gained by a simple NMR measurement. The experiment is based on measuring the shift of the resonance frequency of an indicator compound caused by introducing a known concentration of the paramagnetic compound into the solution. The "doped" solution is prepared in a capillary tube so that the shift can be measured directly.

2. Literature

[1] D. F. Evans, *J. Chem. Soc.* **1958**, 2003–2005.
[2] J. L. Deutsch, S. M. Poling, *J. Chem. Educ.* **1969**, *46*, 167–168.
[3] J. Löliger, R. Scheffold, *J. Chem. Educ.* **1972**, *49*, 646–647.
[4] K. G. Orrel, V. Sik, *Anal. Chem.* **1980**, *52*, 569–572.
[5] A. Furuhashi, I. Ono, A. Yamasaki, *Magn. Reson. Chem.* **1991**, *29*, 1175–1180.
[6] D. H. Grant, *J. Chem. Educ.* **1995**, *72*, 39–40.

3. Pulse Scheme and Phase Cycle

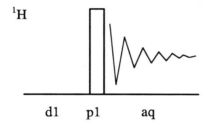

^{1}H

p1: x, x, -x, -x, y, y, -y, -y
aq: x, x, -x, -x, y, y, -y, -y

d1   p1   aq

4. Acquisition

Time requirement: 20 min

Sample: Weigh and dissolve 7 mg $FeSO_4 \cdot 7H_2O$ (p. a.) in 0.5 ml D_2O in a volumetric flask, add 30 µl *t*-butanol and adjust the solution with D_2O to exactly 1 ml. Fill a standard melting-point capillary with this solution and flame-seal the capillary. Prepare an identical solution containing no iron salt and transfer it to a normal 5 mm NMR tube.

Adjust and control the probehead temperature at 298 K. Load standard ^{1}H NMR acquisition parameters, adjust the homogeneity and record a spectrum of the solution in the NMR tube without the capillary. Introduce the capillary and record the spectrum again. The sample should be spun so as to center the capillary in the NMR tube.

Measure the frequency difference between the *t*-butanol signals in the two compartments.

5. Processing

Use standard 1D processing as described in Experiment 3.1

6. Result

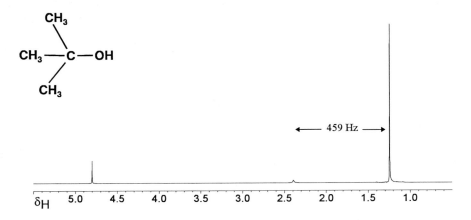

The figure shows the result obtained on an AM-400 spectrometer. The frequency difference between the *t*-butanol signals was 459 Hz using 7.2 mg $FeSO_4 \cdot 7H_2O$ for the solution in the capillary.

Note that the equations and spectra shown in the early literature apply to iron magnets where the magnetic field is perpendicular to the the axis of the NMR tube. For measurements using superconducting magnets the factor $2\pi/3$ must be replaced by $-4\pi/3$; thus the effect is larger and has the opposite sign. The difference between the frequencies of the signals in the outer compartment (v_o) and in the capillary (v_i) is related to the volume susceptibilities X by Equation (1).

$$\frac{v_o - v_i}{v_o} = -\frac{4\pi}{3}(X_i - X_o) \qquad (1)$$

The volume susceptibilities X are usually replaced by the mass susceptibilities χ, where $\chi = X/\rho$, and the density ρ is equal to the mass m of the paramagnetic compound in 1 ml of solution. Thus (1) rearranges to give Equation (2). Here χ_o is approximately equal to the mass susceptibility of water, which is $-0.72 \cdot 10^{-6}$ cm^3g^{-1}.

$$\chi_i = -\frac{3}{4\pi m}\frac{v_o - v_i}{v_o} + \chi_o \qquad (2)$$

The molar susceptibility χ_m is finally obtained by multiplying χ_i by the molar mass, in our case 278. Thus a χ_m-value for $FeSO_4 \cdot 7H_2O$ of $10374 \cdot 10^{-6}$ in c.g.s units was obtained in this experiment from the measured shift difference of 459 Hz, a result which compares reasonably well with the tabulated value of $11200 \cdot 10^{-6}$.

7. Comments

The literature [1–5] gives a variety of methods for measuring paramagnetic susceptibility with NMR. The experiment demonstrated here seems to be the easiest with current NMR instruments. Note that the value obtained is temperature dependent and that the Curie constant can be determined from the temperature dependence.

For the transition metals, where the spin-only approximation for the paramagnetism is valid, the number of unpaired electrons can be calculated from the molar susceptibility. Other indicator compounds may be used, and organometallic paramagnetic compounds can also be investigated.

8. Own Observations

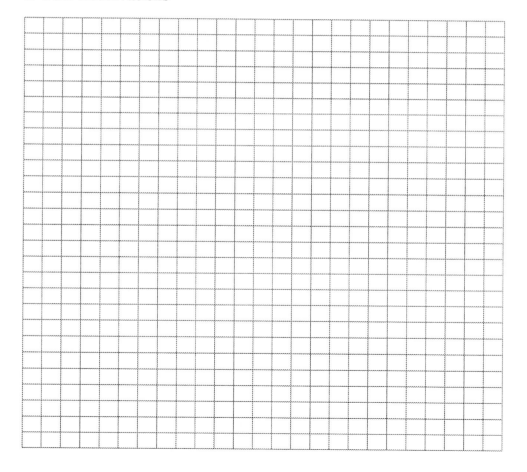

Experiment 8.9

The CIDNP Effect

1. Purpose

This experiment demonstrates the technique used to observe the Chemically Induced Dynamic Nuclear Polarization. Although the name CIDNP based on an early misinterpretation is somewhat misleading, it has become established in the literature. The effect has been widely used to prove the existence of a radical *pair* intermediate during a chemical reaction. Other applications include the signal assignment of aromatic amino acids in proteins, which uses the photochemical CIDNP technique.

2. Literature

[1] J. Bargon, H. Fischer, U. Johnson, *Z. Naturforsch. A* **1967**, *22*, 1551–1555.
[2] H. R. Ward, R. G. Lawler, *J. Am. Chem. Soc.* **1967**, *89*, 5518–5519.
[3] R. Kaptein, *Adv. Free Radical Chem.* **1975**, *5*, 319–380.
[4] G. L. Closs, R. J. Miller, O. D. Redwine, *Acc. Chem. Res.* **1985**, *18*, 196–202.
[5] P. J. Hore, R. W. Broadhurst, *Prog. NMR Spectrosc.* **1993**, *25*, 345–402.

3. Pulse Scheme and Phase Cycle

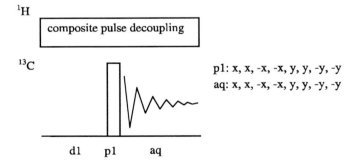

4. Acquisition

Time requirement: 30 min

Sample: 40 mg benzoyl peroxide in cyclohexanone; *remove the cap from the NMR sample tube*

Use the NMR instrument with the *lowest* available field, as even for protons the *net* CIDNP effect cannot be observed on a 200 MHz instrument. However, the effect can be observed for ^{13}C at this magnetic field strength. Raise the probe-head temperature to 90°C, load standard ^{1}H acquisition parameters (Exp. 3.1), turn off the sawtooth field sweep, and shim the magnet on the incoming FID, since the sample provides no lock signal. Switch to ^{13}C operation and record a standard ^{13}C NMR spectrum as a reference. Load an automatic acquisition routine, which measures and subsequentially stores 20 standard ^{13}C spectra with broad-band ^{1}H-decoupling, each with 16 scans. Set the temperature unit to 120°C and immediately start the automatic program. The peroxide decomposes, which results in the CIDNP effect being visible in a few of the recorded spectra. A kinetic diagram can be constructed from the peak heights of the various signals as a function of time.

5. Processing

Use standard 1D processing for ^{13}C NMR as described in Experiment 3.2 with exponential multiplication (lb = 2 Hz).

6. Result

The figure shows the result obtained on an ARX-200 spectrometer. Spectrum **a** is the initial ^{13}C spectrum at 90°C (128 transients). Only the CH signals of the aromatic rings of benzoyl peroxide can be seen under these conditions. Spectrum **b** shows the CIDNP effect at 120°C (16 transients). The emission line of the escape product, benzene, and the two enhanced absorption signals from the carboxyl nucleus and the *ipso* carbon nucleus of the cage recombination product phenyl benzoate are clearly visible. The signals of the initial benzoyl peroxide are hardly visible, which demonstrates the enhancement factor experienced by the other signals.

7. Comments

Other well known examples of the CIDNP effect include organometallic reactions, the decomposition of diazonium salts, 1.2 rearrangements, aromatic nitration, and many photochemically induced reactions. Besides the *net* effect demonstrated in this experiment there exists a *multiplet* effect, where the different lines within one spin multiplet show enhanced absorption and emission. The complex theory of CIDNP can be studied in the literature cited.

8. Own Observations

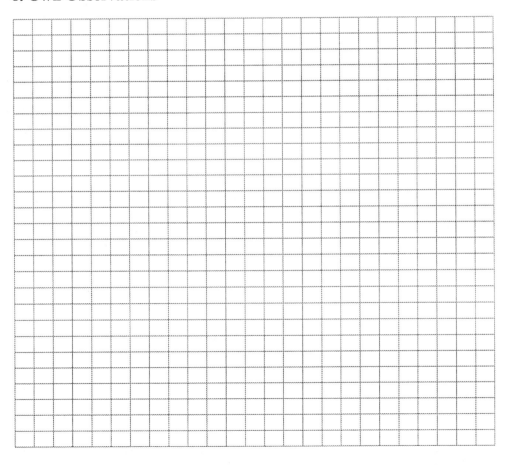

Chapter 9

Heteronuclear NMR Spectroscopy

Nearly all the experiments demonstrated in this book are performed by recording an ^{1}H or a ^{13}C NMR spectrum. However, the world of NMR is much more fascinating if the whole Periodic System is considered, and many of the experiments given can be carried out with other nuclides. Nearly all elements possess at least one isotope with a magnetic moment which is observable, at least in principle, by NMR. However, there are some factors which may prevent routine observations. The main problems arise from low natural abundance and/or a low γ-value giving poor NMR sensitivity and from the existence of a significant electric quadrupolar moment for nuclides with $I >$ 1/2, which leads to very broad lines or even prevents any observations at all. Since the natural abundance and NMR sensitivity of an isotope are constant parameters, they can be combined in a single parameter, the "receptivity" which indicates how difficult it is to obtain a signal in comparison to ^{13}C. In this chapter we provide some basic examples of NMR spectroscopy of the heteroelements to give the beginner an easy start in this field.

For these experiments the spectrometer must be equipped with a frequency synthesizer to provide the necessary frequencies, the appropriate amplifier, and a multinuclear probe-head with a broad-band preamplifier. The following tables give the essential information regarding the resonance frequencies of the NMR-active nuclides together with the recommended reference compounds.

Referencing, however, is a frequently discussed problem in heteronuclear NMR spectroscopy. Whereas there is an accepted common internal standard for ^{1}H, ^{13}C, and ^{29}Si, namely tetramethylsilane, which is easily removable, comparable universal standards do not exist for the other nuclides. The chemical reactivity often prohibits the use of an internal reference. One way out is to use the reference compound in a capillary, though it does result in a loss of sensitivity and a susceptibility correction has to be made.

A common alternative solution is external referencing, where the reference compound is measured before and after the actual experiment and precautions are taken so that the magnetic field is not changed in between. This can work well when using modern instruments, which use digital lock circuits to shift the lock frequency instead of the magnetic field.

A third method uses the Ξ-scale, which does not depend on any nuclide-specific reference compound. Here the chemical shift of TMS is defined to be 100.000000 MHz. The Ξ-value of interest is given by Equation (1).

$$\Xi_X = \frac{100 \, \gamma_X}{\gamma_H} \cdot \frac{1 - \sigma_X}{1 - \sigma_H} \tag{1}$$

Table of Nuclides with $I = 1/2$

Nuclide	Natural abundance N [%]	Gyromagnetic ratio γ [10^7 rad T^{-1}s^{-1}]	NMR frequency[a] Ξ [MHz]	Standard	Receptivity D[b]
^{1}H	99.985	26.7522	100.000 000	Me$_4$Si	$5.68 \cdot 10^3$
^{3}H	-	28.5335	106.663	Me$_4$Si	-
^{3}He	$1.3 \cdot 10^{-4}$	-20.378	76.178		$3.26 \cdot 10^{-3}$
^{13}C	1.108	6.7283	25.145 004	Me$_4$Si	1.00
^{15}N	0.37	-2.7126	10.136 767	MeNO$_2$ (neat)	$2.19 \cdot 10^{-2}$
^{19}F	100.0	25.1815	94.094 003	CCl$_3$F	4.73
^{29}Si	4.70	-5.319	19.867 184	Me$_4$Si	2.09
^{31}P	100.0	10.8394	40.480 747	85% H$_3$PO$_4$	$3.77 \cdot 10^2$
^{57}Fe	2.19	0.8687	3.237 798	Fe(CO)$_5$	$4.19 \cdot 10^{-3}$
^{77}Se	7.58	5.101	19.091 523	Me$_2$Se	2.98
^{89}Y	100.0	-1.3163	4.920	Y(NO$_3$)$_3$/H$_2$O	0.668
^{103}Rh	100.0	-0.8468	3.17		0.177
^{109}Ag	48.18	-1.2519	4.653 623	Ag$^+$/ H$_2$O	0.276
^{113}Cd	12.26	-5.99609	22.193 173	CdMe$_2$	7.59
^{119}Sn	8.58	-10.0318	37.290 665	Me$_4$Sn	25.2
^{125}Te	6.99	-8.453	31.549 802	Me$_2$Te	12.5
^{129}Xe	26.44	-7.3995	27.661	XeOF$_4$	31.8
^{169}Tm	100.0	-2.21	8.272		3.21
^{171}Yb	14.31	4.7117	17.613		4.44
^{183}W	14.28	1.1283	4.151 888	W(CO)$_6$	$5.89 \cdot 10^{-2}$
^{187}Os	1.64	0.6193	2.282 343	OsO$_4$	$1.14 \cdot 10^{-3}$
^{195}Pt	33.8	5.8383	21.414 376	[Pt(CN)$_6$]$^{2-}$	19.1
^{199}Hg	16.84	4.8458	17.910 841	Me$_2$Hg (neat)	5.42
^{205}Tl	70.50	15.6922	57.633 833	TlNO$_3$/ aq.	$7.69 \cdot 10^2$
^{207}Pb	22.6	5.56264	20.920 597	Me$_4$Pb	11.8

a) values given in 9 digits as measured for the standard compounds, other data calculated from the γ-values in column 3. b) receptivity relative to ^{13}C

Thus, by measuring the digital frequency of the resonance signal in question and that of TMS, the corresponding Ξ_X-value can be calculated. In comparison with ^{1}H and ^{13}C the chemical shifts of heteronuclides are much more dependent on concentration, temperature, and solvent.

For setting up an NMR experiment with a heteronuclide you have to tune a multinuclear probe-head to the nuclide in question and, if desired, the proton channel in order to use ^{1}H-decoupling or to perform multi-pulse experiments such as DEPT which require ^{1}H pulses in the decoupler channel. Note that the ^{1}H pulse-length in the decoupler channel can differ from the setting value used, if the observe channel was tuned on ^{13}C.

On modern instruments these [1]H-decoupler pulses do not differ much from the ^{1}H pulses in the observe channel, but for older instruments it is best to use special samples which allow the determination of the [1]H-decoupler pulse while the observe channel is tuned to a heteronuclide, e.g. formamide for [15]N.

The signal of a heteronuclide should then first be located with a strong and well-known sample, so as to determine the correct offset and the required spectral width for the subsequent measurements on the unknown samples. Since heteronuclear NMR spectra often consist of only one signal, it is mandatory to check whether the signal is still present without the sample inserted in the probe-head in order to exclude instrumental artefacts.

We have selected for this chapter examples from spin I = 1/2 nuclei such as ^{15}N, ^{19}F, [29]Si, and [119]Sn. The measurement of quadrupolar nuclei is demonstrated with ^{2}H, [11]B, and [17]O. For a 2D example using [6]Li as the detected nucleus see Experiment 10.19.

Literature

[1] R. K. Harris, B. E. Mann (eds.), *NMR and the Periodic Table*, Academic Press, New York, **1978**.
[2] C. Brevard, P. Granger, *Handbook of High Resolution Multinuclear NMR*, Wiley, Chichester, **1981**.
[3] J. Mason (ed.), *Multinuclear NMR*, 2nd Edition, Plenum Press, London, **1989**.
[4] S. Berger, S. Braun, H.-O. Kalinowski, NMR von Nichtmetallen, Vol. 1-4, Thieme, Stuttgart, **1992–1994**, English edition: Wiley, Chichester, **1996**.

Table of Selected Quadrupolar Nuclei with $I > 1/2$

Nuclide	Spin I	Quadrupole moment Q $[10^{-28} m^2]$	Natural abundance N [%]	Gyromagnetic ratio γ $[10^7 rad\ T^{-1}s^{-1}]$	NMR frequency Ξ [MHz][a]	Standard	Receptivity D[b]
^2H	1	$2.7 \cdot 10^{-3}$	0.015	4.1064	15.351	$CDCl_3$	$8.2 \cdot 10^{-3}$
^6Li	1	$-6.4 \cdot 10^{-4}$	7.42	3.9371	14.717	Li^+/aq.	3.58
^7Li	3/2	$-3.7 \cdot 10^{-2}$	92.58	10.396	38.864	Li^+/aq.	$1.54 \cdot 10^3$
^9Be	3/2	$5.2 \cdot 10^{-2}$	100	-3.7594	14.053	Be^{2+}/aq.	78.8
^{11}B	3/2	$3.6 \cdot 10^{-2}$	80.42	8.5827	32.084	$BF_3.OEt_2$	$7.54 \cdot 10^2$
^{14}N	1	$1.6 \cdot 10^{-2}$	99.63	1.9324	7.224	CH_3NO_2	5.69
^{17}O	5/2	$2.6 \cdot 10^{-2}$	0.037	-3.6266	13.557	H_2O	$6.1 \cdot 10^{-2}$
^{23}Na	3/2	0.1	100	7.0704	26.429	Na^+/aq.	$5.25 \cdot 10^2$
^{25}Mg	5/2	0.22	10.13	-1.6389	6.126	Mg^{2+}/aq.	1.54
^{27}Al	5/2	0.14	100	6.9762	26.077	$Al(H_2O)_6^{3+}$	$1.17 \cdot 10^3$
^{33}S	3/2	$-6.4 \cdot 10^{-2}$	0.76	2.0517	7.670	Cs_2SO_4/aq	$9.7 \cdot 10^{-2}$
^{35}Cl	3/2	$-7.9 \cdot 10^{-2}$	75.53	2.6212	9.798	Cl^-/aq.	20.2
^{37}Cl	3/2	$-6.2 \cdot 10^{-2}$	24.47	2.182	8.156	Cl^-/aq.	3.77
^{39}K	3/2	$-5.5 \cdot 10^{-2}$	93.1	1.2484	4.672	K^+/aq.	2.69
^{43}Ca	7/2	0.2	0.145	-1.7999	6.728	Ca^{2+}/aq.	$5.3 \cdot 10^{-2}$
^{45}Sc	7/2	-0.22	100	6.4989	24.294	Sc^{3+}/aq.	$1.71 \cdot 10^3$
^{47}Ti	5/2	0.29	7.28	-1.5106	5.62476	$TiCl_4$ (neat)	0.864
^{49}Ti	7/2	0.24	5.51	-1.5110	5.638	$TiCl_4$ (neat)	1.18
^{51}V	7/2	$-5.2 \cdot 10^{-2}$	99.76	7.0492	26.350	$VOCl_3$ (neat)	$2.16 \cdot 10^3$
^{53}Cr	3/2		9.55	-1.5120	5.652		0.49
^{55}Mn	5/2	0.55	100	6.598	24.67	$KMnO_4$/aq.	$9.94 \cdot 10^2$

Isotope	Spin					Standard	Receptivity
59Co	7/2	0.42	100	6.3015	23.727118	K$_3$ Co(CN)$_6$	1.57·10^3
63Cu	3/2	-0.22	69.09	7.1088	26.515473	[Cu(NCMe)$_4$]$^+$	3.65·10^2
65Cu	3/2	-0.195	30.91	7.6104	28.403659	[BF$_4$]$^-$	2.01·10^2
67Zn	5/2	0.15	4.11	1.6726	6.252		0.665
71Ga	3/2	0.112	39.6	8.1578	30.495	Ga^{3+}/aq.	3.19·10^2
73Ge	9/2	-0.2	7.76	-0.9332	3.488	GeMe$_4$	0.617
75As	3/2	0.3	100	4.5816	17.127	KAsF$_6$	1.43·10^2
81Br	3/2	0.28	49.46	7.2245	27.006	Br$^-$/aq.	2.77·10^2
83Kr	9/2	0.15	11.55	-1.029	3.848		1.23
87Rb	3/2	0.13	27.85	8.7851	32.839	Rb$^+$/aq.	2.77·10^2
87Sr	9/2	0.36	7.02	-1.1594	4.334	Sr^{2+}/aq.	1.07
93Nb	9/2	-0.32	100	6.5674	24.549	Nb(O)Cl$_3$	2.74·10^3
95Mo	5/2	-1.5·10^{-2}	15.72	1.7514	6.547	MoO$_4$$^{2-}$/aq.	2.88
115In	9/2	1.16	95.72	5.8622	21.914		1.89·10^3
121Sb	5/2	-0.5	57.25	6.4016	23.930	SbCl$_6$$^-$	5.2·10^2
127I	5/2	-0.7	100	5.3521	20.007	I$^-$/aq.	5.3·10^2
131Xe	3/2	-0.12	21.18	2.1935	8.200	XeOF$_4$	3.31
133Cs	7/2	-3·10^{-3}	100	3.5089	13.117	Cs$^+$/aq.	2.69·10^2
137Ba	3/2	0.28	11.32	2.9729	11.113	Ba^{2+}/aq.	4.41
139La	7/2	0.21	99.911	3.7789	14.126		3.36·10^2
181Ta	7/2	3	99.988	3.202	11.97	TaF$_6$$^-$	2.04·10^2
187Re	5/2	2.6	62.93	6.0844	22.744	ReO$_4$$^-$	4.9·10^2
189Os	3/2	0.8	16.1	2.0756	7.759	OsO$_4$	2.13
201Hg	3/2	0.5	13.22	-1.7655	6.600		1.08
209Bi	9/2	-0.4	100	4.2988	16.070		7.77·10^2

a) values given in 9 digits as measured for the standard compounds, other data calculated from the γ-values in column 3. b) receptivity relative to ^{13}C

Experiment 9.1

^{1}H-Decoupled ^{15}N NMR Spectra with DEPT

1. Purpose

For the observation of nitrogen ^{15}N with $I = 1/2$ is the isotope of choice, despite its low natural abundance (0.37 %) and low NMR sensitivity; its receptivity as compared to ^{13}C is only 0.022. Additionally one has to take into account that under the conditions of ^{1}H-broad-band decoupling a decrease in intensity may occur due to a negative NOE effect resulting from the negative gyromagnetic ratio of ^{15}N. This problem may be circumvented using the inverse gated ^{1}H-decoupling technique (see Exp. 4.11). However, the preferred methods are those with polarization transfer, such as the INEPT [1] or DEPT sequences (see Exps. 6.7 and 6.9, respectively), which may be performed with or without ^{1}H-broad-band decoupling and can be tuned either to $^1J(^{15}$N,^{1}H) or to $^2J(^{15}$N,^{1}H) / $^3J(^{15}$N,^{1}H). Here we describe the DEPT experiment on formamide with ^{1}H-broad-band decoupling.

2. Literature

[1] G. A. Morris, *J. Am. Chem. Soc.* **1980**, *102*, 428–429.
[2] W. Witanowski, L. Stefaniak, G. A. Webb, *Annu. Rep. NMR Spectrosc.* **1993**, *25*, 1–480.
[3] S. Berger, S. Braun, H.-O. Kalinowski, *NMR-Spektroskopie von Nichtmetallen*, Vol. 2, *^{15}N-NMR-Spektroskopie*, Thieme, Stuttgart, **1992**; English edition: Wiley, Chichester, **1996**.
[4] W. v. Philipsborn, R. Müller, *Angew. Chem. Int. Ed. Engl.* **1986**, *25*, 383–413.

3. Pulse Scheme and Phase Cycle

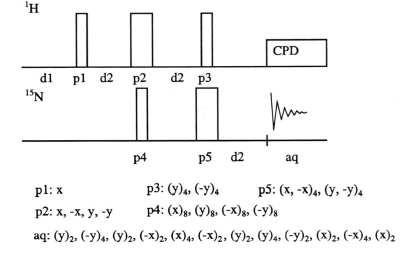

p1: x   p3: (y)$_4$, (-y)$_4$ p5: (x, -x)$_4$, (y, -y)$_4$

p2: x, -x, y, -y   p4: (x)$_8$, (y)$_8$, (-x)$_8$, (-y)$_8$

aq: (y)$_2$, (-y)$_4$, (y)$_2$, (-x)$_2$, (x)$_4$, (-x)$_2$, (y)$_2$, (y)$_4$, (-y)$_2$, (x)$_2$, (-x)$_4$, (x)$_2$

4. Acquisition

Time requirement: 5 min

Sample: 90% formamide in [D_6]dimethylsulfoxide

Set up your spectrometer to ^{15}N, find the signal, and determine the 90° transmitter pulse-length. The reference compound is CH_3NO_2, and formamide has $\delta_N = -268$. Load the DEPT program with ^1H-decoupling; the settings for a 90° ^1H decoupler pulse must be known. You have to set:

td: 32 k
sw: 350 ppm (chemical shift range of NH-groups)
o1: 220 ppm upfield from CH_3NO_2 (middle of NH region)
o2: middle of ^1H NMR spectrum
p1: 90° ^1H decoupler pulse
p2: 180° ^1H decoupler pulse
p3: 45° ^1H decoupler pulse (optimum for NH_2)
p4: 90° ^{15}N transmitter pulse
p5: 180° ^{15}N transmitter pulse
d1: 2s
d2: $1/[2J(^{15}N,{}^1H)] = 5.6$ ms, calculated from $^1J(^{15}N,{}^1H) = 90$ Hz
decoupler attenuation and 90° pulse for CPD
ns: 4

5. Processing

Use standard 1D processing as described in Experiment 3.2

6. Result

The figure on page 249 shows the 30.4 MHz ^{15}N NMR DEPT spectrum obtained on an ARX-300 spectrometer with a 5 mm multinuclear probe-head. As an exercise you may perform an inverse gated experiment (without NOE, see Exp. 4.11) and one with the normal procedure (Exp. 3.2); theoretically, the gain in intensity using DEPT instead of the inverse gated method is given by $|\chi(^1H)/\chi(^{15}N)| = 9.86$.

7. Comments

For a description of the experiment using the the product operator formalism see Experiment 6.9; the choice of the pulse duration of p5 (angle θ) is discussed in Experiment 9.4. An even greater gain in sensitivity can be achieved by performing a 2D inverse ^{1}H,^{15}N correlation experiment (see Exp. 10.11 and 10.12 for ^{1}H,^{13}C).

8. Own Observations

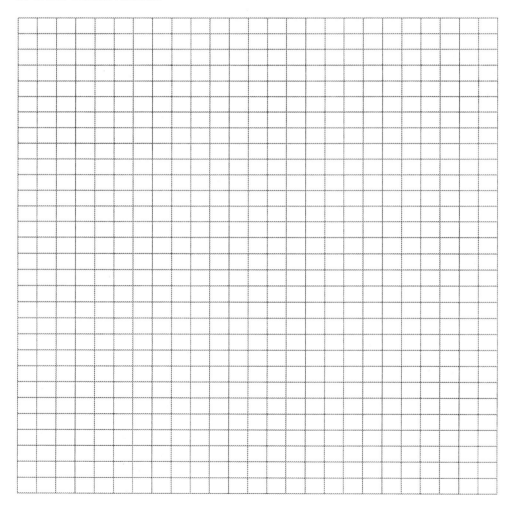

Experiment 9.2

^{1}H-Coupled ^{15}N NMR Spectra with DEPT

1. Purpose

N,H coupling constants are powerful tools in the structure elucidation of nitrogen-containing compounds [1–3] and can be determined by observing ^{15}N at natural abundance using INEPT or DEPT without ^{1}H decoupling. Because of the unusual line intensities associated with the basic INEPT sequence, the use of INEPT$^+$ is recommended. Similarly for DEPT (basic sequence: Exp. 6.9), modifications exist, which are introduced to eliminate spectral distortions [4]. The experiments may be tuned to $^1J(^{15}N, ^1H)$, if present, or to $^{15}N, ^1H$ couplings over two or three bonds. Here we describe the basic DEPT experiment on formamide without ^{1}H-decoupling.

2. Literature

[1] W. Witanowski, L. Stefaniak, G. A. Webb, *Annu. Rep. NMR Spectrosc.* **1993**, *25*, 1–480.
[2] S. Berger, S. Braun, H.-O. Kalinowski, *NMR-Spektroskopie von Nichtmetallen*, Vol. 2, *^{15}N-NMR-Spektroskopie*, Thieme, Stuttgart, **1992**; English edition: Wiley, Chichester, **1996**.
[3] G. C. Levy, R. L. Lichter, *Nitrogen-15 NMR Spectroscopy*, Wiley, New York **1979**.
[4] O. W. Sørensen, R. R. Ernst, *J. Magn. Reson.* **1983**, *51*, 477–489.

3. Pulse Scheme and Phase Cycle

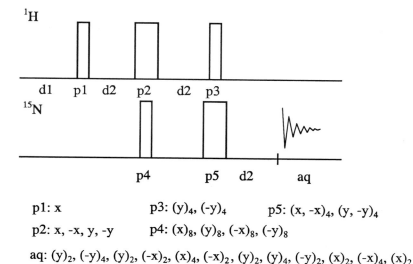

p1: x   p3: $(y)_4$, $(-y)_4$ p5: $(x, -x)_4$, $(y, -y)_4$
p2: x, -x, y, -y   p4: $(x)_8$, $(y)_8$, $(-x)_8$, $(-y)_8$

aq: $(y)_2$, $(-y)_4$, $(y)_2$, $(-x)_2$, $(x)_4$, $(-x)_2$, $(y)_2$, $(y)_4$, $(-y)_2$, $(x)_2$, $(-x)_4$, $(x)_2$

4. Acquisition

Time requirement: 5 min

Sample: 90% formamide in [D_6]dimethylsulfoxide

Set up your spectrometer to ^{15}N and load the DEPT program without ^1H-decoupling. You have to set:

> td: 32 k
> sw: 350 ppm
> o1: 220 ppm upfield from CH_3NO_2
> o2: middle of ^1H NMR spectrum
> p1: 90° ^1H decoupler pulse
> p2: 180° ^1H decoupler pulse
> p3: 45° ^1H decoupler pulse (optimum for NH_2)
> p4: 90° ^{15}N transmitter pulse
> p5: 180° ^{15}N transmitter pulse
> d1: 2 s
> d2: $1/[2J(^{15}N,{}^1H)] = 5.6$ ms, calculated from $^1J(^{15}N,{}^1H) = 90$ Hz
> ns: 32

5. Processing

Use standard 1D processing as described in Experiment 3.2 with lb = 1 Hz

6. Result

In the figure on page 252 **a** is the 30.4 MHz ^{15}N NMR DEPT spectrum obtained on an ARX-300 spectrometer with a 5 mm multinuclear probe-head. From the pattern, which represents a doublet of doublets of doublets, the following coupling constants can be deduced [2,3]: $^1J(^{15}N,H^{syn})$ = 87.9 Hz, $^1J(^{15}N,H^{anti})$ = 90.3 Hz, and $^2J(^{15}N,H)$ = 14.0 Hz. As an exercise you may record the spectrum using INEPT$^+$ (Exp. 6.6), leading to the same result. With the basic INEPT (Exp. 6.5), however, you will obtain spectrum **b**.

7. Comments

A description of the DEPT pulse sequence including the product operator formalism is given in Experiment 6.9.

8. Own Observations

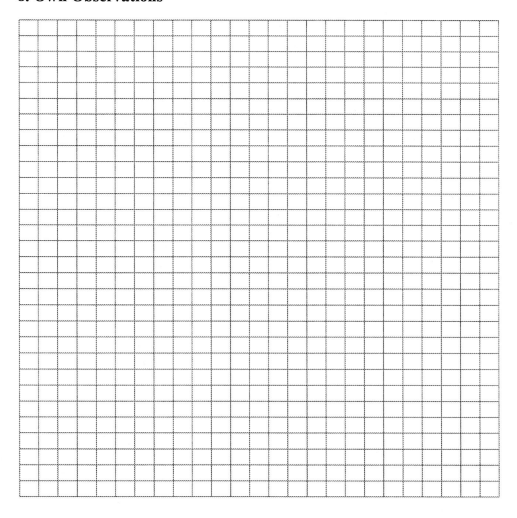

Experiment 9.3

^{19}F NMR Spectroscopy

1. Purpose

The ^{19}F nucleus ($I = 1/2$, natural abundance 100%) has nearly the same NMR sensitivity as the proton and may occupy the equivalent positions in an organic molecule. However, fluorine is much less widely distributed than hydrogen and hardly occurs at all in natural compounds, and therefore it does not have the same importance for NMR spectroscopy, however. On the other hand, it is exactly for this reason that the nuclide is very well suited for biochemical and medical applications, so that ^{19}F NMR spectroscopy plays an increasing role in these areas [4,5]. Because of the proximity of the resonance frequencies of ^{1}H and ^{19}F it is often possible to tune a proton probe-head to the ^{19}F frequency, so that no special equipment, other than an ^{19}F preamplifier, is needed for the standard experiment described here.

2. Literature

[1] J. W. Emsley, L. Phillipps, *Prog. Nucl. Magn. Reson.* **1971**, *7*, 1–526.
[2] J. W. Emsley, L. Phillipps, V. Wray, *Prog. Nucl. Magn. Reson.* **1976**, *10*, 83–756.
[3] V. Wray, *Annu. Rep. NMR Spectrosc.* **1980**, *10B*, 1–507; ibid. **1983**, *14*, 1–406.
[4] M. J. W. Prior, R. J. Maxwell, J. R. Griffith, *NMR–Basic Principles and Progress* **1992**, *28*, 101–130.
[5] J. T. Gerig, *Prog. Nucl. Magn. Reson.* **1994**, *26*, 293–370.
[6] S. Berger, S. Braun, H.-O. Kalinowski, *NMR-Spektroskopie von Nichtmetallen*, Vol. 4, *^{19}F-NMR-Spektroskopie*, Thieme, Stuttgart, **1992**; English edition: Wiley, Chichester, **1996**.

3. Pulse Scheme and Phase Cycle

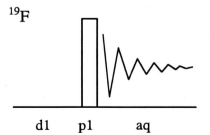

p1: x, x, -x, -x, y, y, -y, -y

aq: x, x, -x, -x, y, y, -y, -y

4. Acquisition

Time requirement: 5 min

Sample: 1% CCl$_3$F (one drop) in CDCl$_3$

Set up your spectrometer to ^{19}F, find the signal, and determine the 90° transmitter pulse-length. CCl_3F serves as reference compound for ^{19}F NMR. You have to set:

td: 64 k
sw: 300 ppm (typical range for fluorine bound to carbon)
o1: about 100 ppm upfield from CCl_3F (center of that range)
p1: 30° ^{19}F transmitter pulse
d1: 1 s
ns: 1

5. Processing

Use standard 1D processing as described in Experiment 3.1

6. Result

The figure shows the 282.1 MHz ^{19}F NMR spectrum obtained on an ARX-300 spectrometer with a 5 mm $^{1}H/^{13}C$ dual probe-head tuned to the ^{19}F resonance frequency and using a ^{19}F preamplifier for that frequency. In order to achieve better resolution the experiment was repeated with improved digital resolution (see inset). As an exercise you may record an $^{19}F,^{19}F$-COSY spectrum on a mixture of *cis/trans* perfluorodecalin (commercially available) or a 2D *J*-resolved ^{19}F NMR spectrum on

2,4,5-trifluoroaniline. Both experiments may be performed in the above configuration, since they don't need an ^{1}H channel.

7. Comments

The fine structure of the ^{19}F signal of CCl_3F results from the different chlorine iso-topomers; $C^{35}Cl_2^{37}ClF$ is used for the calibration of high precision ^{19}F NMR spec-tra. Although isotopes have the same electronic properties within the Born–Oppenheimer approximation, they cause slightly different chemical shifts for an nearby nucleus. This is due to a different ground state vibrational energy which alters the average bond lengths; the heavier isotope usually causes the lower resonance fre-quency.

8. Own Observations

Experiment 9.4

29Si NMR Spectroscopy with the DEPT Sequence

1. Purpose

^{29}Si ($I = 1/2$, natural abundance 4.7%) is a nucleus with a small negative gyromagnetic ratio. This means that under normal ^1H broad-band decoupling conditions the nuclear Overhauser effect can lead to a reduction in signal intensity or even a cancellation of the signal. It is therefore better to use one of the polarization transfer methods such as INEPT (Exp. 6.5–6.7) or DEPT (Exp. 6.9) which can result in a sensitivity enhancement up to a factor of 5, depending on the number of protons which are responsible for the polarization transfer [1]. In addition the signal of the glassware surrounding the receiver coil is suppressed. Cross-polarization techniques with spin-locking can also be used [5].

2. Literature

[1] T. A. Blinka, B. J. Helmer, R. West, *Adv. Organomet. Chem.* **1984**, *23*, 193–218.
[2] H. Marsmann, *NMR–Basic Principles and Progress* **1981**, *17*, 65–235.
[3] E. A. Williams, *Annu. Rep. NMR Spectrosc.* **1982**, *15*, 235–289.
[4] J. Schraml, *Prog. NMR Spectrosc.* **1990**, *22*, 289–348.
[5] R. Wagner and S. Berger, *Phosphorus, Sulfur, Silicon, and Rel. Elements* **1994**, *91*, 213–218.

3. Pulse Scheme with Phasecycle

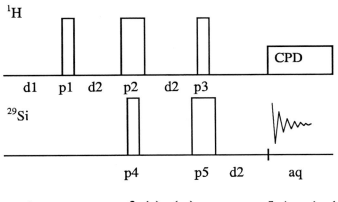

p1: x   p3: (y)$_4$, (-y)$_4$ p5: (x, -x)$_4$, (y, -y)$_4$

p2: x, -x, y, -y   p4: (x)$_8$, (y)$_8$, (-x)$_8$, (-y)$_8$

aq: (y)$_2$, (-y)$_4$, (y)$_2$, (-x)$_2$, (x)$_4$, (-x)$_2$, (-y)$_2$, (y)$_4$, (-y)$_2$, (x)$_2$, (-x)$_4$, (x)$_2$

4. Acquisition

Time requirement: 15 min

Sample: 50% TMS in $CDCl_3$

A multinuclear probe-head is required for the measurement of ^{29}Si spectra. After tuning the probe-head to ^{29}Si on the observe channel and to ^1H on the decoupler channel, determine the 90° pulse for ^{29}Si. Load the DEPT pulse sequence (see Exp. 6.9) and record a DEPT spectrum. You have to set:

> td: 64 k
> sw: 250 ppm
> o1: 70 ppm upfield from ^{29}Si signal of TMS
> o2: middle of ^1H NMR spectrum
> p1: 90° ^1H decoupler pulse
> p2: 180° ^1H decoupler pulse
> p3: 16.8° ^1H decoupler pulse corresponding to the 12 equivalent protons of the sample
> p4: 90° ^{29}Si transmitter pulse
> p5: 180° ^{29}Si transmitter pulse
> d1: 1 s
> d2: $0.5/J = 0.07s$, calculated from $^2J\,(^{29}Si,{}^1H) = 7$ Hz
> decoupler attenuation and 90° pulse for CPD
> ds: 2
> ns: 32

5. Processing

Use standard 1D processing as described in Experiment 3.2 with exponential multiplication (lb = 3 Hz).

6. Result

The figure on page 259 shows the 79.44 MHz ^{29}Si NMR spectrum obtained for TMS with an AM-400 spectrometer. Spectrum **a** is a normal spectrum, which shows in addition to the TMS signal a broad signal at approximately −110 ppm. This signal is due to the glass NMR tube and the quartz insert surrounding the receiver coil. Spectrum **b** was taken with the DEPT sequence under otherwise identical conditions. Note the improvement in the signal-to-noise ratio. The signal of the glass is suppressed.

7. Comments

To understand the DEPT sequence you can follow the discussion in Experiment 6.9. In the INEPT experiment (see Exps. 6.5–6.7) the optimum polarization transfer is controlled by the last delay d2. The optimum value of this delay is a function of the scalar coupling constant J and the number of coupled nuclei n which are responsible for the polarization transfer [1] and is given by Equation (1):

$$d2_{opt} = (\pi J)^{-1} \arcsin (n)^{-1/2} \tag{1}$$

As n increases the value of $d2_{opt}$ decreases and the enhancement factor E becomes more sensitive to a variation in d2.

Number of protons n:	1	2	3	6	9	12
Enhancement E:	5.03	5.03	5.82	7.83	9.44	10.82
Delay $d2_{opt}$: (in units of J^{-1})	0.5	0.25	0.196	0.134	0.108	0.093

In the DEPT experiment the optimal polarization transfer is controlled by the angle α of the last pulse. The optimum pulse angle α_{opt} is independent of J and depends only on the number of coupled nuclei n of the polarization source, usually protons, as given in Equation (2):

$$\alpha_{opt} = \arcsin (n)^{-1/2} \text{ radians} \tag{2}$$

Number of protons n:	1	2	3	6	9	12
Pulse angle α_{opt} (in degrees):	90	45	35	24.1	19.5	16.8

Therefore the DEPT sequence is less sensitive to variations in J. In contrast the NOE enhancement is independent of the number of protons and has a theoretical limit of $\eta = 1 + \gamma_H / 2\gamma_{Si} = -1.5$ for ^{29}Si. Spin-lock experiments as an alternative to INEPT or DEPT are described in Ref. [5].

8. Own Observations

Experiment 9.5

119Sn NMR Spectroscopy

1. Purpose

For the observation of Sn by NMR the isotope ^{119}Sn with $I = 1/2$ and a natural abundance of 8.6% is usually chosen; the alternative is ^{117}Sn with $I = 1/2$, 7.6%. For both isotopes γ has a negative sign, as for ^{15}N and ^{29}Si, so that the comments given in Experiments 9.1 and 9.4 also apply to Sn. Because of the high receptivity of ^{119}Sn (25 relative to ^{13}C) it may be observed by the standard experiment with ^{1}H broad-band decoupling as described here (see Exp. 3.2). For low concentrations the DEPT method is recommended.

2. Literature

[1] B. Wrackmeyer, *Chem. Br.* **1990**, *26*, 48–51.
[2] B. Wrackmeyer, *Ann. Rep. NMR Spectrosc.* **1985**, *16*, 73–186.
[3] V. S. Petrosyan, *Prog. NMR Spectrosc.* **1977**, *11*, 115–148.

3. Pulse Scheme and Phase Cycle

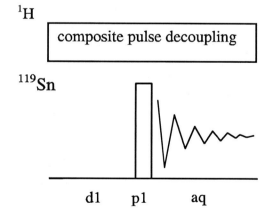

^{1}H

composite pulse decoupling

^{119}Sn

p1: x, x, -x, -x, y, y, -y, -y
aq: x, x, -x, -x, y, y, -y, -y

d1   p1   aq

4. Acquisition

Time requirement: 5 min

Sample: 50% Sn(CH$_3$)$_4$ in CDCl$_3$

Set up your spectrometer to ^{119}Sn, find the signal, and determine the 90° transmitter pulse. This compound serves as standard, so reference the signal to $\delta_{Sn} = 0$. You have to set:

> td: 32 k
> sw: 600 ppm (Sn chemical shift range typical for $R_{4-n}SnX_n$)
> o1: 100 ppm upfield from $Sn(CH_3)_4$ (center of that chemical shift range)
> o2: middle of ^{1}H NMR spectrum
> p1: 30° ^{119}Sn transmitter pulse
> d1: 1 s
> decoupler attenuation and 90° pulse for CPD
> ns: 8

5. Processing

Use standard 1D processing as described in Experiment 3.2 with lb = 3 Hz.

6. Result

The figure shows the 111.9 MHz ^{119}Sn NMR spectrum recorded on an ARX-300 spectrometer; the ^{13}C satellites are clearly visible. For a more precise determination of the coupling constant, a spectrum with a higher digital resolution has been recorded (see inset, $^1J(^{119}Sn, ^{13}C) = 336.9$ Hz).

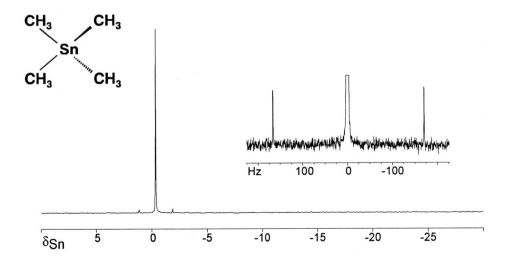

7. Comments

Note the fourfold higher intensity of the ^{13}C satellites (about 2%) because of the four equivalent carbon nuclei.

    As an exercise and as an example of what is called multinuclear NMR spectroscopy you may record a standard ^1H and a standard ^{13}C NMR spectrum. In these spectra you can determine the ^1H and ^{13}C chemical shifts and from the satellites the two-bond couplings of ^{117}Sn and ^{119}Sn with the protons and the one-bond couplings of the two Sn isotopes with the ^{13}C nuclei. It is also interesting to record a ^1H-coupled spectrum from the sample to observe the spin coupling pattern caused by the twelve equivalent protons (gated ^1H-decoupling, see Exp. 4.10).

8. Own Observations

Experiment 9.6

^{2}H NMR Spectroscopy

1. Purpose

This experiment demonstrates the technique used to observe deuterium (^{2}H, $I = 1$) by NMR spectroscopy in natural abundance (0.015%). As an example we have chosen pure ethanol, since this is currently routinely used in food analysis. Since the isotope distribution in ethanol is dependent on the sugar source and its geographic origin, quantitative ^{2}H NMR spectroscopy can be used to detect fraud [3].

2. Literature

[1] C. Brevard, J. P. Kintzinger, in: *NMR and the Periodic Table*, R. K. Harris, B. E. Mann (eds.), Academic Press, London, **1978**, 107–128.
[2] J. W. Akitt, in: *Multinuclear NMR*, J. Mason (ed.), Plenum Press, New York, **1987**, 171–187.
[3] M. L. Martin, G. J. Martin, *NMR–Basic Principles and Progress* **1991**, *23*, 1–62.

3. Pulse Scheme and Phase Cycle

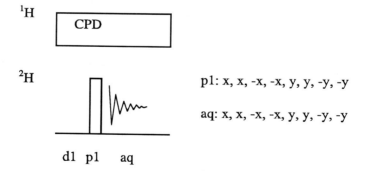

^{1}H   CPD

^{2}H

p1: x, x, -x, -x, y, y, -y, -y

aq: x, x, -x, -x, y, y, -y, -y

d1 p1   aq

4. Practical Procedure

Time requirement: 30 min

Sample: pure ethanol

A multinuclear probe-head is required for the measurement of ^{2}H spectra. Disconnect the ^{2}H lock channel and remove any ^{2}H-stop filter from the transmitter line (which is sometimes hidden in the preamplifier). Use an ^{19}F lock, if available; alternatively the magnet must be stable enough to hold its field position for the duration of the measurement. After tuning the multinuclear probe-head to deuterium on the observe channel and to ^{1}H on the decoupler channel, it is best to use a sample of CDCl$_3$ to detect the

^{2}H resonance and to determine the 90° pulse. First record a standard ^{1}H NMR spectrum of the sample, center on the ethanol resonances, and note the offset. This value should be used for the decoupler offset in the following experiment. The chemical shifts of isotopes are essentially identical, and therfore you can reference the ^{2}H resonance of the secondary standard CDCl$_3$ to $\delta_H = 7.25$. You have to set:

td : 8 k
sw: 8 ppm
o1: middle of ^{2}H-NMR spectrum
o2: middle of ^{1}H-NMR spectrum
p1: 90° ^{2}H transmitter pulse
d1: 100 ms
decoupler attenuation and 90° pulse for CPD
ns: 256

5. Processing

Use standard 1D processing as described in Experiment 3.2 with exponential multiplication (lb = 2 Hz).

6. Result

CH$_3$—CH$_2$—OH

Integral			
	72.89	178.25	300.0

δ_H 5   4   3   2   1   0

The figure on page 265 shows the result obtained on an AMX-500 spectrometer with a 5 mm multinuclear probe-head. The integrals indicate that the deuterium is not distributed in the expected 3:2:1 ratio. For a reliable quantitative evaluation, however, the signal-to-noise ratio must be much better. Furthermore, a certified standard with a known deuterium content is required. Note that the chemical shift of the OD signal is temperature dependent.

7. Comments

Although deuterium is a quadrupolar nucleus, its relaxation behavior frequently resembles that of spin 1/2 nuclei in small molecules, due to the very small quadrupole moment. Therefore it is necessary to use a sufficiently long repetition time for quantitative work. As well as the application illustrated here, ^{2}H NMR spectroscopy of labeled compounds is widely used for mechanistic studies in organic chemistry.

8. Own Observations

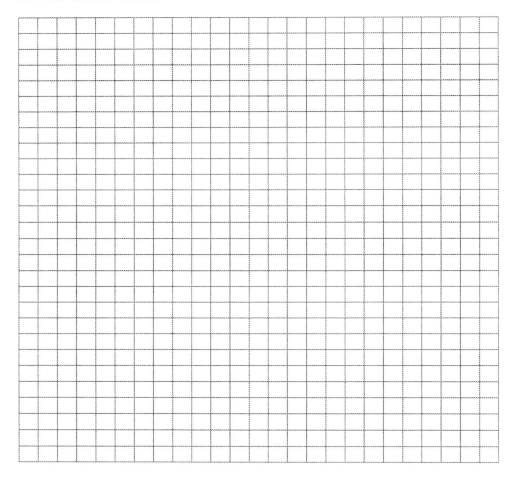

Experiment 9.7

11B NMR Spectroscopy

1. Purpose

This experiment demonstrates the technique used to obtain ^{11}B NMR spectra ($I = 3/2$, natural abundance 80.42%). As an example we have chosen the commercially available 1,7-dicarba-*closo*-dodecaborane, since this compound gives a spectrum containing four different signals. Furthermore, the spectrum can be recorded with or without proton decoupling; thus a spin–spin coupling ^1J(B,H) can be observed.

2. Literature

[1] D. Reed, *Chem. Soc. Rev.* **1993**, 109–116.
[2] B. Wrackmeyer, *Annu. Rep. NMR Spectrosc.* **1988**, *20*, 61–203.
[3] A. R. Siedle, *Annu. Rep. NMR Spectrosc.* **1988**, *20*, 205–314.

3. Pulse Scheme and Phase Cycle

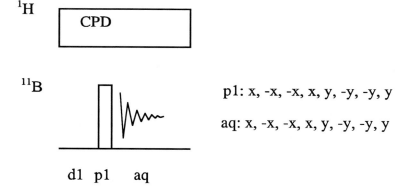

p1: x, -x, -x, x, y, -y, -y, y

aq: x, -x, -x, x, y, -y, -y, y

4. Acquisition

Time requirement: 5 min

Sample: 100 mg 1,7-dicarba-*closo*-dodecaborane in 0.7 ml CDCl$_3$

A multinuclear probe-head is required for the measurement of ^{11}B spectra. There are special ^{11}B probe-heads available which dont have a glass insert resulting in a smaller background signal. After tuning the multinuclear probe-head to ^{11}B on the observe channel and to ^{1}H on the decoupler channel, use a sample of BF$_3$·O(C$_2$H$_5$)$_2$ to detect the ^{11}B resonance and to determine the 90° pulse. The δ_B value of this standard is referenced to 0. To obtain the spectrum displayed below you have to set:

td : 4 k
sw: 36 ppm
o1: middle of ^{11}B NMR spectrum
o2: middle of ^{1}H NMR spectrum
d1: 100 ms
p1: 90° ^{11}B transmitter pulse
decoupler attenuation and 90° pulse for CPD
ns: 8

5. Processing

Use standard 1D processing with exponential multiplication (lb = 2 Hz) and a baseline correction. For referencing use the external reference of the standard; be sure not to change the magnetic field between the two measurements.

6. Result

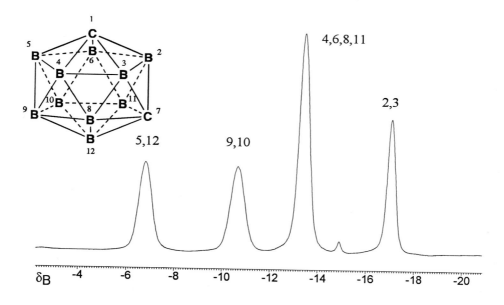

The figure shows the 96.23 MHz ^{11}B NMR spectrum obtained on an AC-300 spectrometer with a 5 mm special boron probehead.

7. Comments

^{11}B is a quadrupolar nucleus and can give very broad signals depending on the molecular environment. The repetition time of the experiment can be selected according to the sample used, so that much faster pulsing than used here is often possible.

To obtain ^{11}B spectra without any background signal both the insert of the probe-head and the NMR sample tube must be from boron-free material, such as quartz or teflon.

8. Own Observations

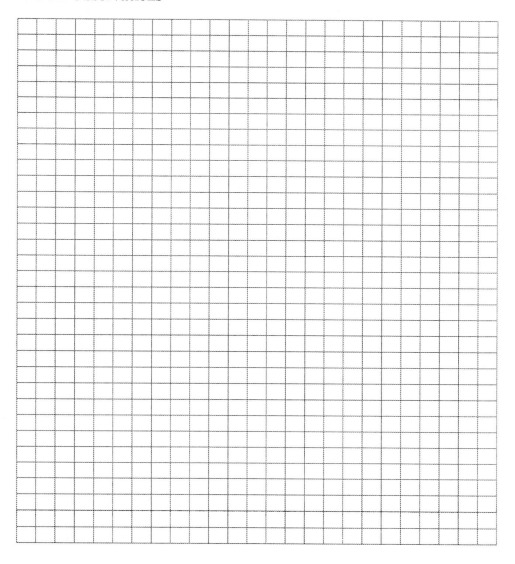

Experiment 9.8

17O NMR Spectroscopy with RIDE

1. Purpose

This experiment demonstrates the technique used to obtain ^{17}O NMR spectra ($I = 5/2$, natural abundance 0.037%). ^{17}O is a quadrupolar nucleus with a relatively low γ-value. Probe-head ringing poses an experimental problem for these types of nuclei, resulting in extensive baseline roll. One possible solution is the RIDE (**RI**ng **D**own **E**limination) pulse sequence which is demonstrated here.

2. Literature

[1] P. S. Belton, I. J. Cox, R. K. Harris, *J. Chem. Soc. Faraday Trans. 2* **1985**, *81*, 63–75.
[2] I. P. Gerothannassis, *Prog. Nucl. Magn. Reson. Spectrosc.* **1987**, *19*, 267–329.
[3] J. P. Kintzinger, *NMR–Basic Principles and Progress*, **1981**, *17*, 1–64.
[4] D. W. Boykin (ed.), *^{17}O-NMR in Organic Chemistry*, CRC Press, Boca Raton, Florida, **1991**, 1–325.
[5] S. Berger, S. Braun, H.-O. Kalinowski, *NMR von Nichtmetallen*, Vol. 1, Ch.4, Thieme, Stuttgart, **1992**, English edition: Wiley, Chichester, **1996**.

3. Pulse Scheme and Phase Cycle

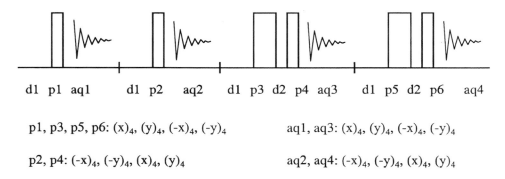

d1 p1 aq1   d1 p2   aq2   d1 p3 d2 p4 aq3   d1 p5 d2 p6   aq4

p1, p3, p5, p6: $(x)_4$, $(y)_4$, $(-x)_4$, $(-y)_4$ aq1, aq3: $(x)_4$, $(y)_4$, $(-x)_4$, $(-y)_4$

p2, p4: $(-x)_4$, $(-y)_4$, $(x)_4$, $(y)_4$ aq2, aq4: $(-x)_4$, $(-y)_4$, $(x)_4$, $(y)_4$

4. Acquisition

Time requirement: 5 min

Sample: ethyl crotonate (neat)

A multinuclear probe-head is required for the measurement of ^{17}O spectra. Be sure to remove any ^{2}H stop filter from the transmitter line, since ^{17}O and ^{2}H NMR frequencies are rather similar at lower field strengths. Tune the probe-head to ^{17}O on the observe channel and locate the ^{17}O signal using a sample of D_2O, since the ^{17}O content of D_2O is higher than that of normal water. Determine the 90° pulse for ^{17}O with this sample and use it as reference standard. After loading the RIDE pulse sequence you have to set:

td : 4 k
sw: 500 ppm
o1: 200 ppm downfield from ^{17}O water signal
p1, p2, p4, p6: 90° ^{17}O transmitter pulse
p3, p5: 180° ^{17}O transmitter pulse
d1: 10 ms
d2: 0.5 µs
preacquisition delay: 15 µs
ns: 4·128

5. Processing

Use standard 1D processing as described in Experiment 3.2 with exponential multiplication (lb = 200 Hz)

6. Result

The figure shows the 54.24 MHz ^{17}O NMR spectrum obtained on an AM-400 spectrometer with a 5 mm inverse multinuclear probe-head. A carboxylic ester gives two signals, one for the C=O oxygen (here at δ_O = 336) and one for the C-O oxygen (here at δ_O = 162). As an exercise record a normal ^{17}O NMR spectrum and compare the baseline roll.

7. Comments

One can aim to minimize ring-down effects by using a relatively high preacquisition delay, although this method may also suppress broad signals which decay rapidly. The reasoning behind the RIDE sequence shown here is that probe-head ring-down is dependent of the phase of the r.f. pulses, but independent of any previous pulses. Thus, the ring-down of the first acquisition period is cancelled by the ring-down of the third, which is where the NMR signals first become inverted by an 180° pulse. The ring-down from the second acquisition period is similarily cancelled by the last. Four acquisitions are needed to provide the ringdown elimination both for the 90° and 180° pulses. Note, however, that since the sequence uses 180° pulses it only works well for relatively small spectral widths.

8. Own Observations

Chapter 10

The Second Dimension

2D NMR spectra are obtained by recording a series of 1D NMR spectra. These individual spectra differ only by a time increment which is introduced within the pulse sequence. It is helpful to distinguish four time periods for these spectra. In the *preparation* period the spin system relaxes and is then excited by at least one r.f. pulse. In the *evolution* period t_1 the chemical shifts and spin–spin couplings evolve; this is the time domain which is incremented during a 2D experiment. In the *mixing* period one or several r.f. pulses are applied and create an observable transverse magnetization. This is recorded in the *detection* period (which in 1D NMR spectroscopy is called the acquisition time); here it is usually labeled with t_2.

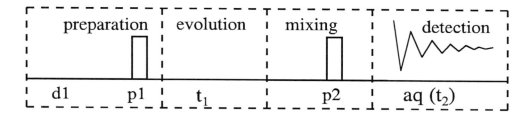

Thus the primary 2D matrix consists of a series of FIDs, from which a set of 1D NMR spectra is obtained by Fourier transformation with respect to t_2. The signals of each transformation may differ in amplitude and/or phase. A second Fourier transformation with respect to t_1 yields the final 2D matrix with frequency axes F_1 and F_2.

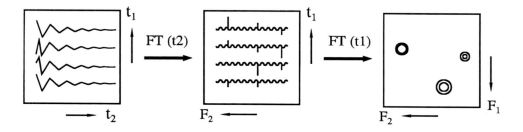

In setting up a 2D experiment one first has to consider the appropriate amount of data that can be acquired and processed. A typical routine set-up for standard 2D spectra in organic chemistry (COSY, C,H correlation) would consist of 128 FIDs, each of 1 k data points, yielding a primary serial file of 128 k data points. The number of FIDs determines the total experiment time and the resolution in F_1, while their data length determines the resolution in F_2.

From both the theoretical and experimental points of view it is important to distinguish whether 2D spectra are recorded and processed in the phase-sensitive mode or not phase-sensitive.

In 1D NMR all spectra are usually taken with quadrature phase detection. The transmitter offset is placed in the middle of the spectrum. The original NMR signal is split and detected by two phase detectors which are 90° out of phase with respect to each other, producing a sine and a cosine component. By either *simultaneous* or *sequential* acquisition of the sine and cosine components of the NMR signal one can then determine the sign of the frequency difference relative to the transmitter offset. This can be visualized by looking at the figure, where the sine and cosine functions, their transforms, and the final result after addition are shown.

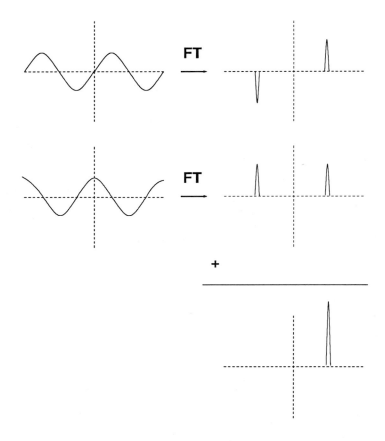

In 2D NMR spectroscopy there is no detector in the F_1 dimension; therefore the signs of the frequencies in F_1 must be determined beforehand during the acquisition in F_2. A specific phase cycling for the individual FIDs obtained in F_2 for each t_1 increment provides the necessary basis for this.

There are two different approaches. In the *phase-sensitive mode* sine and cosine components with respect to the t_1 evolution are created by the phase cycle and stored separately. Subsequent real Fourier transformation detects the signs of the frequencies and the phase of the signals. This is almost equivalent to the procedure used in 1D NMR spectroscopy and can be performed in either the *simultaneous* or the *sequential* mode; the former is called the Ruben–States–Haberkorn procedure and the latter the TPPI (**T**ime **P**roportional **P**hase **I**ncrement) or Redfield method.

The other method is based on subtracting or adding the sine and cosine components (N or P type, or echo/anti-echo selection) created by the phase cycle within the FIDs recorded in t_2; thus they are not stored separately. The subsequent complex Fourier transformation again detects the signs of the frequencies. However, here the signal shapes are skewed, consisting of cosine and sine components in both dimensions. These signals are usually processed in magnitude mode.

There have been numerous debates about the advantages and disadvantages of the two principal approaches. The phase-sensitive approach is clearly the more modern concept and yields Lorentzian lineshapes in both dimensions. However, it requires larger data matrices for processing and, since the full phase information is retained, twice the amount of time. The N or P type mode gives crude information in half the time and requires a smaller data matrix for transformation. However, exact spin coupling constants cannot be extracted from the resulting spectra due to the skewed line shape. Clearly, the choice of method depends upon the information required. In the following examples we use both methods.

Pulsed field gradients can select the coherence pathways directly without the need of phase cycling. If the field gradients are applied during the t_1 period, echo or anti-echo selection results. Various phase sensitive approaches using field gradients also have recently been developed (see Ch. 11).

For a phase-sensitive experiment the NMR spectroscopist has to set the t_1 increment to $1/[2 \cdot \text{sw}1]$, where sw1 is the spectral width [Hz] in the F_1 dimension. If the t_1 period is split by a 180° pulse this increment is set to $1/[4 \cdot \text{sw}1]$. For non-phase-sensitive measurements these increments are $1/\text{sw}1$ and $1/[2 \cdot \text{sw}1]$ respectively. In the following experiments (except the *J*-resolved methods) we have given the parameter sw1 in ppm so that it does not depend on the field strength. Of course, the software calculates these increments from sw1 values given in Hz.

Before processing 2D NMR data one first has to consider the data matrix. Usually one performs a zero-filling in F_1 by a factor of at least 2, in order to give nearly symmetrical data matrices. Zero-filling in F_2 is uncommon, it is always better to use more data points in F_2 from the beginning.

The processing of 2D NMR spectra must take into account the phase mode under which the recording was performed and the correct FT procedure has to be chosen. After baseline correction on the FIDs in F_2, the appropriate window functions need to be chosen. For phase-sensitive spectra the usual exponential or gaussian functions should be used; for N or P type spectra sinusoidal windows are popular, as they narrow the skewed line-shape. It is advisable to select the best window function interactively, and this is possible by modern software. After Fourier transformation in F_2, a data column in F_1 (the "FID" in t_1) can be downloaded and inspected as for a 1D spectrum. After a baseline correction the appropriate window function must again be found. Generally the same remarks as for the F_2 dimension hold. N or P type spectra are finally displayed in magnitude mode, so that a phase correction is not necessary.

Phase-sensitive spectra have to be corrected at least in the F_2 dimension, and for some techniques a phase correction in F_1 is also required.

The final processing steps of a 2D NMR spectrum include calibration, integration by calculating volume integrals, aligning of the corresponding 1D high-resolution spectra (as shown throughout in this chapter), and choosing correct contour levels for plotting.

This chapter first introduces the basic J-resolved methods for the homonuclear and heteronuclear case. A description of the common variants of COSY spectroscopy follows. A large part of the chapter is devoted to the different techniques of C,H correlation, both forward and inverse including correlations via $^1J(C,H)$ and long-range spin coupling. Pulse sequences using a spin-lock as TOCSY and ROESY are demonstrated and examples for homonuclear and heteronuclear 2D NOE spectroscopy are provided. The 2D-INADEQUATE experiment (Exp. 10.19) is the most time consuming experiment described in this book.

Three 2D experiments using a selective pulse are found in Chapter 7 and those which work with pulsed field gradients are described in Chapter 11.

Literature

[1] R. R. Ernst, G. Bodenhausen, A. Wokaun, *Principles of Nuclear Magnetic Resonance in One and Two Dimensions*, Clarendon Press, Oxford, **1987**.

[2] W. E. Hull, in: W. R. Croasmun, R. M. K. Carlson (eds.), *Two Dimensional NMR Spectroscopy*, VCH, Weinheim, **1994**, 67–456.

[3] A. E. Derome, *Modern NMR Techniques for Chemistry Research*, Pergamon, Oxford, **1987**, Chs. 8, 9, 10.

[4] J. K. M. Sanders, B. K. Hunter, *Modern NMR Spectroscopy*, 2nd Edition, Oxford University Press, **1993**, Ch. 4.

Experiment 10.1

2D *J*-Resolved ^1H NMR Spectroscopy

1. Purpose

In a normal 1D ^1H NMR spectrum chemical shift and spin–spin coupling information may be obscured by overlapping multiplets. In the 2D *J*-resolved experiment these two parameters are separated and displayed on different axes of the 2D matrix. On the F_2-axis only chemical shift information is present, and on the F_1-axis, only spin–spin coupling information. The projection of the 2D spectrum onto the F_2-axis is effectively a "^1H broad-band decoupled" proton spectrum. Another advantage of the experiment is the separation of homonuclear spin couplings from heteronuclear spin couplings (such as couplings to ^{31}P or ^{19}F), since the latter are confined to the F_2-axis.

2. Literature

[1] W. P. Aue, J. Karhan, R. R. Ernst, *J. Chem. Phys.* **1976**, *64*, 4226–4227.
[2] A. E. Derome, *Modern NMR Techniques for Chemistry Research*, Pergamon, Oxford, **1991**, 270–275.
[3] R. Freeman, *A Handbook of NMR*, Longman, Harlow, **1987**, 106–110.

3. Pulse Scheme and Phase Cycle

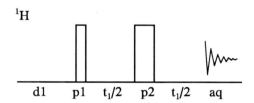

^1H

d1 p1 $t_1/2$ p2 $t_1/2$ aq

p1: $(x)_4$, $(y)_4$, $(-x)_4$, $(-y)_4$
p2: x, -x, y, -y, (y, -y, -x, x)$_2$, -x, x, -y, y
aq: $(x)_2$, $(-x)_2$, $(y)_2$, $(-y)_2$

4. Acquisition

Time requirement: 20 min.

Sample: 5% ethyl crotonate in $CDCl_3$

Record a normal ^1H NMR spectrum and optimize the spectral width. Change to the 2D mode of the spectrometer software and load the pulse program for *J*-resolved spectroscopy. You have to set:

td2: 1 k data points in F_2
td1: 128 data points in F_1
sw2: 8 ppm

swl: 40 Hz
o1: middle of ^{1}H NMR spectrum
p1: 90° ^{1}H transmitter pulse
p2: 180° ^{1}H transmitter pulse
d1: 2 s
initial value for t_1 evolution: 3 μs
increment for t_1 evolution: 1/[2·swl]
preacquisition delay: as small as possible
ds: 2
ns: 4

5. Processing

Apply zero filling in F_1 to 256 real data points. Use unshifted sinusoidal windows in both dimensions. Apply complex Fourier transformation corresponding to the N type signal selection using the quadrature off mode in F_1. Phase correction is not necessary, since the data are processed in magnitude mode. After the Fourier transformation the spectrum is tilted, since the signals are also modulated by J in F_2. This tilt can be eliminated by a software command. Finally the data may be symmetrized with respect to the horizontal through the center of F_1.

6. Result

The figure on page 279 shows the 2D spectrum obtained on an ARX-200 spectrometer after the tilt and symmetrization operation. The high resolution spectrum is shown in the F_2 axis, the internal projection (not shown) would give the ^{1}H decoupled proton spectrum. In F_1 the individual proton multiplets are observed.

7. Comments

The sequence is, in principle, identical to that in the spin-echo technique as described in Experiment 6.2, but differs in that now the spin-echo delay 2τ is incremented, thus creating the second dimension. At the end of t_1 the chemical shift information is refocused. However, the echo is modulated by the spin–spin coupling which evolved during t_1, and thus a 2D Fourier transformation will separate these two signal components. Well-resolved multiplet are obtained in F_1, because line broadening due to field inhomogeneity is refocused. On low-field spectrometers artefacts due to higher-order spin systems may occur. There also exist selective and doubly selective variants of this technique, see Experiment 7.12.

8. Own Observations

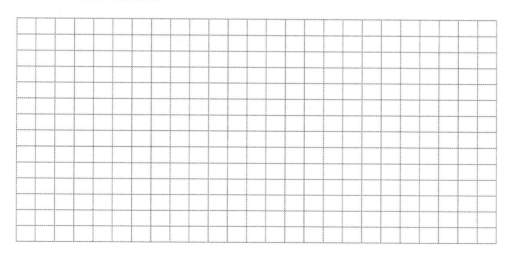

Experiment 10.2

2D *J*-Resolved ^{13}C NMR Spectroscopy

1. Purpose

In a ^{1}H coupled ^{13}C NMR spectrum (see Exp. 4.10) chemical shift and spin–spin coupling information may be obscured by overlapping multiplets. In the 2D *J*-resolved experiment these two parameters are separated and displayed on different axes of the 2D matrix. On the F_2-axis only chemical shift information is present, and on the F_1-axis only C,H coupling information. If the experiment is performed with high resolution in F_1, the C,H multiplets can be observed with their natural line-width. There are several variants; here we demonstrate a method in which the decoupler is gated. Note, however, that it results in splittings which are only half the actual spin coupling constants J(C,H).

2. Literature

[1] W. P. Aue, E. Bartholdi, R. R. Ernst, *J. Chem. Phys.* **1976**, *64*, 2229–2246.
[2] G. Bodenhausen, R. Freeman, R. Niedermeyer, D. L. Turner, *J. Magn. Reson.* **1977**, *26*, 133–164.
[3] A. E. Derome, *Modern NMR Techniques for Chemistry Research*, Pergamon, Oxford, **1991**, 259–268.
[4] J. K. M. Sanders, B. M. Hunter, *Modern NMR Spectroscopy*, 2nd Edition, Oxford University Press, **1993**, 117–120.

3. Pulse Scheme and Phase Cycle

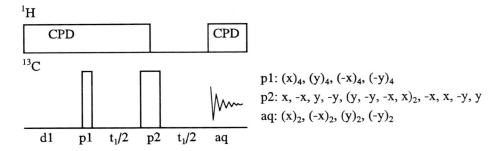

p1: (x)$_4$, (y)$_4$, (-x)$_4$, (-y)$_4$
p2: x, -x, y, -y, (y, -y, -x, x)$_2$, -x, x, -y, y
aq: (x)$_2$, (-x)$_2$, (y)$_2$, (-y)$_2$

4. Acquisition

Time requirement: 1.5 h

Sample: 20% ethyl crotonate in CDCl$_3$

Record a normal ^{13}C NMR spectrum and optimize the spectral width. Change to the 2D mode of the spectrometer software and load the pulse program for heteronuclear *J*-resolved spectroscopy. You have to set:

> td2: 1 k data points in F_2
> td1: 64 data points in F_1
> sw2: 175 ppm
> sw1: 250 Hz
> o1: middle of ^{13}C NMR spektrum
> o2: middle of ^1H NMR spectrum
> p1: 90° ^{13}C transmitter pulse
> p2: 180° ^{13}C transmitter pulse
> d1: 2 s
> initial value for t1 evolution: 3 μs
> increment for t1 evolution: 1/[2·sw1]
> preacquisition delay: as short as possible
> ds: 2
> ns: 32

5. Processing

Apply zero filling in F_1 to 256 real data points. Use squared $\pi/2$ shifted sinusoidal windows in both dimensions. Apply complex Fourier transformation corresponding to the N type signal selection using the quadrature-off mode in F_1. Phase correction is not necessary, since the data are processed in magnitude mode. The data can be symmetrized with respect to the horizontal through the middle of the spectrum.

6. Result

The figure on page 282 shows the 2D spectrum obtained on an ARX-200 spectrometer; symmetrization has been performed. Note that the splittings observed in F_1 are only half the actual C,H spin coupling constants.

7. Comments

The sequence is, in principle, identical to the spin-echo technique as described in Experiment 6.3, but differs in that now the spin-echo delay τ is incremented, thus creating the second dimension. At the completion of t_1, the chemical shift information is refocused. The echo, however, contains the spin–spin coupling information, which evolved during the second half of t_1, when the decoupler was switched off. Therefore, these two signal components can be separated by 2D Fourier transformation and the splittings are half of the actual spin coupling constants. There are selective variants of this technique (see Experiment 7.10).

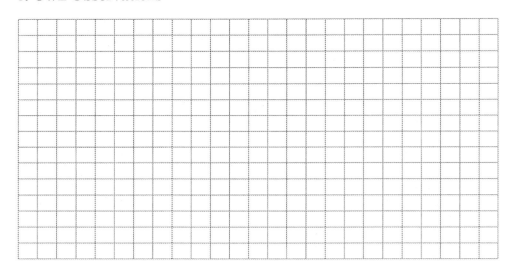

8. Own Observations

Experiment 10.3

The Basic H,H-COSY Experiment

1. Purpose

The COSY (**CO**rrelation **S**pectroscop**Y**) pulse sequence generates a 2D NMR spectrum in which the signals of a normal ^{1}H NMR spectrum are correlated with each other. Cross-peaks appear if spin coupling is present; thus the COSY sequence detects coupled pairs of protons (or pairs of other nuclei such as ^{19}F or ^{31}P). Since coupled protons are usually separated by two or three bonds, the connectivity and very often a chemical structure can be derived from the COSY spectrum. The COSY sequence is the most important and most frequently used 2D NMR experiment. We describe here the basic COSY technique with two 90° pulses and phase cycling for magnitude processing; other versions are given in Experiments 10.4–10.7.

2. Literature

[1] J. Jeener, *Ampère International Summer School*, Basko Polje, **1971**, (proposal).
[2] W. P. Aue, E. Bartholdi, R. R. Ernst, *J. Chem. Phys.* **1975**, *64*, 2229–2246.
[3] A. E. Derome, *Modern NMR Techniques for Chemistry Research*, Pergamon, Oxford, **1991**, 183–234.

3. Pulse Scheme and Phase Cycle

^{1}H

p1: $(x)_4$, $(y)_4$, $(-x)_4$, $(-y)_4$
p2: x, y, -x, -y
aq: $(x, -x)_2$, $(-y, y)_2$, $(-x, x)_2$, $(y, -y)_2$

d1   p1 t_1 p2   aq

4. Acquisition

Time requirement: 20 min

Sample: 5 % ethyl crotonate in CDCl$_3$

Record a standard ^{1}H NMR spectrum and optimize the spectral width. Change to the 2D mode of the spectrometer software and load the COSY pulse program. You have to set:

> td2: 1 k data points in F_2
> td1: 128 data points in F_1
> sw2: 8 ppm
> sw1: 8 ppm

o1: middle of ^1H NMR spectrum
p1, p2: 90° ^1H transmitter pulse
d1: 2 s
initial value for t_1 evolution: 3 μs
increment for t_1 evolution: 1/sw1
ds: 2
ns: 4

5. Processing

Apply zero filling in F_1 to 512 real data points to obtain a symmetrical matrix of 512·512 real points. Use unshifted sinusoidal windows in both dimensions. Apply complex Fourier transformation corresponding to the N type signal selection using the quadrature-off mode in F_1. Phase correction is not necessary, since the data are processed in magnitude mode. Finally the data may be symmetrized.

6. Result

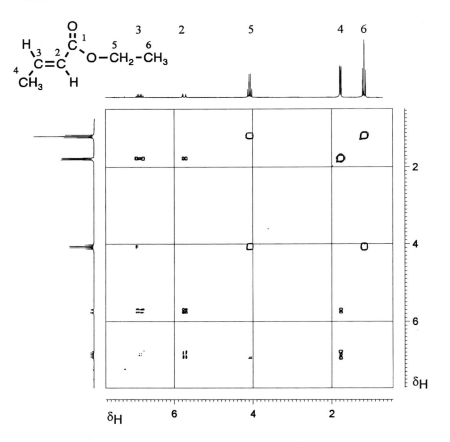

The Figure shows the H,H-COSY spectrum obtained on an ARX-200 spectrometer with symmetrization. Note that a cross peak connecting the hydrogen nucleus at C-2

with those at C-4 appears, although these hydrogens are not in a vicinal relationship. The cross peak results from an allylic coupling.

7. Comments

For the product operator formalism we consider a spin system of two protons. The key to any COSY protocol is the transformation of antiphase magnetization of proton 1 with respect to proton 2 into antiphase magnetization of proton 2 with respect to proton 1. The first r.f. pulse transforms z magnetization into transverse magnetization. Then the chemical shift develops during t_1, which is written here only for proton 1, giving Equation (1). In addition, spin–spin coupling develops; thus a term $2I_{1y}I_{2z}$ with antiphase magnetization of proton 1 with respect to proton 2 appears, as in Equation (2). Other terms are neglected.

$$I_{1z} + I_{2z} \xrightarrow{\quad I_x \quad} -I_{1y} - I_{2y} \xrightarrow{\quad \Omega_1 t_1 I_{1z} \quad} I_{1x}\sin\Omega_1 t_1 - I_{1y}\cos\Omega_1 t_1 \tag{1}$$

$$\xrightarrow{\quad \pi J t_1 2I_{1z}I_{2z} \quad} 2I_{1y}I_{2z}\sin\Omega_1 t_1 \sin\pi J\, t_1 \tag{2}$$

The second r.f. pulse transforms this into antiphase magnetization $2I_{1z}I_{2y}$, as in Equation (3). During the acquisition time t_2, chemical shift and spin-spin coupling develop once again, giving Equation (4).

$$\xrightarrow{\quad I_x \quad} 2I_{1z}I_{2y}\sin\Omega_1 t_1 \sin\pi J\, t_1 \tag{3}$$

$$\xrightarrow{\quad \Omega_2 t_2 I_{1z} \quad} \xrightarrow{\quad \pi J t_2\, 2I_{1z}I_{2z} \quad} I_{2y}\sin\Omega_1 t_1 \sin\pi J\, t_1\, \sin\Omega_2 t_2\, \sin\pi J\, t_2 \tag{4}$$

The last expression describes a cross-peak in the COSY matrix.

With the pulse sequence and phase cycling used the sign of the frequencies in F_1 is determined by adding together the sine and cosine terms, which leads to distorted lineshapes. Extraction of spin–spin coupling constants from this type of COSY spectrum is not recommended (see Exp. 10.5).

8. Own Observations

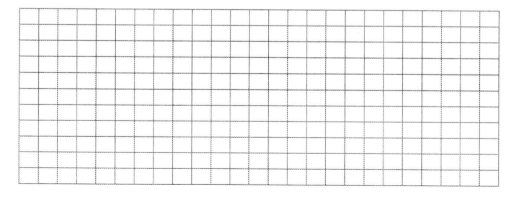

Experiment 10.4

Long-Range COSY

1. Purpose

The standard COSY pulse sequence (see Exp. 10.3) works best for spin–spin coupling constants of 3 to 15 Hz. With the long-range variant it is possible to observe cross-signals between protons which are connected by a very small coupling constant (as in allylic, homoallylic, or W-coupling). The method succeeds even in cases where the spin coupling is not resolved in the normal 1D ^{1}H NMR spectrum.

2. Literature

[1] A. Bax, R. Freeman, *J. Magn. Reson.* **1981**, *44*, 542–561.
[2] A. E. Derome, *Modern NMR Techniques for Chemistry Research*, Pergamon, Oxford, **1991**, 227–230.

3. Pulse Scheme and Phase Cycle

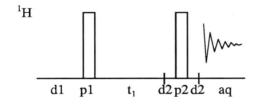

¹H

d1   p1   t₁   d2 p2 d2   aq

p1: $(x)_4$, $(y)_4$, $(-x)_4$, $(-y)_4$
p2: x, y, -x, -y
aq: $(x, -x)_2$, $(-y, y)_2$, $(-x, x)_2$, $(y, -y)_2$

4. Acquisition

Time requirement: 25 min

Sample: 5% ethyl crotonate in CDCl₃

Record a normal ^{1}H NMR spectrum and optimize the spectral width. Change to the 2D mode of the spectrometer software and load the long-range COSY pulse program. You have to set:

> td2: 1 k data points in F_2
> td1: 128 data points in F_1
> sw2: 8 ppm
> sw1: 8 ppm
> o1: middle of ^{1}H NMR spectrum
> p1: 90° [1]H pulse
> p2: 90° [1]H pulse
> d1: 2 s

d2: 200 ms
initial value for t_1 evolution: 3 μs
increment for t_1 evolution: 1/sw1
ds: 2
ns: 4

5. Processing

Apply zero filling in F_1 to 512 real data points to obtain a symmetrical matrix of
512·512 real points. Use unshifted sinusoidal windows in both dimensions. Apply
complex Fourier transformation corresponding to the N type signal selection using the
quadrature-off mode in F_1. Phase correction is not necessary, since the data are
processed in magnitude mode. Finally the data may be symmetrized.

6. Result

The figure shows a long-range COSY spectrum obtained on a ARX-200 spectrometer
with symmetrization of the matrix. Note that the cross peak connecting the hydrogen
nucleus at C-2 with those at C-4 is now of similar height to that connecting the
hydrogen atoms of C-4 with the proton at C-3. This can best be seen from the

corresponding row which was taken from the 2D matrix and displayed on the F_2-axis. Furthermore, the cross signals between the olefinic hydrogen nuclei arising from the large *trans* vicinal coupling virtually disappear at the contour level used.

7. Comments

The sequence differs from the standard version by the insertion of an additional fixed delay before and after the second r.f. pulse. This allows the small spin coupling constants to develop sufficiently to give detectable cross-signals. Values from 0.1 s to 0.4 s may be tried. For sensitivity reasons it is advisable to use two 90° pulses in the long range version of COSY. The first delay d2 can also be inserted directly after the first pulse p1.

8. Own Observations

Experiment 10.5

Phase-Sensitive COSY

1. Purpose

The standard COSY experiment (see Exp. 10.3) yields skewed line shapes due to the N type peak selection, arising from the adding together cosine and sine components within the same FID followed by magnitude processing. Therefore spin coupling constants cannot be measured from COSY spectra of this type. To obtain this information it is desirable to have Lorentzian lineshapes in both dimensions; thus the sign of frequencies in F_1 must be determined by separate storing of the sine and cosine components followed by a real Fourier transformation. There are several methods for achieving this goal [1, 2]. In the experiment described here the TPPI method of quadrature detection in F_1 is used.

2. Literature

[1] D. Marion, K. Wüthrich, *Biochem. Biophys. Res. Commun.* **1983**, *113*, 967–974.
[2] D. J. States, R. A. Haberkorn, D. J. Ruben, *J. Magn. Reson.* **1982**, *48*, 286–292.
[3] A. E. Derome, *Modern NMR Techniques for Chemistry Research*, Pergamon, Oxford, **1991**, 201–221.
[4] M. Eberstadt, G. Gemmecker, D. F. Mierke, H. Kessler, *Angew. Chem. Int. Ed. Engl.* **1995**, *34*, 1671-1695.

3. Pulse Scheme and Phase Cycle

^{1}H

d1   p1 t_1 p2   aq

p1: x, -x, -x, x, y, -y, -y, y
p2: x, -x, -x, x, y, -y, -y, y
aq: x, -x, -x, x, y, -y, -y, y
phase cycle for p1 incremented
according to TPPI

4. Acquisition

Time requirement: 2 h

Sample: 5% 2,3-dibromopropionic acid in [D_6]benzene

Record a standard ^{1}H NMR spectrum and optimize the spectral width. Change to the 2D mode of the spectrometer software and load the pulse program for phase-sensitive COSY with TPPI mode. You have to set:

td2: 2 k data points in F_2
td1: 256 data points in F_1
sw2: 1.5 ppm
sw1: 1.5 ppm
o1: middle of ^{1}H NMR spectrum
p1: 90° ^{1}H transmitter pulse
p2: 90° ^{1}H transmitter pulse
d1: 2 s
initial value for t_1 evolution: 3 μs
increment for t_1 evolution: 1/[2·sw1]
ds: 2
ns: 4

5. Processing

Apply zero filling in F_1 to 1 k real data points to obtain a symmetrical matrix of 1024·1024 real points. Use Gaussian windows in both dimensions. Apply real Fourier transformation corresponding to the TPPI mode of data acquisition in F_1. Phase correction for phase-sensitive COSY spectra can be performed in two ways. If one has measured a 1D ^{1}H NMR spectrum under the same conditions as for the 2D file (same probe-head tuning, same spectral width, time domain and preacquisition delay) one can phase the 1D spectrum and use the phase correction parameters in the F_2 dimension of the 2D file. Otherwise, using the 2D phase correction routines of the NMR software, one adjusts strong diagonal peaks at the left and right of the spectrum in dispersion, which yields the cross signals in pure antiphase.

6. Result

The figure on page 291 shows an expansion of the phase sensitive COSY spectrum obtained on an AC-300 spectrometer for the two crosspeaks connecting H-3b with H-2 and H-3b with H-3a. The dotted contour lines represent negative signals, the solid contourlines positive signals. In this type of COSY spectrum the active coupling (the one which causes the cross-peak) is in antiphase, whereas the passive one remains inphase. Thus from the cross peak at $\delta_H = 3.85$ it can be seen that J(H-3b,H-2) is small (4.6 Hz), whereas the absolute value of J(H-3b,H-3a) is larger (−10.1 Hz). The cross peak at $\delta_H = 3.35$ displays the active coupling J(H-3b,H-3a) and the passive coupling J(H-3a,H-2) = 11.0 Hz. For the sign determination see Experiments 4.5 and 10.6.

7. Comments

The TPPI (time proportional phase increment) method in 2D resembles somewhat the sequential quadrature detection of 1D spectra. Thus, for each t_1 increment the phase of the first pulse is incremented by 90°, leading to sine, cosine, −sine, −cosine character of the corresponding FIDs. For the same resolution twice the number of FIDs have to be recorded compared with the standard COSY. In the RSH (Ruben–States–Habercorn) method the FID is recorded twice for each t_1 increment with a 90° phase shift of p1.

To evaluate spin coupling constants from phase sensitive COSY spectra the digital resolution must be set appropriately high to avoid cancellation of signal components with opposite phases.

8. Own Observations

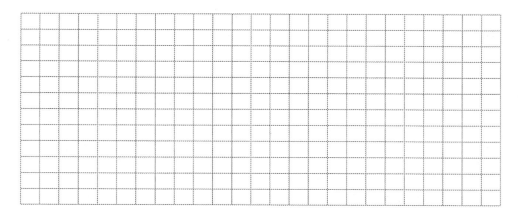

Experiment 10.6

Phase-Sensitive COSY-45

1. Purpose

The second pulse in a COSY experiment can be set to a smaller angle than the usual 90°. Two effects can be achieved by this measure. Firstly, the intensities of the autocorrelation signals, which are the cross-signals *within* the multiplets, become smaller; the diagonal will be narrower and cross signals near the diagonal can be observed more easily. Secondly the cross-signals become tilted and from the slope of this tilt the relative signs of spin coupling constants can be derived. Thus the COSY-45 experiment serves to distinguish between a ^2J and a ^3J spin coupling constant. The effect is, of course, best seen if the COSY spectrum is recorded with high digital resolution and in the phase-sensitive mode as shown here.

2. Literature

[1] W. P. Aue, E. Bartholdi, R. R. Ernst, *J. Chem. Phys.* **1975**, *64*, 2229–2246.
[2] A. Bax, R. Freeman, *J. Magn. Reson.* **1981**, *44*, 542–561.
[3] W. E. Hull, in: W. R. Croasmun, R. M. K. Carlson (eds.), *Two Dimensional NMR Spectroscopy*, VCH, Weinheim, **1994**, 301–303.

3. Pulse Scheme and Phase Cycle

^{1}H

d1   p1 t_1 p2   aq

p1: x, -x, -x, x, y, -y, -y, y
p2: x, -x, -x, x, y, -y, -y, y
aq: x, -x, -x, x, y, -y, -y, y
phase cycle for p1 incremented
according to TPPI

4. Acquisition

Time requirement: 3 h

Sample: 5% 2,3-dibromopropionic acid in [D$_6$]benzene

Record a normal ^{1}H NMR spectrum and optimize the spectral width. Change to the 2D mode of the spectrometer software and load the pulse program for phase-sensitive COSY with TPPI mode. You have to set:

td2: 2 k data points in F_2
td1: 256 data points in F_1

sw2: 1.5 ppm
sw1: 1.5 ppm
o1: middle of ^{1}H NMR spectrum
p1: 90° ^{1}H transmitter pulse
p2: 45° ^{1}H transmitter pulse
d1: 2 s
initial value for t_1 evolution: 3 μs
increment for t_1 evolution: 1/[2·sw1]
ds: 2
ns: 4

5. Processing

Apply zero filling in F_1 to 1 k real data points to obtain a symmetrical matrix of 1024·1024 real points. Use Gaussian windows in both dimensions. Apply real Fourier transformation corresponding to the TPPI mode of data acquisition in F_1. Phase correction as described in Experiment 10.5 for phase-sensitive COSY spectra must be performed.

6. Result

The figure on page 294 shows an expansion of the phase sensitive COSY-45 spectrum obtained on an AC-300 spectrometer for the same two cross-peaks connecting H-3b with H-2 and H-3b with H-3a as given in Experiment 10.5. Note that specific contours are missing, and the tilt of both cross-peaks has a different slope, since the cross-peak at δ_H = 3.85 is caused by a vicinal spin coupling whereas the cross-peak at δ_H = 3.35 is caused by a geminal spin coupling.

7. Comments

In a two-spin system the intensity of the cross peaks is proportional to $\sin^2\alpha$, where α is the pulse angle of the second pulse in the COSY sequence. In multi-spin systems, however, the situation is more complex. In the three-spin system of the example shown the cross-peaks are reduced from a 4·4 matrix to two 2·2 matrices which are offset both in F_1 and F_2 by the passive coupling. Thus, if the sign of active and passive couplings are the same, one obtains a different slope of the cross-peak compared with the situation when the signs differ.

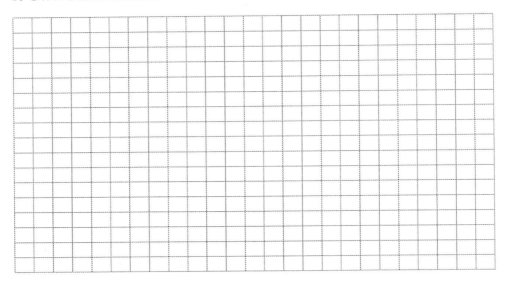

8. Own Observations

Experiment 10.7

Double Quantum Filtered COSY With Presaturation

1. Purpose

The NMR spectra of proteins, peptides, and carbohydrates are usually measured in water solution. Only 10% D_2O is added to provide a lock signal, since otherwise exchangeable NH protons would disappear; thus a huge water signal is present in these samples. In order to get reasonable COSY spectra one first uses a water suppression technique, such as presaturation (see Exp. 6.15) and, in addition, the COSY variant with a double quantum filter. Since water has no double quantum transitions, its signal is further suppressed. Since one wants to analyze the spin systems of the different amino acids in detail, this experiment is usually run in the phase-sensitive mode. An additional asset is the circumstance that the diagonal peaks of the DQF–COSY spectrum can be phased into absorption; thus one avoids having to cope with the tailing of the dispersion diagonal peaks as in the normal phase-sensitive COSY.

2. Literature

[1] U. Piantini, O. W. Sørensen, R. R. Ernst, *J. Am. Chem. Soc.* **1982**, *104*, 6800–6801.
[2] M. Rance, O. W. Sørensen, G. Bodenhausen, G. Wagner, R. R. Ernst, K. Wüthrich, *Biochem. Biophys. Res. Commun.* **1983**, *117*, 479–485.
[3] A. E. Derome, M. P. Williamson, *J. Magn. Reson.* **1990**, *88*, 177–185.

3. Pulse Scheme and Phase Cycle

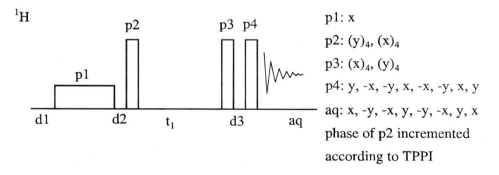

p1: x
p2: $(y)_4$, $(x)_4$
p3: $(x)_4$, $(y)_4$
p4: y, -x, -y, x, -x, -y, x, y
aq: x, -y, -x, y, -y, -x, y, x
phase of p2 incremented according to TPPI

4. Acquisition

Time requirement: 11 h

Sample: 2 mmol sucrose in 90% H_2O/10% D_2O + 0.5 mmol DSS (2,2-dimethyl-2-silapentan-5-sulfonate, sodium salt) including a trace of NaN_3 against bacteria growth.

The probe-head must be tuned to the water sample. Record a normal ^{1}H NMR spectrum and redetermine the 90° pulse. Record a 1D spectrum with water presaturation and optimize the transmitter power for presaturation (Exp. 6.15). Change to the 2D mode of the spectrometer software and load the pulse program for phase-sensitive double quantum COSY with presaturation. You have to set:

> td2: 2 k data points in F_2
> td1: 256 data points in F_1
> sw2: 10 ppm
> sw1: 10 ppm
> o1: on resonance of water signal
> p1: 2 s at transmitter attenuation corresponding to $\gamma B_1 \approx 25$ Hz, 90° pulse ≈ 10 ms, typically 65 dB, see Experiments 2.6 and 6.15
> d1: 30 ms
> d2: 20 μs
> d3: 4 μs
> initial value for $t1$ evolution: 3 μs
> increment for $t1$ evolution: $1/[2 \cdot sw1]$
> ds: 2
> ns: 64

5. Processing

Apply zero-filling in F_1 to 1 k real data points to obtain a symmetrical matrix of 1024·1024 real points. Use Gaussian window in both dimensions. Apply real Fourier transformation corresponding to the TPPI mode of data acquisition in F_1.

6. Result

The figure on page 297 shows an expansion of the DQF–COSY spectrum obtained on an AMX-500 spectrometer. Note that the water signal of the 1D spectrum, which was obtained by presaturation, is much larger than the residual water signal of the 2D file. At the contour level chosen the cross-peak of the anomeric proton at $\delta_H = 5.41$ can be seen only in the upper left part of the matrix.

7. Comments

The sequence employs a third 90° pulse acting in combination with p2 as the double quantum filter. The second pulse of a COSY sequence not only generates antiphase magnetization as described in Experiment 10.3, but also creates double quantum terms depending on its phase. In the product operator formalism we can first repeat the findings of Experiment 10.3 with regard to the actual pulse phases used. The first r.f. pulse transforms z-magnetization into transverse magnetization. Then the chemical shift develops during t_1, which is written in Equation (1) only for proton 1. In addition, spin–spin coupling develops; thus a term $2I_{1y}I_{2z}$ with antiphase magnetization of proton 1 with respect to proton 2 appears, as indicated in Equation (2). Other terms are neglected.

$$I_{1z} + I_{2z} \xrightarrow{\;I_y\;} I_{1x} + I_{2x} \xrightarrow{\;\Omega_1 t_1 I_{1z}\;} I_{1x}\cos\Omega_1 t_1 - I_{1y}\sin\Omega_1 t_1 \tag{1}$$

$$\xrightarrow{\;\pi J t_1 2 I_{1z} I_{2z}\;} -2 I_{1x} I_{2z}\sin\Omega_1 t_1 \sin\pi J t_1 \tag{2}$$

The second r.f. pulse now creates double quantum magnetization $2 I_{1x} I_{2y}$. This is transformed back into antiphase magnetization of proton 2 with respect to proton 1 by the pulse p4 as indicated in Equation (3). During the acquisition time $t2$ chemical shift and spin–spin coupling develop once again, as indicated in Equation (4). However, due to the full phase cycle used, only those signals are observed which have passed through the double quantum state, whereas all others are suppressed.

$$\xrightarrow{\;I_x\;} 2 I_{1x} I_{2y}\sin\Omega_1 t_1 \sin\pi J t_1 \xrightarrow{\;I_y\;} -2 I_{1z} I_{2y}\sin\Omega_1 t_1 \sin\pi J t_1 \tag{3}$$

$$\xrightarrow{\;\Omega_2 t_2 I_{1z}\;} \xrightarrow{\;\pi J t_2 2 I_{1z} I_{2z}\;} I_{2y}\sin\Omega_1 t_1 \sin\pi J t_1 \; \sin\Omega_2 t_2 \; \sin\pi J t_2 \tag{4}$$

8. Own Observations

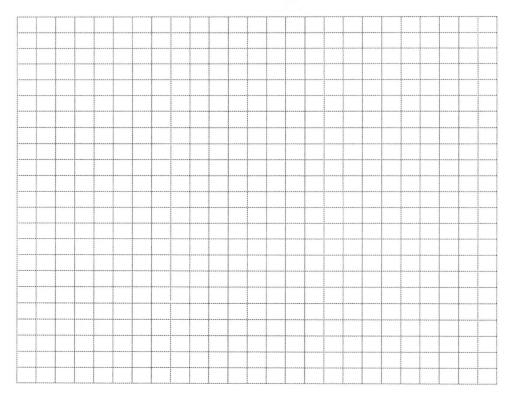

Experiment 10.8

C,H Correlation by Polarization Transfer (HETCOR)

1. Purpose

A two dimensional C,H correlation experiment yields cross signals for all protons and ^{13}C nuclei which are connected by a ^{13}C,^{1}H coupling over one bond. The assignment of one member of a spin-coupled pair leads immediately to the assignment of the other. A C,H correlation experiment may be performed in many ways. The experiment described here encodes the proton chemical shift information into the ^{13}C signals and can be performed on most older instruments, since the observed nucleus is ^{13}C. The 1D equivalent of this correlation technique is described in Experiment 4.11.

2. Literature

[1] R. Freeman, G. A. Morris, *J. Chem. Soc. Chem. Commun.* **1978**, 684–686.
[2] A. Bax, G. A. Morris, *J. Magn. Reson.* **1981**, *42*, 501–505.
[3] G. E. Martin, A. S. Zektzer, *Two Dimensional NMR Methods for Establishing Molecular Connectivity*, VCH, Weinheim, **1988**, Ch. 3.

3. Pulse Scheme and Phase Cycle

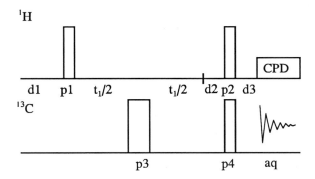

p1: x   p3: $(x)_4$, $(-x)_4$

p2: x, -x, y, -y   p4: $(x)_8$, $(y)_8$, $(-x)_8$, $(-y)_8$

aq: $(x, -x, y, -y)_2$, $(y, -y, -x, x)_2$ $(-x, x, -y, y)_2$, $(-y, y, x, -x)_2$

4. Acquisition

Time requirement: 2.5 h

Sample: 20% ethyl crotonate in CDCl$_3$

Record normal ^{13}C and ^{1}H NMR spectra and optimize the spectral widths. Change to the 2D mode of the spectrometer software and load the pulse program for X,H correlation. You have to set:

td2: 1 k data points in F_2
td1: 128 data points in F_1
sw2: 175 ppm
sw1: 8 ppm
o1: middle of ^{13}C NMR spectrum
o2: middle of ^{1}H NMR spectrum
p1, p2: 90° ^{1}H decoupler pulse
p3: 180° ^{13}C transmitter pulse
p4: 90° ^{13}C transmitter pulse
d1: 2 s
d2: $1/[2J(C, H)] = 3.45$ ms, calculated from $^{1}J(C,H) = 145$ Hz
d3: $1/[3J(C,H)] = 2.29$ ms, calculated from $^{1}J(C, H) = 145$ Hz
initial value for t_1 evolution: 3 µs
increment for t_1 evolution $= 1/[2 \cdot sw1]$
decoupler attenuation and 90° pulse for CPD
ns: 32

5. Processing

Apply zero filling in F_1 to 256 real data points. Use squared $\pi/2$ shifted sinusoidal windows in both dimensions. Apply complex Fourier transformation corresponding to the N type signal selection using the quadrature-off mode in F_1. Phase correction is not necessary, since the data are processed in magnitude mode.

6. Result

The figure on page 301 shows the 2D spectrum obtained on an ARX-200 spectrometer. Note that the heteronuclear spin coupling is removed in both dimensions. This is achieved by CPD decoupling in F_2 and by the 180° ^{13}C pulse in case of F_1.

7. Comments

The first proton pulse creates $-I_{Hy}$ magnetization, which subsequently develops ^{1}H chemical shift during t_1 as shown in Equation (1). The 180° ^{13}C pulse p3 in the middle of t_1 removes heteronuclear spin coupling during t_1.

$$I_{Hz} \xrightarrow{ I_{Hx} } -I_{Hy} \xrightarrow{ \Omega_H t_1 I_{Hz} } I_{Hx}\sin\Omega_H t_1 - I_{Hy}\cos\Omega_H t_1 \qquad (1)$$

C,H spin coupling evolves during the delay τ, leading to an antiphase magnetization of proton with respect to carbon, as indicated in Equation (2). If the delay τ is set equal to d2 $= 1/[2J(C,H)]$ the corresponding cosine terms become zero.

$$\xrightarrow{ \pi J\tau\, 2I_{Hz}I_{Cz} } 2I_{Hy}I_{Cz}\sin\Omega_H t_1 + 2I_{Hx}I_{Cz}\cos\Omega_H t_1 \qquad (2)$$

The two simultaneous pulses p2 and p4 transform this into antiphase magnetization of carbon with respect to proton, as shown in Equation (3). Since this magnetization was originally a proton magnetization, bearing γ_H, we call this a polarization transfer.

$$\xrightarrow{\;I_{Hx}, I_{Cx}\;} \quad -2I_{Hz}I_{Cy}\sin\Omega_H t_1 \tag{3}$$

The antiphase magnetization is refocused during the delay d3 to give an observable in-phase magnetization. The delay d3 is chosen so as to obtain the maximum signal for all multiplicities. During acquisition the ^{13}C chemical shift develops, while proton decoupling ensures that no spin coupling appears in F_2.

8. Own Observations

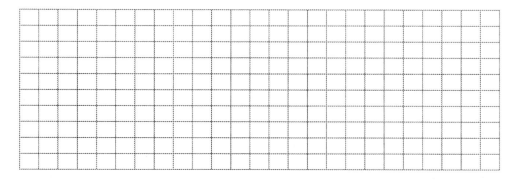

Experiment 10.9

Long-Range C,H Correlation by Polarization Transfer

1. Purpose

The normal C,H correlation procedure as described in Experiment 10.8 yields cross-signals for all ^{1}H and ^{13}C nuclei that are connected by a one-bond coupling constant ^1J(C,H). However, it is often desirable to be able to observe cross-signals for C,H spin pairs connected by two- or three-bond couplings ^2J(C,H) or ^3J(C,H). This can be achieved with the same pulse sequence by adjusting the appropriate delays. Other alternatives are the COLOC (Exp. 10.10) and HMBC (Exp. 10.13) experiments. The experiment described here incorporates the proton chemical shift information into the carbon signals and can be performed on most older instruments since the observed nuclide is ^{13}C. The 1D equivalent of this correlation technique is described in Experiment 4.13.

2. Literature

[1] C. Bauer, R. Freeman, S. Wimperis, *J. Magn. Reson.* **1984,** *58,* 526–532.
[2] A. S. Zektzer, B. K. John, G. E. Martin, *Magn. Reson. Chem.* **1987,** *25,* 752–756.
[3] G. E. Martin, A. S. Zektzer, *Two Dimensional NMR Methods for Establishing Molecular Connectivity*, VCH, Weinheim, **1988,** 221–255.

3. Pulse Scheme and Phase Cycle

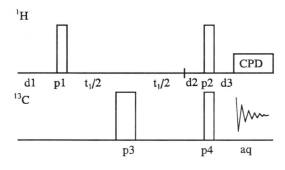

p1: x   p3: (x)$_4$, (-x)$_4$
p2: x, -x, y, -y   p4: (x)$_8$, (y)$_8$, (-x)$_8$, (-y)$_8$
aq: (x, -x, y, -y)$_2$, (y, -y, -x, x)$_2$ (-x, x, -y, y)$_2$, (-y, y, x, -x)$_2$

4. Acquisition

Time requirement: 5 h

Sample: 20% ethyl crotonate in CDCl$_3$

Record normal ^{13}C and ^{1}H NMR spectra and optimize the spectral widths. Change to the 2D mode of the spectrometer software and load the pulse program for X,H correlation. You have to set:

td2: 1 k data points in F_2
td1: 128 data points in F_1
sw2: 175 ppm
sw1: 8 ppm
o1: middle of ^{13}C NMR spectrum
o2: middle of ^{1}H NMR spectrum
p1, p2: 90° ^{1}H decoupler pulse
p3: 180° ^{13}C transmitter pulse
p4: 90° ^{13}C transmitter pulse
d1: 2 s
d2: $1/[2J(C,H)]$ = 50 ms, calculated from $^nJ(C,H)$ = 10 Hz
d3: $1/[3J(C,H)]$ = 33 ms, calculated from $^nJ(C,H)$ = 10 Hz
initial value for t_1 evolution: 3 µs
increment for t_1 evolution = $1/[2 \cdot sw1]$
decoupler attenuation and 90° pulse for CPD
ds: 2
ns: 64

5. Processing

Apply zero filling in F_1 to 256 real data points. Use squared $\pi/2$ shifted sinusoidal windows in both dimensions. Apply complex Fourier transformation corresponding to the N type signal selection using the quadrature-off mode in F_1. Phase correction is not necessary, since the data are processed in magnitude mode.

6. Result

The figure on page 304 shows the 2D spectrum obtained on an ARX-200 spectrometer. Of interest are the weak cross-signals of H-5, H-3, and H-2 to the carboxyl ^{13}C nucleus C-1, and the large intensity difference between the cross-signals of H-4 to C-2 and C-3. Note, however, that the noise is considerably greater than that obtained for $^1J(C,H)$ in Experiment 10.8 and that there is some breakthrough of axial signals. Furthermore, most of the cross-signals corresponding to $^1J(C,H)$ can still be observed.

7. Comments

The product operator description of the experiment is given in Experiment 10.8. The selection of delays d2 and d3 is frequently difficult and is discussed extensively in the literature. A good initial value for d2 is usually 50 ms (corresponding to a coupling constant of 10 Hz), although ^2J- and ^3J-values are seldom as large as 10 Hz. Relaxation times and homonulear spin–spin coupling of protons must also be taken into account.

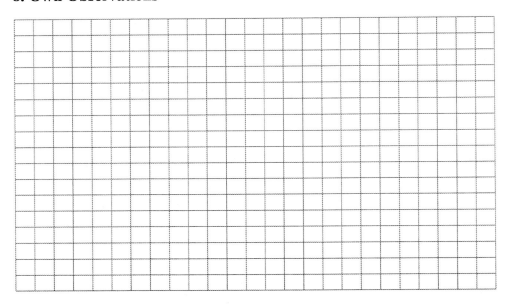

8. Own Observations

Experiment 10.10

C,H Correlation via Long-Range Couplings (COLOC)

1. Purpose

The long-range C,H correlation procedure as described in Experiment 10.9 is not always satisfactory. With increasing t_1 values homonuclear spin coupling of the protons evolves, and proton relaxation reduces the sensitivity of the experiment. A constant time method called COLOC (**CO**rrelation spectroscopy via **LO**ng range **C**oupling) has therefore been developed. In this experiment the t_1 evolution and the polarization transfer period are combined in one constant time interval and the separation of the two is achieved by incrementally shifted 180° pulses. As in Experiment 10.9, COLOC incorporates the proton chemical shift information into the carbon signals and can be performed on most older instruments since the observed nuclide is ^{13}C. The version shown here is not phase-sensitive.

2. Literature

[1] H. Kessler, C. Griesinger, J. Zarbock, H. R. Loosli, *J. Magn. Reson.* **1984**, *57*, 331–336.
[2] H. Kessler, C. Griesinger, K. Wagner, *J. Am. Chem. Soc.* **1987**, *109*, 6927–6933.
[3] G. E. Martin, A. S. Zektzer, *Two Dimensional NMR Methods for Establishing Molecular Connectivity*, VCH, Weinheim, **1988**, 255–267.

3. Pulse Scheme and Phase Cycle

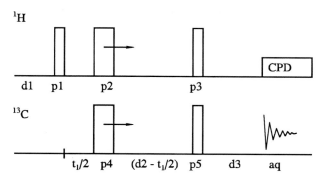

p1: $(x)_{16}$, $(y)_{16}$, $(-x)_{16}$, $(-y)_{16}$ p2, p4: x

p3: $(x, y)_8$, $(-x, -y)_8$ aq: $(x)_2$, $(-x)_2$, $(y)_2$, $(-y)_2$

p5: x, y, -x, -y, y, -x, -y, x, -x, -y, x, y, -y, x, y, -x ,

　　y, -x, -y, x, -x, -y, x, y, -y, x, y, -x, x, y, -x, -y,

　　-x, -y, x, y, -y, x, y, -x, x, y, -x, -y, y, -x, -y, x,

　　-y, x, y, -x, x, y, -x, -y, y, -x, -y, x, -x, -y, x, y

4. Acquisition

Time requirement: 5 h

Sample: 20% ethyl crotonate in $CDCl_3$

Record normal ^{13}C and ^{1}H NMR spectra and optimize the spectral widths. Change to the 2D mode of the spectrometer software and load the COLOC pulse program. You have to set:

> td2: 1 k data points in F_2
> td1: 64 data points in F_1
> sw2: 175 ppm
> sw1: 8 ppm
> o1: middle of ^{13}C NMR spectrum
> o2: middle of ^{1}H NMR spectrum
> p1, p3: 90° ^{1}H decoupler pulse
> p2: 180° ^{1}H decoupler pulse
> p4: 180° ^{13}C transmitter pulse
> p5: 90° ^{13}C transmitter pulse
> d1: 2 s
> d2: 25 ms
> d3: $1/[3J(C,H)] = 33$ ms, calculated from $^{n}J(C,H) = 10$ Hz
> initial value for t_1 evolution: 3 μs
> increment for t_1 evolution: $1/[2 \cdot sw1]$
> decrement for d2: $1/[2 \cdot sw1]$; note that d2 must be larger than td1 times $1/[2 \cdot sw1]$
> decoupler attenuation and 90° pulse for CPD
> ds: 2
> ns: 128

5. Processing

Apply zero filling in F_1 to 256 real data points. Use squared $\pi/2$ shifted sinusoidal windows in both dimensions. Apply complex Fourier transformation corresponding to the N type signal selection using the quadrature off mode in F_1. Phase correction is not necessary, since the data are processed in magnitude mode.

6. Result

The figure on page 307 shows the 2D spectrum obtained on an ARX-200 spectrometer. Compared with the result of Experiment 10.9, which was obtained under otherwise identical conditions, there is less noise and the cross-peaks from H-4 to C-2 and C-3, as well the cross peak from H-5 to C-1, are much stronger; however, the correlations of H-3 and H-2 to C-1 are completely missing. Most of the cross-signals corresponding to $^{1}J(C,H)$ can still be observed. Careful adjustment of d2 and d3 is necessary; this can be optimized by a 1D INEPT experiment.

7. Comments

The experiment is of the constant-time type as the time period of the chemical shift evolution is held constant while 180° pulses are moved through this period. The product operator description as given in Experiment 10.8 still holds in principle. The advantages of this approach are that the evolution of homonuclear spin coupling of the protons is held constant during the experiment, and that the protons are given less time to relax, since t_1 evolution and transfer delay d2 are combined. Several modifications of the original experiment are known [3].

8. Own Observations

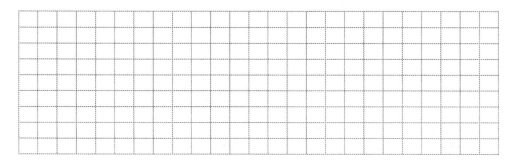

Experiment 10.11

The Basic HMQC Experiment

1. Purpose

The experiment described is the simplest form of an inverse H,X correlation technique. HMQC stands for **H**eteronuclear **M**ultiple **Q**uantum **C**oherence. The suppression of unwanted signals is performed only by the phase cycle; no ^{13}C broad-band decoupling is applied during acquisition and the 2D spectrum is recorded without quadrature detection in F_1, which requires the magnitude mode of data processing. Using only four different r.f. pulses it demonstrates the sensitivity advantage of the inverse detection method.

2. Literature

[1] L. Müller, *J. Am. Chem. Soc.* **1979**, *101*, 4481–4484.
[2] A. Bax, R. H. Griffey, B. L. Hawkins, *J. Magn. Reson.* **1983**, *55*, 301–315.
[3] G. E. Martin, A. S. Zektzer, *Two Dimensional NMR Methods for Establishing Molecular Connectivity*, VCH, Weinheim, **1988**, 213–221.

3. Pulse Scheme and Phase Cycle

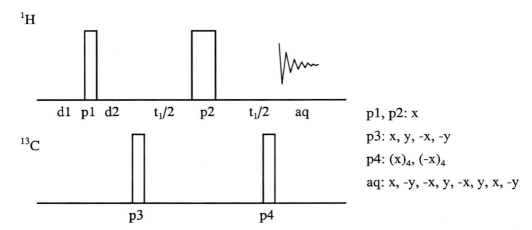

p1, p2: x

p3: x, y, -x, -y

p4: (x)$_4$, (-x)$_4$

aq: x, -y, -x, y, -x, y, x, -y

4. Acquisition

Time requirement: 40 min

Sample: 5% ethyl crotonate in CDCl$_3$

Record normal 1D ^{1}H and ^{13}C NMR spectra, optimize the spectral widths, and note the offsets. Switch to the 2D mode of the spectrometer software, load the HMQC pulse program, and, if required, change the spectrometer to the inverse set-up. You have to set:

> td2: 1 k data points in F_2
> td1: 128 data points in F_1
> sw2: 8 ppm
> sw1: 175 ppm
> offset of ^{1}H frequency: middle of ^{1}H NMR spectrum
> offset of ^{13}C frequency: middle of ^{13}C NMR spectrum
> p1: 90° ^{1}H transmitter pulse
> p2: 180° ^{1}H transmitter pulse
> p3, p4: 90° ^{13}C decoupler pulse
> d1: 2 s
> d2: $1/[2J(C,H)] = 3.5$ ms, calculated from $^1J(C,H) = 145$ Hz
> initial value for t_1 evolution: 3 μs
> increment for t_1 evolution: $1/[2 \cdot sw1]$
> ds: 2
> ns: 8

5. Processing

Apply zero filling in F_1 to 256 real data points to obtain a matrix of 512·256 real data points. Use π/2 shifted squared sinusoidal windows in both dimensions. Apply complex Fourier transformation corresponding to the N type signal selection using the quadrature-off mode in F_1. Phase correction is not necessary, since the data are processed in magnitude mode.

6. Result

The figure on page 310 shows the HMQC spectrum obtained on an ARX-200 spectrometer in a normal forward dual probe-head. This demonstrates that a special inverse probe-head is not an absolute necessity. Note that the spectrum displays in F_2 doublets with the spin coupling constant $^1J(C,H)$, and in addition the homonuclear splittings caused by H,H spin couplings. These also broaden the signals in the F_1 dimension. There is considerable signal breakthrough from the protons bound to ^{12}C, which is seen mostly at the methyl group signals.

7. Comments

The first 90° proton pulse creates a transverse proton magnetization $-I_{Hy}$ as in Equation (1). During the delay $\tau = $ d2 C,H spin coupling develops and creates antiphase magnetization $2I_{Hx}I_{Cz}$. Since τ was set to $1/[2J(C,H)]$ the cosine term becomes zero and the sine term unity.

$$I_{Hz} + I_{Cz} \xrightarrow{I_{Hx}} -I_{Hy} + I_{Cz} \xrightarrow{\pi J \tau I_{Hz}I_{Cz}} 2I_{Hx}I_{Cz} \tag{1}$$

The first 90° ^{13}C pulse p3 transforms the antiphase magnetization is into double quantum magnetization $-2I_{Hx}I_{Cy}$ as in Equation (2). During t_1 this term develops ^{13}C chemical shift as in Equatiuon (3). Of course, ^{1}H chemical shift and H, H spin coupling evolve also during t_1. The former is removed by the 180° proton pulse p2 which for simplicity is not shown in the equations. Furthermore, this 180° proton pulse interchanges double quantum and zero quantum terms.

$$2I_{Hx}I_{Cz} \xrightarrow{\;I_{Cx}\;} -2I_{Hx}I_{Cy} \tag{2}$$

$$\xrightarrow{\;\Omega_C\, t_1\, I_{Cz}\;} -2I_{Hx}I_{Cy}\cos\Omega_C t_1 + 2I_{Hx}I_{Cx}\sin\Omega_C t_1 \tag{3}$$

$$\xrightarrow{\;I_{Cx}\;} -2I_{Hx}I_{Cz}\cos\Omega_C t_1 + 2I_{Hx}I_{Cx}\sin\Omega_C t_1 \tag{4}$$

The last ^{13}C pulse p4 transforms the magnetization back into antiphase terms as shown in Equation (4). During the acquisition time aq C,H spin coupling again evolves, leading to the observable proton signal which is modulated with the ^{13}C chemical shift information during t_1 as in Equation (5).

$$\xrightarrow{\;\pi J\, \mathrm{aq}\, I_{Hz}I_{Cz}\;} -I_{Hy}\cos\Omega_C t_1 \sin\pi J\mathrm{aq} \tag{5}$$

8. Own Observations

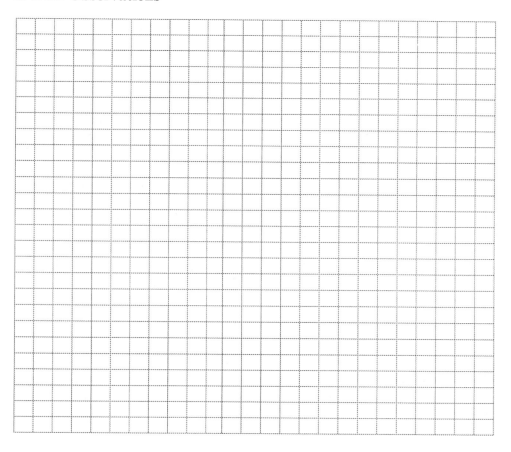

Experiment 10.12

Phase-Sensitive HMQC with BIRD Selection and GARP Decoupling

1. Purpose

The basic HMQC sequence as described in Experiment 10.11 gives rather poor signal suppression for protons bound to ^{12}C or ^{14}N. A considerable improvement [1] can be achieved by using the BIRD sandwich [2] (see Exp. 6.12) prior to the HMQC sequence. Furthermore, decoupling all ^{13}C nuclei with the GARP technique (**G**lobally optimized **A**lternating-phase **R**ectangular **P**ulses) [3] improves the signal-to-noise ratio. Here we describe the phase sensitive version which yields Lorentzian line shapes in both dimensions. Prior to the introduction of gradient-selected spectroscopy (see Exp. 11. 5), this experiment was the first choice for inverse H,C correlation.

2. Literature

[1] A. Bax, S. Subramanian, *J. Magn. Reson.* **1986**, *67*, 565–569.
[2] J. R. Garbow, D. P. Weitekamp, A. Pines, *Chem. Phys. Lett.* **1982**, *93*, 504–508.
[3] A. J. Shaka, P. B. Barker, R. Freeman, *J. Magn. Reson.* **1985**, *64*, 547–552.

3. Pulse Scheme and Phase Cycle

pl, p2, p4, p5, p6: x   p8: x, -x   p7: (x)$_4$, (-x)$_4$
p3: -x   p9: (x)$_2$, (-x)$_2$ aq: x, -x, -x, x
phase cycle for p8 incremented according to TPPI

4. Acquisition

Time requirement: 40 min

Sample: 5% ethyl crotonate in CDCl$_3$

Record normal 1D ^{1}H and ^{13}C NMR spectra, optimize the spectral widths and note the offsets. Switch to the 2D mode of the spectrometer software, load the pulse program and, if required, change the spectrometer to the inverse configuration. For the experiment you have to determine the 90° ^{13}C pulse for GARP decoupling (see Exp. 2.5). You have to set:

> td2: 1 k data points in F_2
> td1: 128 data points in F_1
> sw2: 8 ppm
> sw1: 175 ppm
> offset of ^{1}H frequency: middle of ^{1}H NMR spectrum
> offset of ^{13}C frequency: middle of ^{13}C NMR spectrum
> p1, p3, p4: 90° ^{1}H transmitter pulse
> p2, p5: 180° ^{1}H transmitter pulse
> p7, p8, p9: 90° ^{13}C decoupler pulse
> p6: 180° ^{13}C decoupler pulse
> d1: 1 s
> d2: $1/[2J(C,H)] = 3.5$ ms, calculated from $^1J(C,H) = 145$ Hz
> d3: BIRD delay to be optimized for minimum FID, ca 1 s; observe in the set-up mode the incoming FID and adjust d3 for minimum intensity (see Exp. 6.12).
> initial value for t_1 evolution: 3 μs
> increment for t_1 evolution: $1/[4 \cdot sw1]$
> ^{13}C decoupler attenuation and 90° pulse width for GARP
> ds: 2
> ns: 8

5. Processing

Apply zero filling in F_1 to 256 real data points to obtain a matrix of 512·256 real points. Use exponential or Gaussian windows in both dimensions. Apply real Fourier transformation corresponding to the TPPI type signal selection using the quadrature mode in F_1. Phase correction is required; it is often sufficient to correct the phase only in F_2.

6. Result

The figure on page 314 shows the HMQC spectrum obtained on an ARX-200 spectrometer with a normal dual probe-head. This demonstrates that special inverse probe-heads are not an absolute necessity. Note that the spectrum displays only singlets in F_2 which are further split by the homonuclear spin couplings. These also broaden the signals in the F_1 dimension. The breakthrough of the signals from protons bound to ^{12}C is dramatically reduced in comparison with Experiment 10.11.

7. Comments

The description of the HMQC and BIRD part of the sequence in the product operator formalism has been given in Experiments 10.11 and 6.12. The dashed pulse p7 in the pulse sequence removes artefacts caused by residual longitudinal ^{13}C magnetization [1]. For the conditions given we have obtained identical results from experiments in which this pulse was used and those in which it was omitted.

8. Own Observations

Experiment 10.13

Phase-Sensitive HMBC with BIRD Selection

1. Purpose

The HMQC (**H**etero **M**ultinuclear **Q**uantum **C**oherence) sequence as described in Experiments 10.11 and 10.12 was designed to correlate proton and carbon nuclei via $^1J(C,H)$. To obtain long-range H,C correlations via $^2J(C,H)$ and $^3J(C,H)$ one can simply set the delay d2 to 50 ms, corresponding to a spin coupling constant of 10 Hz. Alternatively, one can use a special pulse sequence called HMBC (**H**eteronuclear **M**ultiple **B**ond **C**orrelation) [1], the purpose of which is to suppress correlations via $^1J(C,H)$. Since this suppression is not perfect, one usually does not apply ^{13}C-decoupling, so that cross peaks caused by ^1J and $^{2/3}J(C,H)$ coupling constants can be distinguished. The gradient selected version is given in Experiment 11.6.

2. Literature

[1] A. Bax, M. F. Summers, *J. Am. Chem. Soc.* **1986**, *108*, 2093–2094.
[2] G. E. Martin, A. S. Zektzer, *Two Dimensional NMR Methods for Establishing Molecular Connectivity*, VCH, Weinheim, **1988**, 267–273.

3. Pulse Scheme and Phase Cycle

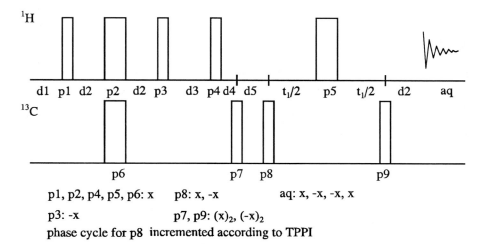

p1, p2, p4, p5, p6: x   p8: x, -x   aq: x, -x, -x, x

p3: -x   p7, p9: $(x)_2$, $(-x)_2$

phase cycle for p8   incremented according to TPPI

4. Acquisition

Time requirement: 9 h

Sample: 5% ethyl crotonate in CDCl$_3$

Record normal 1D ^{1}H and ^{13}C NMR spectra, optimize the spectral widths and note the offsets. Switch to the 2D mode of the spectrometer software, load the phase-sensitive HMBC pulse program including the BIRD filter, and if required, change the spectrometer to the inverse set-up. You have to set:

td2: 1 k data points in F_2
td1: 128 data points in F_1
sw2: 8 ppm
sw1: 175 ppm
offset of ^{1}H frequency: middle of ^{1}H NMR spectrum
offset of ^{13}C frequency: middle of ^{13}C NMR spectrum
p1, p3, p4: 90° ^{1}H transmitter pulse
p2, p5: 180° ^{1}H transmitter pulse
p7, p8, p9: 90° ^{13}C decoupler pulse
p6: 180° ^{13}C decoupler pulse
d1: 1 s
d2: $1/[2J(C,H)] = 50$ ms, calculated from $^nJ(C,H) = 10$ Hz
d3: BIRD delay to be optimized for minimum FID, ca. 1 s; observe in the set-up mode the incoming FID and adjust d3 for minimum intensity (see Exp. 6.12)
d4: $1/[2J(C,H)] = 3.5$ ms, calculated from $^1J(C,H) = 145$ Hz
d5: 46.5 ms (d5 = d2 – d4)
initial value for t_1 evolution: 3 µs
increment for t_1 evolution: $1/[4 \cdot sw1]$
ds: 2
ns: 128

5. Processing

Apply zero-filling in F_1 to 256 real data points to obtain a matrix of 512·256 real data points. Use exponential or Gaussian windows in both dimensions. Apply real Fourier transformation corresponding to the TPPI type signal selection using the quadrature mode in F_1. Phase correction in both dimensions is required.

6. Result

The figure on page 317 shows the HMBC spectrum obtained on an ARX-200 spectrometer in a normal forward dual probe-head. This demonstrates that a special inverse probe-head is not an absolute necessity. Note that the 2D spectrum shown is split into two different ranges, since it is often difficult to display cross-peaks of broad multiplets with the same treshold value as used for the sharp singlets. The cross-signals caused by $^1J(C,H)$ of C-6 and C-3 are still observable, but those arising from $^3J(C,H)$ or $^2J(C,H)$ are predominant.

7. Comments

The description of the HMQC and BIRD parts of the sequence in the product operator formalism has been given in Experiments 10.11 and 6.12. The pulse p7 in the pulse sequence acts as a low-pass filter. Coherences stemming from $^1J(C,H)$ are suppressed by the phase cycle of p7. This, however, does not work equally well for all protons; therefore it is advisable not to use GARP decoupling in this sequence, so that one can distinguish between signals arising from ^1J and those from ^2J or ^3J.

8. Own Observations

Experiment 10.14

The Basic HSQC Experiment

1. Purpose

Whereas the HMQC experiment 10.11 performs the H,C correlation via the ^{13}C chemical shift evolution of a *double* quantum coherence, this can also be achieved by the HSQC (Heteronuclear *Single* Quantum Coherence) method. This is sometimes superior in the case of a crowded ^{13}C NMR spectrum, as in this sequence the signals are not broadened by homonuclear H,H coupling in F_1. The HSQC scheme is included as a building block in many 3D sequences. The following example describes the phase-sensitive technique, which is also known as the "Overbodenhausen experiment" in the NMR jargon. A gradient selected version including a sensitivity enhancement is given in Experiment 11.7.

2. Literature

[1] G. Bodenhausen, D. J. Ruben, *Chem. Phys. Lett.* **1980**, *69*, 185–188.

3. Pulse Scheme and Phase Cycle

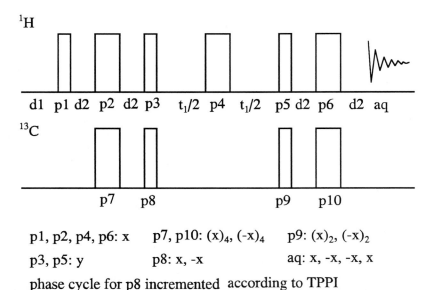

p1, p2, p4, p6: x   p7, p10: (x)$_4$, (-x)$_4$ p9: (x)$_2$, (-x)$_2$

p3, p5: y   p8: x, -x   aq: x, -x, -x, x

phase cycle for p8 incremented according to TPPI

4. Acquisition

Time requirement: 40 min

Sample: 5% ethyl crotonate in $CDCl_3$

Record normal 1D ^1H and ^{13}C NMR spectra, optimize the spectral widths and note the offsets. Switch to the 2D mode of the spectrometer software, load the HSQC pulse program, and if required, change the spectrometer to the inverse set-up. You have to set:

> td2: 1 k data points in F_2
> td1: 128 data points in F_1
> sw2: 8 ppm
> sw1: 175 ppm
> offset of ^1H frequency: middle of ^1H NMR spectrum
> offset of ^{13}C frequency: middle of ^{13}C NMR spectrum
> p1, p3, p5: 90° ^1H transmitter pulse
> p2, p4, p6: 180° ^1H transmitter pulse
> p8, p9: 90° ^{13}C decoupler pulse
> p7, p10: 180° ^{13}C decoupler pulse
> d1: 2 s
> d2: $1/[4J(C,H)] = 1.72$ ms, calculated from $^1J(C,H) = 145$ Hz
> initial increment for t_1 evolution: 3 μs
> increment for t_1 evolution: $1/[4 \cdot sw1]$
> ds: 2
> ns: 8

5. Processing

Apply zero filling in F_1 to 256 real data points to obtain a matrix of 512·256 real data points. Use exponential windows in both dimensions. Apply real Fourier transformation corresponding to the TPPI mode signal selection using the quadrature mode in F_1. Phase correction in both dimensions is necessary.

6. Result

The figure on page 320 shows the HSQC spectrum obtained on an ARX-200 spectrometer in a normal forward dual probe-head. This demonstrates that a special inverse probe-head is not an absolute necessity. Note that the spectrum displays in F_2 doublets with the $^1J(C,H)$ spin coupling constant and, in addition, the homonuclear splittings caused by H,H spin couplings. There is considerable breakthrough of signals from the protons bound to ^{12}C since no additional filter was used.

7. Comments

The sequence consists of an INEPT transfer from proton to ^{13}C (see Exp. 6.5), a t_1 period with a 180° pulse on the protons, and a reverse INEPT transfer (see Exp. 6.8) from ^{13}C to proton. As described in Experiment 6.5, the first INEPT transfer results in antiphase magnitization of ^{13}C with respect to proton, $-2I_{Hz}I_{Cy}$ single quantum coherence is present. During t_1 this term develops ^{13}C chemical shift as described by Equation (1). The 180° proton pulse p4 (in the middle of t_1) decouples $J(C,H)$ spin coupling which develops in F_1 and for simplicity is not shown in the equations. The last 90° ^{13}C pulse p9 together with the 90° proton pulse p5 transfers the cosine term back into antiphase of the proton with respect to ^{13}C as in Equation (2). During the subsequent refocusing period, an observable in-phase magnetization develops.

$$-2I_{Hz}I_{Cy} \cdot \xrightarrow{\Omega_C \, t_1 \, I_{Cz}} -2I_{Hz}I_{Cy}\cos\Omega_C t_1 + 2I_{Hz}I_{Cx}\sin\Omega_C t_1 \qquad (1)$$

$$\xrightarrow{I_{Cx}} \xrightarrow{I_{Hy}} -2I_{Hx}I_{Cz}\cos\Omega_C t_1 + 2I_{Hx}I_{Cx}\sin\Omega_C t_1 \qquad (2)$$

With regard to sensitivity, the HMQC and HSQC sequences should be identical, since both start with a proton coherence which is transfered to carbon and back to proton. However, HSQC uses 10 r.f. pulses and is therefore more sensitive to experimental error. Nevertheless, in protein research this sequence is of primary importance for N,H correlation, since the correlation signals are not broadened in F_1 by homonuclear coupling.

8. Own Observations

Experiment 10.15

The HOHAHA or TOCSY Experiment

1. Purpose

Homonuclear correlation as described for the COSY technique (see Exps. 10.3–10.7) generally correlates protons via a geminal or vicinal spin coupling. Relayed methods have been proposed to step further along a scalar-coupled spin system. The HOHAHA (**HO**monuclear **HA**rtmann **Ha**hn) or TOCSY (**TO**tal **C**orrelation **S**pectroscop**Y**) method [1, 2], can in principle give a total correlation of all protons of a chain with each other. The technique is therefore mostly used for peptides or oligosaccharides, since here it serves for the identification of single residues. In this experiment the basic phase-sensitive method using an MLEV-17 spin-lock is described; many variations, including a selective method (see Exp. 7.8) and a gradient-selected method (see Exp. 11.8) are known.

2. Literature

[1] L. Braunschweiler, R. R. Ernst, *J. Magn. Reson.* **1983**, *53*, 521–528.
[2] A. Bax, D. G. Davis, *J. Magn. Reson.* **1985**, *65*, 355–360.
[3] G. E. Martin, A. S. Zektzer, *Two Dimensional NMR Methods for Establishing Molecular Connectivity*, VCH, Weinheim, **1988**, 303–316.

3. Pulse Scheme and Phase Cycle

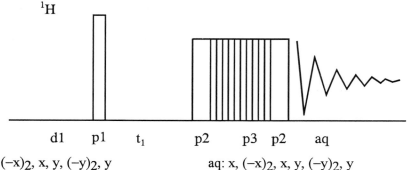

p1: x, (–x)$_2$, x, y, (–y)$_2$, y   aq: x, (–x)$_2$, x, y, (–y)$_2$, y
p2: (x, –x)$_2$, (y, –y)$_2$ (trim pulses)
p3: spinlock out of composite 180° pulses (90°, 180°, 90°); sequence:

90 (ph1), 180 (ph2), 90 (ph1)   ph1: (–y, y)$_2$, (x, –x)$_2$
[90 (ph3), 180 (ph4), 90 (ph3)]$_2$ ph2: (x, –x)$_2$, (y, –y)$_2$
90 (ph1), 180 (ph2), 90 (ph1)   ph3: (y, –y)$_2$, (–x, x)$_2$
[90 (ph3), 180 (ph4), 90 (ph3)]$_2$ ph4: (–x, x)$_2$, (–y, y)$_2$
[90 (ph1), 180 (ph2), 90 (ph1)]$_2$

90 (ph3), 180 (ph4), 90 (ph3)
[90 (ph1), 180 (ph2), 90 (ph1)]$_2$
90 (ph3), 180 (ph4), 90 (ph3)
[90 (ph1), 180 (ph2), 90 (ph1)]$_2$
[90 (ph3), 180 (ph4), 90 (ph3)]$_2$
60 (ph2)

4. Acquisition

Time requirement: 20 min

Sample: 10% strychnine in CDCl$_3$

Prior to the experiment the 90° pulse-width and transmitter attenuation for the spin-lock pulses must be calibrated (see Exp. 2.6). For optimum results one should make allowance for the phase difference between the hard pulse p1 and the spin-lock pulses, either in the pulse program or in the adjustable parameter set if the software allows (see Exp. 7.1). Run a normal ^{1}H NMR spectrum of the sample and optimize the spectral width. The duration of the spin-lock is an adjustable parameter. You have to set:

> td2: 1 k data points in F_2
> td1: 128 data points in F_1
> sw2: 10 ppm
> sw1: 10 ppm
> o1: middle of ^{1}H NMR spectrum
> p1: 90° ^{1}H transmitter pulse
> p2: ^{1}H trim pulse, 2.5 ms at transmitter attenuation of spin-lock (12 dB)
> p3: series of composite 180° ^{1}H pulses (90°, 180°, 90°) at transmitter attenuation of spin-lock; 90° pulse-width and transmitter attenuation typically in the order of 40 µs and 12 dB, corresponding to an effective spin-lock field of ca. 7000 Hz (magnetic field dependent). Total length of spin-lock set to 200 ms by 2· p2 + loop parameter of spin-lock sequence. The loop parameter must be an even number; 76 was used here.
> d1: 2 s
> initial value for t_1 evolution: 3 µs
> increment for t_1 evolution: 1/[2·sw1]
> ds: 2
> ns: 4

5. Processing

Apply zero filling in F_1 to 512 real data points to obtain a symmetrical matrix of 512· 512 real data points. Use exponential windows in both dimensions corresponding to the digital resolution. Apply real Fourier transformation corresponding to the TPPI mode of data acquisition in F_1. Phase correction in both dimensions is necessary.

6. Result

The figure shows the result obtained on an AMX-500 spectrometer. Note that the olefinic proton H-22 displays cross-peaks to many other protons and even to the H-11 pair, although H-12 and H-13 are not reached. The geminal protons H-20 give a weak correlation signal of opposite phase rather than a TOCSY correlation. This is probably a ROESY transfer because of the relatively long spin-lock duration used in this experiment.

7. Comments

During the spin-lock time the spins "see" only B_1 as the effective field; therefore their chemical shift differences become negligible and the spin systems are all of higher order, leading to cross signals of all protons with each other along a chain of connected CH_x groups. It is possible to adjust the length of the spin-lock for different results. Thus, rather short spin-lock times (30 ms) give roughly the equivalent of a COSY spectrum, intermediate spin-lock times may display results similar to a relayed COSY, and, finally, long spin-lock times result in the desired total correlation. Another adjustable parameter is the individual 90° pulse within the spin-lock defined by the transmitter attenuation which determines the spectral width covered by the spin-lock (see Exp. 2.6).

8. Own Observations

Experiment 10.16

The NOESY Experiment

1. Purpose

The NOESY (Nuclear **O**verhauser **E**nhancement **S**pectroscop**Y**) experiment is the two-dimensional equivalent of the NOE difference experiment (see Exp. 4.7) and yields correlation signals which are caused by dipolar cross-relaxation between nuclei in a close spatial relationship. Quantitatively, however, the results differ from NOE difference spectroscopy, since the latter is a steady-state experiment, whereas NOESY is a transient experiment. In a qualitative way, the NOESY technique gives answers to many stereochemical problems such as *exo/endo*, *E/Z* and similar assignment questions. Exchanging spins also give cross-signals, see the EXSY experiment 10.20. In NMR studies of peptides and proteins NOESY is the essential method for determining peptide conformations or tertiary structure of proteins. Here we describe the basic phase-sensitive 2D method.

2. Literature

[1] J. Jeener, B. H. Meier, P. Bachmann, R. R. Ernst, *J. Chem. Phys.* **1979**, *71*, 4546–4563.
[2] D. J. States, R. A. Haberkorn, D. J. Ruben, *J. Magn. Reson.* **1982**, *48*, 286–292.
[3] G. Bodenhausen, H. Kogler, R. R. Ernst, *J. Magn. Reson.* **1984**, *58*, 370–388.
[4] D. Neuhaus, M. Williamson, *The Nuclear Overhauser Effect in Structural and Conformational Analysis*, VCH, Weinheim, **1989**, 253–305.

3. Pulse Scheme and Phase Cycle

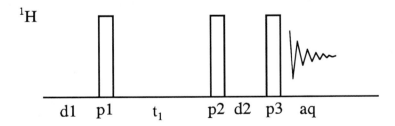

$$p1: x, -x \quad p2: (x)_8, (-x)_8 \quad p3: (x)_2, (-x)_2, (y)_2, (-y)_2$$

$$aq: x, (-x)_2, x, y, (-y)_2, y, -x, (x)_2, -x, -y, (y)_2, -y$$

phase cycle for p1 incremented according to TPPI

4. Acquisition

Time requirement: 4.5 h

Sample: 10% strychnine in $CDCl_3$; for the best results the sample should be degassed.

Run a normal ^1H NMR spectrum of the sample and optimize the spectral width. Change to the 2D mode of the spectrometer software and load the NOESY pulse program. The length of the mixing time d2 is an adjustable parameter. For small organic molecules a trial value of 1–2 s is reasonable. You have to set:

> td2: 1 k data points in F_2
> td1: 256 data points in F_1
> sw2: 10 ppm
> sw1: 10 ppm
> o1: middle of ^1H NMR spectrum
> d1: 2 s
> d2: 2 s
> p1, p2, p3: 90° ^1H transmitter pulse
> initial value for t_1 evolution: 3 μs
> increment for t_1 evolution: $1/[2 \cdot sw1]$
> ds: 2
> ns: 16

5. Processing

Apply zero filling in F_1 to 512 real data points to obtain a symmetrical matrix of $512 \cdot 512$ real data points. Use exponential windows in F_2 and F_1. Apply real Fourier transformation corresponding to the TPPI mode of data acquisition in F_1. Phase correction is usually only necessary in F_2. Adjust the phase of the diagonal signals so that they are negative. The NOESY correlation signals will then be positive if the compound has a molar mass below 1000. Correlation signals caused by chemical exchange will have the same phase as the diagonal signals.

6. Result

The figure on page 328 shows the result obtained on an AMX-500 spectrometer. Note that the phase of the diagonal signals is opposite to that of the cross-peaks as can be seen from the dotted contours. There is a wealth of information to be taken from the spectrum which can best be studied using a molecular model. Notice for instance, that only one of the H-20 protons has an NOE contact with one of the H-15 protons, from which a relative assignment of the protons in these methylene groups can be derived.

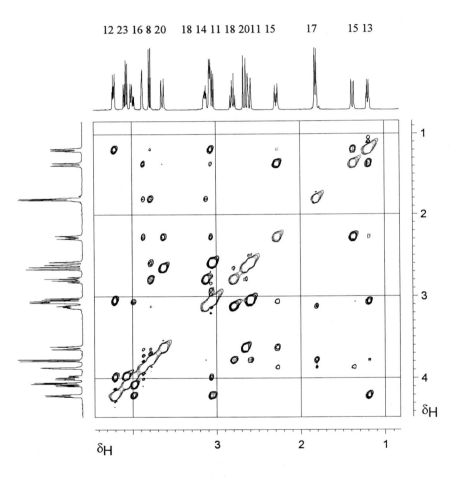

7. Comments

The NOESY sequence can be understood from the vector model. We consider two protons with different chemical shifts and no spin–spin coupling. The first pulse of the NOESY sequence aligns all proton magnetization into the x,y-plane. After this, chemical shift evolution begins during t_1. The second pulse aligns the two vectors, which are by now labeled with their individual chemical shifts into the negative z-direction. During the mixing time d2 both protons are allowed to relax and show cross-relaxation. The final pulse reads the situation at the end of the mixing time and realigns the vectors into the x,y plane, where the FID is recorded.

    A considerable drawback of the NOESY technique is the dependence of the NOE effect on molar mass and viscosity, which can change its sign and may cause it to disappear for certain conditions. The ROESY technique as described in Experiment 10.17 may be more effective in this case.

8. Own Observations

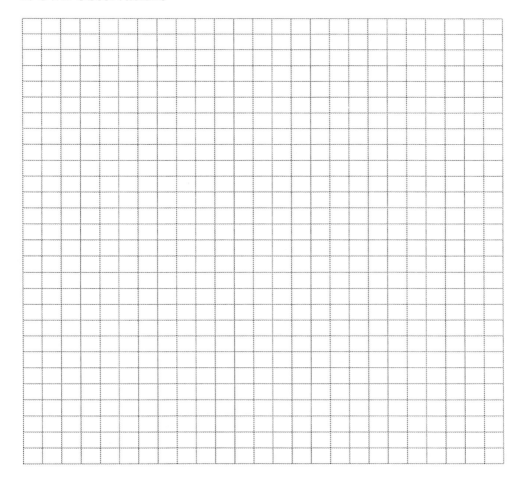

Experiment 10.17

The CAMELSPIN or ROESY Experiment

1. Purpose

The NOESY technique (see Exp. 10.16) has the disadvantage that for molecules with a molar mass in the order of 1000 to 3000 the cross-signals may disappear, since the NOE effect changes its sign depending on the molecular correlation time. However, the nuclear Overhauser effect in the rotating frame under spin-lock conditions is always positive [1,2] and this is used in the ROESY (**R**otating frame **O**verhauser **E**nhancement **S**pectroscop**Y**) experiment. One disadvantage of ROESY is that TOCSY correlations may also break through. This problem has been greatly diminished with a special spin-lock [3,4] which is used here. The experiment described gives identical results to the NOESY technique, but in a shorter time, due to the shorter mixing period during which the spin-lock is used.

2. Literature

[1] A. A. Bothner-By, R. L. Stephens, J.-M. Lee, C. D. Warren, R. W. Jeanloz, *J. Am. Chem. Soc.* **1984**, *106*, 811–813.
[2] A. Bax, D. G. Davis, *J. Magn. Reson.* **1985**, *63*, 207–213.
[3] T.-L. Hwang, A. J. Shaka, *J. Am. Chem. Soc.* **1992**, *114*, 3157–3159.
[4] T.-L. Hwang, M. Kadkhodaei, A. Mohebbi, A. J. Shaka, *Magn. Reson. Chem.* **1992**, *30*, S24–S34.
[5] D. Neuhaus, M. Williamson, *The Nuclear Overhauser Effect in Structural and Conformational Analysis*, VCH, Weinheim, **1989**, 312–327.

3. Pulse Scheme and Phase Cycle

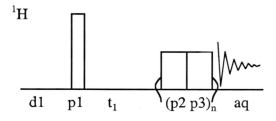

^{1}H

d1   p1 t_1 $(p2\ p3)_n'$ aq

p1: x, $(-x)_2$, x, y, $(-y)_2$, y   p2: $(-y, y)_2$, $(x, -x)_2$

p3: $(y, -y)_2$, $(-x, x)_2$ aq: x, $(-x)_2$, x, y, $(-y)_2$, y

phase cycle for p1 incremented according to TPPI

4. Acquisition

Time requirement: 2.3 h

Sample: 10% strychnine in $CDCl_3$

Prior to the experiment the 90° pulse-width and transmitter attenuation for the spin-lock pulses must be calibrated (see exp. 2.6). For optimum results one should make allowance for the phase difference between the hard pulse p1 and the spin-lock pulses either in the pulse program or in the adjustable parameter set if the software allows (see Exp. 7.1). Run a normal ^1H NMR spectrum of the sample and optimize the spectral width. Change to the 2D mode of the spectrometer software and load the ROESY pulse program. The duration of the spin-lock is an adjustable parameter. You have to set:

td2: 1 k data points in F_2
td1: 256 data points in F_1
sw2: 10 ppm
sw1: 10 ppm
o1: middle of ^1H NMR spectrum
p1: 90° ^1H transmitter pulse
p2, p3: series of 180° pulses at transmitter attenuation of spin-lock; 90° pulse
    width and transmitter attenuation typically in the order of 90 µs and 23 dB. Total duration of spin-lock set to 300 ms by loop parameter n of spin lock sequence. The loop parameter must be an even number, 832 was used here.
d1: 2 s
initial value for t_1 evolution: 3 µs
increment for t_1 evolution: $1/[2 \cdot sw1]$
ds: 2
ns: 16

5. Processing

Apply zero filling in F_1 to 512 real data points to obtain a symmetrical matrix of 512·512 real data points. Use an exponential window in F_2 and a squared $\pi/2$ shifted sinusoidal window in F_1. Apply real Fourier transformation corresponding to the TPPI mode of data acquisition in F_1. Phase correction in both dimensions is necessary. Adjust the phase of the diagonal signals negative so that the ROESY correlation signals are positive. TOCSY breakthrough signals would have the same phase as the diagonal peaks.

6. Result

The figure on page 332 shows the result obtained on an AMX-500 spectrometer. Note that the diagonal signals have a negative phase (dotted contours). No TOCSY breakthrough signals are observed. There is a wealth of information to be taken from the spectrum which can best be studied with a molecular model to hands. Note, for instance, that only one of the H-20 protons is connected with one of the H-15 protons, from which a relative assignment of these methylene protons can be derived.

7. Comments

The ROESY sequence is, in principle, identical to the TOCSY sequence as described in Experiment 10.15. After the first pulse and chemical shift evolution during the t_1 period the spins are locked by the spin-lock field B_1, which is considerably weaker in ROESY than in TOCSY. The explanation of the suppression of TOCSY correlations due to the special spin-lock sequence used here is given in the literature [3, 4]. In spectra with sharp signals near the offset (e.g. methoxy groups) artefacts have been observed.

8. Own Observations

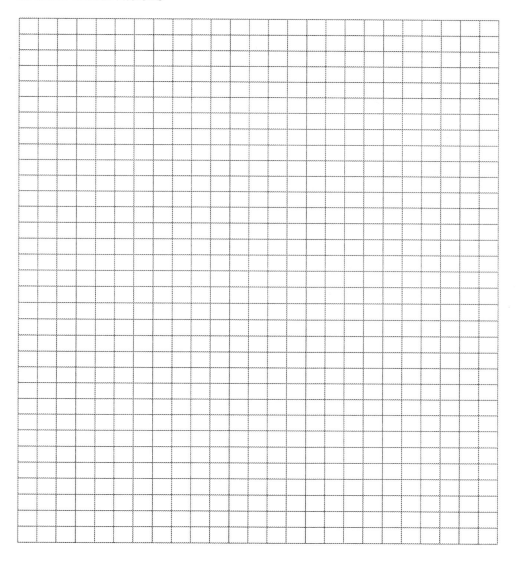

Experiment 10.18

The HOESY Experiment

1. Purpose

The HOESY (**H**eteronuclear **O**verhauser **E**ffect **S**pectroscop**Y**) experiment is the 2D equivalent of Experiment 4.14 and also has many similarities with the NOESY experiment (see Exp. 10.16), yielding information on the spatial relationship between spins in the heteronuclear case. It is therefore used to determine distances between quaternary carbon atoms and protons, especially for cases in which information from spin–spin couplings is unhelpful or unavailable. Although the experiment has been introduced for the C,H and P,H spin pairs, its predominant current application seems to be in the field of organolithium chemistry [4]. The example shown here is therefore taken from this field; the phase-sensitive version is presented.

2. Literature

[1] P. L. Rinaldi, *J. Am. Chem. Soc.* **1983**, *105*, 5167–5168.
[2] C. Yu, G. C. Levy, *J. Am. Chem. Soc.* **1983**, *105*, 6994–6996.
[3] C. Yu, G. C. Levy, *J. Am. Chem. Soc.* **1984**, *106*, 6533–6537.
[4] W. Bauer, P. v. R. Schleyer, *Adv. Carbanion Chem.* **1992**, *1*, 89–175.
[5] W. E. Hull, in: W. R. Croasmun, R. M. K. Carlson (eds.), *Two Dimensional NMR Spectroscopy*, VCH, Weinheim, **1994**, 406–409.

3. Pulse Scheme and Phase Cycle

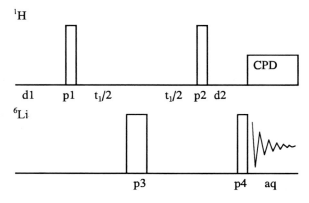

p1: $(x)_2$, $(y)_2$, $(-x)_2$, $(-y)_2$

p2, p4: x, -x, y, -y, -x, x, -y, y

p3: $(x)_8$, $(y)_8$, $(-x)_8$, $(-y)_8$

aq: $(x)_2$, $(y)_2$, $(-x)_2$, $(-y)_2$

phase cycle for p1

incremented according to TPPI

4. Acquisition

Time requirement: 9 h

Sample: commercial 1.4 M n-butyllithium in hexane; add 10% *dry* [D$_8$]THF for locking purposes. Seal the sample with parafilm. The measurement can be done at room temperature.

Since the ^{2}H and ^{6}Li NMR frequencies are very close, remove any lock stop filter from the transmitter channel at the preamplifier and tune the probe-head for ^{6}Li. Record normal ^{1}H and ^{6}Li NMR spectra, change to the 2D mode of the spectrometer, and load the HOESY pulse program. You have to set:

td2: 512 data points in F_2
td1: 128 data points in F_1
sw2: 4 ppm
sw1: 9 ppm
o1: middle of ^{6}Li NMR spectrum
o2: middle of ^{1}H NMR spectrum
p1, p2: 90° ^{1}H decoupler pulse
p3: 180° ^{6}Li transmitter pulse
p4: 90° ^{6}Li transmitter pulse
d1: 6 s
d2: 1.7 s mixing time
initial value for t_1 evolution: 3 μs
increment for t_1 evolution = 1/[4·sw1]
decoupler attenuation and 90° pulse for CPD
ds: 4
ns: 32

5. Processing

Apply zero filling in F_1 to 256 real data points. Use exponential windows in both dimensions. Apply real Fourier transformation corresponding to the TPPI mode of data acquisition in F_1. Phase correction is usually only necessary in F_2.

6. Result

The figure on page 336 shows the result obtained on an AMX-500 spectrometer with a 5 mm multinuclear probe-head. The cross peaks with the α- and β-protons of butyllithium are clearly visible. The resonance of the β-protons ($\delta_H \approx 1.6$) is hidden under one of the resonances of hexane.

7. Comments

The HOESY sequence can be understood from the simple vector analysis. The first pulse creates proton magnetization $-I_{Hy}$. This develops proton chemical shift during t_1. The 180° Li pulse removes any Li,H spin coupling during t_1 and creates $-I_{Liz}$ magnetization. After t_1 the proton pulse p2 changes the proton transverse magnetization into the negative z-direction. Now both spins are in the $-z$-direction, and the proton signal is modulated with its chemical shift information. The spins undergo cross-relaxation during the mixing time d2. The final read pulse p4 creates transverse magnetization of lithium which is detected during t_2. Note that we have chosen a rather long d1 value due to the slow spin–lattice relaxation of ^{6}Li.

8. Own Observations

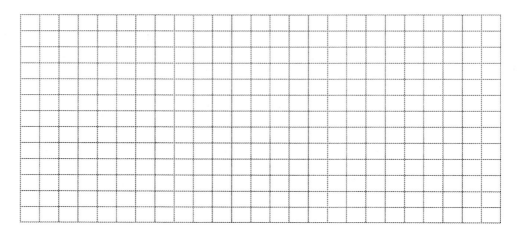

Experiment 10.19

2D-INADEQUATE

1. Purpose

The INADEQUATE procedure (Incredible Natural Abundance DoublE QUAntum Transfer Experiment) is the 2D equivalent of Experiments 6.11 and 7.7. It provides the ultimate form of structure elucidation of organic compounds in solution, since all C,C connectivities can be obtained unequivocally. The main drawback of the method is its very poor sensitivity; many attempts have therefore been made to improve its performance. Nevertheless, there is a rule of thumb by which you can judge whether a 2D-INADEQUATE experiment will be successful. Record a normal ^{13}C NMR spectrum with one transient using a 90° pulse. If the signal-to-noise ratio is better than 30:1 you might invest the time for the experiment. From the many versions known [3] we describe here the method with a 90° transfer pulse using 45° steps of phase cycling. Very recently, a gradient selected ^{1}H detected version was introduced, this is shown in Experiment 11.10.

2. Literature

[1] A. Bax, R. Freeman, T. A. Frenkiel, *J. Am. Chem. Soc.* **1981**, *103*, 2102–2104.
[2] J. Buddrus, H. Bauer, *Angew. Chem. Int. Ed. Engl.* **1987**, *26*, 625–643.
[3] W. E. Hull, in: W. R. Croasmun, R. M. K. Carlson (eds.), *Two Dimensional NMR Spectroscopy*, VCH, Weinheim, **1994**, 353–356.

3. Pulse Scheme and Phase Cycle

p1, p3: 0, 135, 90, 45, 180, 315, 270, 225, 90, 225, 180, 135, 270, 45, 0, 315,
    135, 270, 225, 180, 315, 90, 45, 0, 45, 180, 135, 90, 225, 0, 315, 270
p2: 0, 135, 90, 45, 180, 315, 270, 225, 90, 225, 180, 135, 270, 45, 0, 315,
    135, 270, 225, 180, 315, 90, 45, 0, 45, 180, 135, 90, 225, 0, 315, 270
    180, 315, 270, 225, 0, 135, 90, 45, 270, 45, 0, 315, 90, 225, 180, 135,
    315, 90, 45, 0, 135, 270, 225, 180, 225, 0, 315, 270, 45, 180, 135, 90
p4: x, y, -x, -y   aq: $(x)_8$, $(-x)_8$, $(y)_8$, $(-y)_8$

4. Acquisition

Time requirement: 15 h

Sample: 80% 1-hexanol in $[D_6]$acetone

Tune the probe-head to the actual sample, record a normal ^{13}C NMR spectrum and optimize the spectral width. Determine the ^{13}C observe pulse-width for this sample. For this experiment the instrument must be set so as to obtain optimum performance. Change to the 2D mode of the spectrometer and load the 2D-INADEQUATE pulse program. You have to set:

> td2: 1 k data points in F_2
> td1: 128 data points in F_1
> sw2: 60 ppm
> sw1: 120 ppm (double quantum frequency)
> o1: middle of ^{13}C NMR spectrum
> p1, p3, p4: 90° ^{13}C transmitter pulse
> p2: 180° ^{13}C transmitter pulse
> d1: 3 s
> d2: $1/[4J(C,C)] = 7.6$ ms, calculated from $^1J(C,C) = 33$ Hz
> decoupler attenuation and 90° pulse for CPD
> initial value for t_1 evolution: 3 μs
> increment for t_1 evolution $= 1/sw1$
> ds: 4
> ns: 128

5. Processing

Apply zero filling in F_1 to 256 real data points to obtain a matrix of 512·256 real data points. Use $\pi/2$ shifted sinusoidal windows in both dimensions. Apply complex Fourier transformation corresponding to the N type signal selection using the quadrature-off mode in F_1. Phase correction is not necessary, since the data are processed in the magnitude mode.

6. Result

The figure on page 337 shows an expansion of the 2D-INADEQUATE spectrum obtained on an ARX-200 spectrometer. Each pair of connected ^{13}C nuclei forms an AX or AB spin system, which is found in the same row of the data matrix; the pairs of doublets are symmetrical with respect to the diagonal (dotted line), and spin coupling constants can be obtained from such a row. If one carbon is connected to more than one other carbon, the corresponding doublets are found at the same chemical shift in F_2, but at another double quantum frequency in F_1. Thus the molecular carbon skeleton can be obtained by a criss-cross progression through the 2D spectrum.

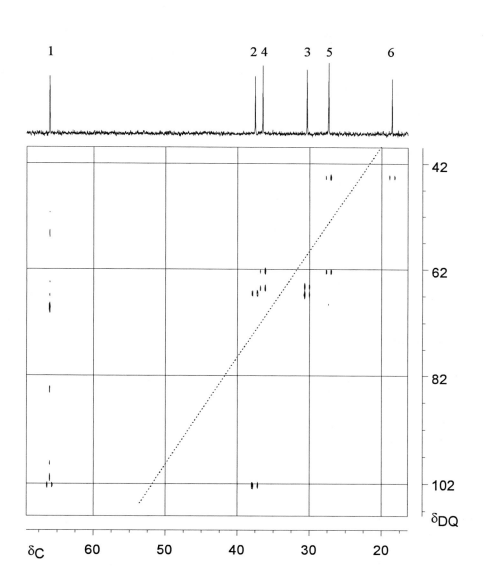

7. Comments

The product operator formalism follows the treatment given in Experiment 6.11. After the pulse p3, which creates double quantum magnetization $2I_{1x}I_{2y}$, chemical shift evolution of $2I_{1x}I_{2y}$ during t_1 yields the double quantum frequencies, of which only one typical term is shown in equation (1) for simplicity.

$$2I_{1x}I_{2y} \xrightarrow{\quad \Omega_1 t_1 I_{1z} \quad} \xrightarrow{\quad \Omega_2 t_2 I_{2z} \quad} 2I_{1x}I_{2y} \cos\Omega_1 t_1 \cos\Omega_2 t_1 \tag{1}$$

The final pulse p4 transforms the double quantum magnetization back into single quantum terms. Evolution of spin coupling between the coupled ^{13}C nuclei creates in-phase magnetization, which is detected during t_2.

On older spectrometers which are not capable of phase cycling in 45° steps, a method equivalent to the experiment shown here uses a 135° pulse for p4 to distinguish between N- and P-type signals.

8. Own Observations

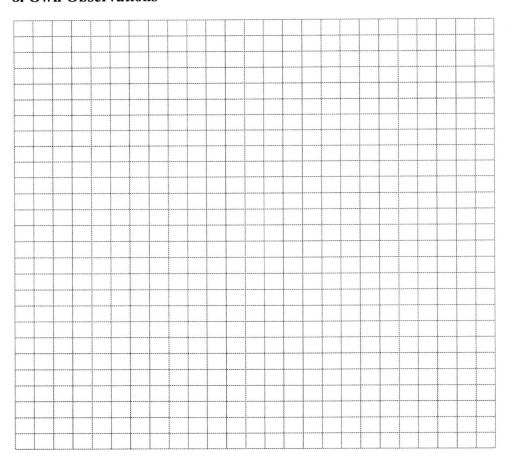

Experiment 10.20

The EXSY Experiment

1. Purpose

For the investigation of dynamic processes 1D spectra are usually recorded at different temperatures (see Exp. 5.3) and the line-broadening and coalescence of signals analyzed. The 2D EXSY (**EX**change Spectroscop**Y**) method can indicate chemical exchange before line-broadening occurs. It can therefore be regarded as the 2D equivalent of the saturation transfer experiment (see Exp. 5.4). For multisite exchange it has the important advantage that cross-signals of all exchanging species can be seen and the nature of the exchange process may be clarified by simple inspection. The pulse sequence is exactly the same as that used for phase-sensitive NOESY (Exp. 10.16).

2. Literature

[1] J. Jeener, B. H. Meier, P. Bachmann, R. R. Ernst, *J. Chem. Phys.* **1979**, *71*, 4546–4563.
[2] C. L. Perrin, T. J. Dwyer, *Chem. Rev.* **1990**, *90*, 935–967.

3. Pulse Scheme and Phase Cycle

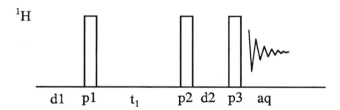

d1   p1 t_1 p2 d2 p3   aq

p1: x, -x   p2: (x)$_8$, (-x)$_8$ p3: (x)$_2$, (-x)$_2$, (y)$_2$, (-y)$_2$

aq: x, (-x)$_2$, x, y, (-y)$_2$, y, -x, (x)$_2$, -x, -y, (y)$_2$, -y

phase cycle for p1 incremented according to TPPI

4. Acquisition

Time requirement: 0.5 h

Sample: 5% DMF in $C_2D_2Cl_4$

Set up your instrument for high temperature measurement, ensure a reasonable nitrogen flow, set the temperature to 363 K, and let the sample equilibrate for at least 5 minutes. Run a normal ^1H NMR spectrum of the sample and optimize the spectral width for the methyl groups only. Change to the 2D mode of the spectrometer and load the NOESY pulse program. The length of the mixing time d2 is an adjustable parameter. You have to set:

> td2: 512 data points in F_2
> td1: 32 data points in F_1
> sw2: 0.7 ppm
> sw1: 0.7 ppm
> o1: middle of methyl group region
> p1, p2, p3: 90° ^{1}H transmitter pulse
> d1: 2 s
> d2: 1 s
> initial increment for t_1 evolution: 3 μs
> increment for t_1 evolution: $1/[2 \cdot \text{sw1}]$
> ds: 2
> ns: 4

5. Processing

Apply zero filling in F_1 to 256 real data points to obtain a symmetrical matrix of 256·256 real data points. Use exponential windows in F_2 and F_1. Apply real Fourier transformation corresponding to the TPPI mode of data acquisition in F_1. Phase correction is usually only necessary in F_2. The cross-signals caused by chemical exchange, unlike the NOESY signals, have the same phase as the diagonal signals.

6. Result

The figure on page 343 shows the result obtained on an AM-400 spectrometer. Note that the cross-signals are very strong, displaying an intensity never reached by NOE signals. In the high-resolution 1D spectrum a dynamic line broadening is not yet present. Note that the coalescence temperature is field-dependent.

7. Comments

Although the occurrence of dynamic processes is easily demonstrated qualitatively by this experiment, the extraction of rate constants is not straightforward. A whole series of EXSY spectra has to be recorded with different mixing times d2 and the volume integrals must be evaluated. Furthermore, the spin–lattice relaxation times of the exchanging spins must be known. From these data a relaxation matrix can be constructed and, using certain assumptions, the rate constants are calculated. For details see Reference [2]. For a qualitative investigation of a two site exchange, the literature gives an optimum mixing time as in Equation (1), where k_{AB} and k_{BA} are the forward and backward rate constants.

$$d2_{opt} \approx \frac{1}{T_1^{-1} + k_{AB} + k_{BA}} \tag{1}$$

8. Own Observations

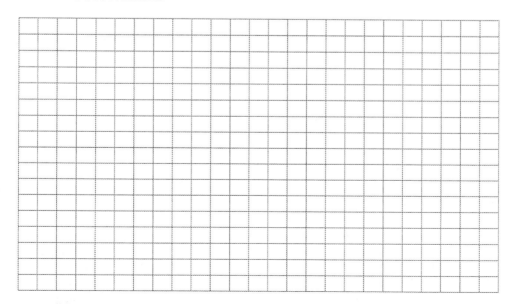

Chapter 11

NMR Spectroscopy With Pulsed Field Gradients

Although pulsed field gradients are used routinely in NMR imaging, in *in-vivo* spectroscopy, and for diffusion measurements, they have only recently been employed extensively in high-resolution NMR spectroscopy. The advantage of experiments with gradient-selection is of fundamental importance for homo- and heteronuclear 2D applications. Nearly all 3D experiments currently published use pulsed field gradients. We therefore dedicate a chapter of this book to experiments employing this technology.

Currently these experiments require special hardware for the spectrometer, however, this hardware will soon be regarded as standard equipment. A special probe-head with self-shielded gradient coils and a gradient amplifier are usually required for the experiments described. Since this field is rapidly developing at the time of writing, many experimental details, such as lock and amplifier blanking, gradient ring-down delays and pre-emphasis, for example, are very dependent on the actual hardware used and must therefore be adapted to the particular instrument of the user. Furthermore, only experiments with *z*-gradients are described, as further developments with three orthogonal gradients are outside the scope of this collection of „basic" experiments.

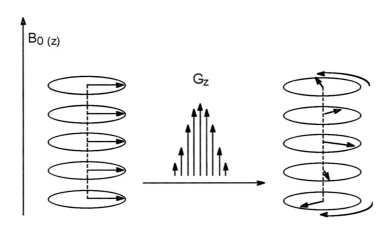

As shown in the figure, a pulsed *z*-field gradient dephases the coherences along the *z*-axis. Gradient-selected experiments rely on the fact that another identical gradient applied at a later stage of the pulse sequence can rephase these coherences if their coherence level was changed, for example by a 180° pulse. Thus one is able to select coherence pathways by combining r.f. pulses and pulsed field gradients in one pulse sequence. This task was previously performed by time-consuming phase cycling. Since the NMR receiver detects now only the desired signals, its gain can be set much higher. Therefore H,C correlations using pulsed field gradients are performed in a fraction of time formerly needed. To help in understanding the experiments described, the coherence pathway diagram is given below the pulse sequences; the pulsed field gradients are depicted with g.

In this chapter we describe how to calibrate gradients (Exp. 11.1) and to measure diffusion constants (Exp 11.2). After demonstrating a number of meanwhile common 2D experiments with gradient selection, such as gs-DQF-COSY, gs-HMQC and gs-TOCSY we also show some advanced experiments including the very recently published ^{1}H detected 2D-INADEQUATE. The chapter concludes with a water suppression technique, called WATERGATE. In addition, Chapter 12 includes a 3D procedure with gradient selection which uses the gs-TOCSY (Exp. 11.8) as a building block.

Literature

[1] T. J. Norwood, *Chem. Soc. Rev.* **1994**, 59–66.

Experiment 11.1

Calibration of Pulsed Field Gradients

1. Purpose

For all experiments working with pulsed field gradients the gradient strength has to be known in order to get meaningful results. This experiment describes a calibration routine.

2. Literature

[1] M. Holz, H. Weingärtner, *J. Magn. Reson.* **1991**, *92*, 115–125.
[2] M. I. Hrovat, C. G. Wade, *J. Magn. Reson.* **1981**, *44*, 62–75.
[3] E. Fukushima, S. B. W. Roeder, Experimental Pulse NMR, Addison–Wesley, London, **1981**, 210–215.

3. Pulse Scheme and Phase Cycle

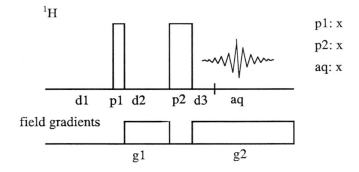

4. Acquisition

Time requirement: 20 min

Sample: Prepare a special calibration sample as shown.
In a 5 mm NMR tube two layers of normal water are separated by a rubber or Teflon disk of 2 mm thickness. The tube should be adjusted in the magnet in such a way that this disk is situated in the center of the r.f . coil. No sample spinning should be applied.

Set the instrument to normal ^{1}H NMR operation and load a pulse program as shown above. You have to set:

td: 2 k
sw: 100 KHz
o1: on resonance of water signal
p1: 90° ^{1}H transmitter pulse
p2: 180° ^{1}H transmitter pulse
d1: 1 s
d2: 10 ms
d3: 8 ms
g1: pulsed field gradient, rectangular shape, duration = 10 ms, strength to be varied
g2: pulsed field gradient, rectangular shape, duration = 20 ms, same strength as g1. Depending on the instrumentation you may in addition have to set a gradient recovery delay (100 µs), gradient coil blanking switch, and loop counters which define the shaped gradients.
ns: 1

First record a normal ^{1}H spectrum without gradients, then increase the gradient strength in several steps and observe the dip in the water signal.

5. Processing

Use standard ^{1}H processing with an exponential window (lb = 20 Hz), however, apply magnitude calculation. Measure the width of the dip [Hz], and calculate the gradient strength G_Z according to the Equation (1).

$$G_Z = \frac{\Delta\omega}{\gamma\,\Delta z} = \Delta\nu\cdot 1.17\cdot 10^{-5} \tag{1}$$

where $\Delta\omega$ is 2π times the width of the dip [Hz], γ is the proton gyromagnetic ratio $(26.751\cdot 10^7 \text{ T}^{-1}\text{s}^{-1})$ and Δz is the thickness of the disk (0.002 m). Equation (1) gives the gradient strength in tesla/m, which may be converted to gauss/cm as often used in the literature by multiplying by 100.

6. Result

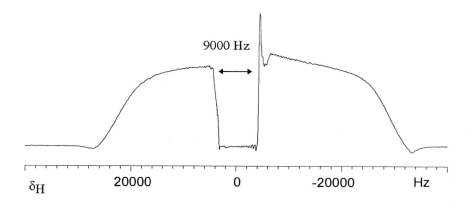

9000 Hz

δH   20000   0   -20000   Hz

The figure on page 347 shows the result obtained on an AMX-500 spectrometer with a BGU (10 A) gradient unit and an inverse gradient probe-head. The measurement of the dip is indicated. In this spectrum a gradient of 0.105 T/m was applied.

7. Comments

The experiment as described works only for superconducting magnets in which the direction of the magnetic field B_0 is vertical, i.e. along the axis of the sample tube, and the field gradient is in the same z-direction. The resonance frequency of a proton in the presence of a z-gradient is given by Equation (2).

$$\omega_z = \gamma B_{eff} = \gamma[B_0 + B_z] \tag{2}$$

Thus the resonance frequency of the proton is dependent on its z-position. A field gradient G_z can be defined as in Equation (3).

$$G_z = \frac{B_{z1} - B_{z2}}{\Delta z} = \frac{\Delta\omega}{\gamma\Delta z} \tag{3}$$

Using a sample such as the one described above with well-defined points $z1$ and $z2$ determined by the thickness of the Teflon disk, one can measure an image of the water distribution in the tube from a gradient spin-echo experiment and calculate from this image the strength of the gradients.

This experiment can be thought as a normal spin-echo sequence (see Exp. 6.2), where in addition a gradient is switched on after the first 90° pulse. For technical reasons, however, the gradient pulse is divided into two, so that the 180° r.f. pulse can be inserted in between. Each spin is spatially labeled by its resonance frequency, thus giving an image of the water distribution within the sample. The 180° pulse refocuses all magnetizations so that the spin-echo builds up to a maximum at a time d2 after the 180° pulse.

8. Own Observations

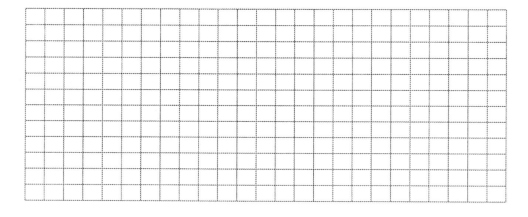

Experiment 11.2

The Pulsed Gradient Spin-Echo Experiment

1. Purpose

The PGSE (**P**ulsed **G**radient **S**pin **E**cho) experiment consists of the normal spin-echo experiment (see Exp. 6.2) with additional pulsed field gradients in both half periods before and after the 180° pulse. It was introduced to measure diffusion constants D for restricted and unrestricted diffusion in liquids. It can also be used to determine the strength of field gradients, if the diffusion constant of the sample is accurately known by other means. The experiment provides important insights into the theory and pratice of pulsed field gradients and can be viewed as one of the basic physical experiments in NMR. Here the determination of diffusion constants is shown.

2. Literature

[1] E. O. Stejskal, J. E. Tanner, *J. Chem. Phys.* **1965**, *42*, 288–292.
[2] J. R. Singer, *J. Phys. E: Sci. Instrum.* **1978**, *11*, 281–291.
[3] P. Stilbs, *Prog. NMR Spectrosc.* **1987**, *19*, 1–45.
[4] H. Weingärtner, *Z. Phys. Chem. (Neue Folge)* **1982**, *132*, 129–149.
[5] M. Holz, H. Weingärtner, *J. Magn. Reson.* **1991**, *92*, 115–125.

3. Pulse Scheme with Phase Cycle

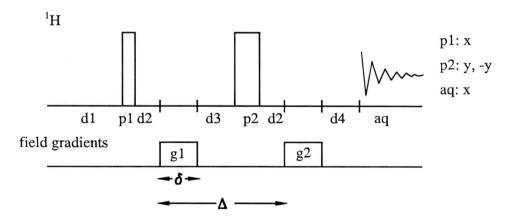

4. Acquisition

Time requirement: 0.5 h

Sample: normal H_2O

Record a normal ^{1}H NMR spectrum of the sample and center the offset at the water resonance; *set and control temperature at 298 K.* In this experiment one can vary either the gradient strength or the gradient length δ. For observation of restricted diffusion Δ would be varied, since Δ is the time during which the diffusion process occurs. In this example we vary the gradient strength. You have to set:

  td: 1 k
  sw: 1000 Hz
  o1: on resonances of water signal
  p1: 90° ^{1}H transmitter pulse
  p2: 180° ^{1}H transmitter pulse
  d1: 2 s
  d2: 1 ms
  d3: 10 ms (dependent on gradient ring-down time)
  d4: d3 minus preacquisition delay
  g1, g2: rectangular shaped field gradients, 4 ms duration and variable strength
      from 0 to 0.2 T/m in 10 steps, with gradient loop counters, ring-down delays (100 μs), lock blanking and gradient coil blanking switches according to the actual instrumentation used. Gradient strength ratio: 1 : 1.
  ns: 1

5. Processing

Process all 10 spectra identically with exponential multiplication using lb = 5 Hz and a baseline correction in order to obtain good integrals. Integrate the water signal in all spectra and refer all integrals to the integral value of the starting spectrum with gradient strength of 0. Compile a table of integral ratios I_g/I_0 vs. gradient strength G used, where the gradient strength is determined as described in Experiment 11.1. Equation (1) relates the integral ratio to the diffusion constant D.

$$\ln (I_g/I_0) = - [\gamma^2\, \delta^2\, G^2\, (\Delta - \delta/3)]\, D \tag{1}$$

Thus, a plot of $\ln(I_g/I_0)$ versus G^2 yields the diffusion constant from the slope, when the values $\gamma = 2.675 \cdot 10^8$ T^{-1}s^{-1}, $\delta = 0.004$ s, and $\Delta = 0.0151$ s are inserted.

6. Result

The table gives the results obtained on an AMX-500 spectrometer equipped with a BGU(10A) gradient unit and an inverse multinuclear gradient p51, giving a value of $D = 2 \cdot 10^{-9}$ m^2/s, which is reasonably close to the accepted literature value of $2.30 \cdot 10^{-9}$ m^2/s [4, 5].

G [T/m]	0	0.022	0.045	0.065	0.089	0.11	0.13	0.15	0.18	0.19	0.22
I_g/I_0	1	0.96	0.92	0.88	0.82	0.73	0.62	0.52	0.40	0.30	0.22

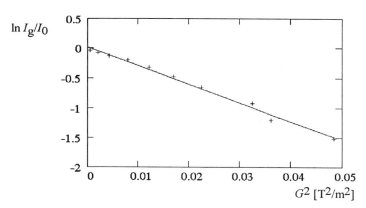

7. Comments

In the normal spin-echo experiment the echo amplitude is dependent on the spin–spin relaxation time and the diffusion constant. If the magnetic field is homogeneous, the latter does not affect the measurement. In the PGSE experiment the pulsed field gradient during the first half period positionally labels the spins with their Larmor frequency. The 180° pulse reverses the coherence order and the second gradient pulse therefore rephases all nuclear spins except those which have diffused during the time period Δ. Thus, the echo amplitude varies strongly with the gradient field strength.

The diffusion constant D is given theoretically by the Stokes–Einstein equation (2), where k_B is the Boltzmann constant, η the viscosity, and r the radius of the molecular sphere.

$$D = \frac{k_B T}{6\pi\eta r} \qquad (2)$$

Often a modification of Equation (2) with a factor 4 instead of 6 in the denominator is used when the surrounding particles are of similar size compared to the solute (slip boundary condition).

8. Own Observations

Experiment 11.3

Gradient Selected H,H-COSY

1. Purpose

In a 2D experiment it is necessary to distinguish the sign of the frequencies in the F_1 dimension. This is usually achieved by phase cycling, which requires up to four transients per t_1 increment including the suppression of axial peaks. Different phase cycling methods are used to perform the required coherence pathway selection. However, by using pulsed field gradients this coherence pathway selection can be achieved with only one scan per t_1 increment. Thus, if enough substance is available, a typical gs-COSY experiment with 256 time increments can be recorded in 10 minutes.

2. Literature

[1] R. E. Hurd, *J. Magn. Reson.* **1990**, *87*, 422–428.
[2] M. von Kienlin, C. T. W. Moonen, A. van der Toorn, P. C. M. van Zijl, *J. Magn. Reson.* **1991**, *93*, 423–429.

3. Pulse Scheme and Phase Cycle

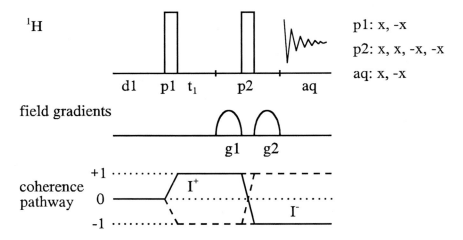

p1: x, -x
p2: x, x, -x, -x
aq: x, -x

4. Acquisition

Time requirement: 10 min

Sample: 10% strychnine in CDCl$_3$

Record a normal ^{1}H NMR spectrum of the sample and optimize the spectral width. For the 2D experiment you have to set:

td2: 1 k data points in F_2
td1: 256 data points in F_1
sw2: 10 ppm
sw1: 10 ppm
o1: middle of ^{1}H NMR spectrum
p1, p2: 90° ^{1}H transmitter pulse
d1: 2 s
initial value for t_1 evolution: 3 μs
increment for t_1 evolution: 1/sw1
g1, g2: sinusoidal shaped field gradients with 1% truncation, 2 ms duration
    and 0.01 T/m strength, with gradient loop counters, ringdown delays (100
    μs), lock blanking and gradient coil blanking switches according to actual
    instrumentation used. Gradient strength ratio 1 : 1.
ds: 4
ns: 1

5. Processing

Apply zero filling in F_1 to 512 words in order to have a symmetrical matrix of 512·512 real data points. Use unshifted sinusoidal windows in both dimensions. Apply complex Fourier transformation as for the standard N or P type COSY. Instead of phase correction use the absolute value mode; symmetrization of the matrix may be performed.

6. Result

The figure on p. 354 shows the expansion of a 2D spectrum obtained on an AMX-500 spectrometer with an inverse multinuclear gradient probe-head and a 10 A gradient unit. Symmetrization has been used. Note that the intensities of the cross peaks reflect to some extent the magnitude of the spin coupling constants.

7. Comments

Gradient experiments are best understood by using shift operators I^+ and I^- and constructing a coherence pathway diagram like the one shown above. The first pulse of the COSY sequence creates $-I_y$ magnetization, which can be written in shift operator terms as in Equation (1).

$$-I_y = -1/2\, i\, (I^+ - I^-) \tag{1}$$

Both coherence levels, the I^+ and the I^- paths are, after t_1 evolution, dephased by the first gradient g1. The second 90° pulse transforms I^+ and I^- according to Equation (2).

$$I^+ \xrightarrow{\ 90°\,I_x\ } 1/2\, I^+ + 1/2\, I^- + iI_z \;;\; I^- \xrightarrow{\ 90°\,I_x\ } 1/2\, I^- + 1/2\, I^+ - iI_z \tag{2}$$

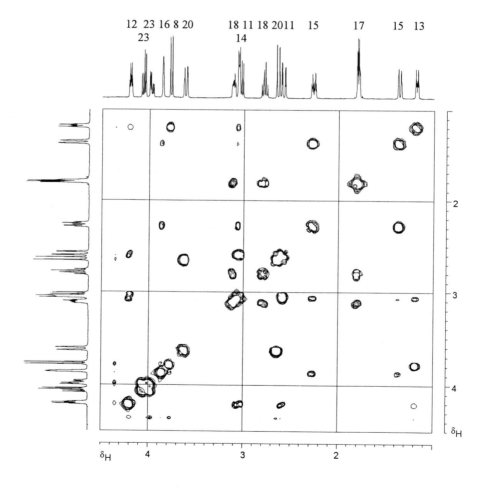

The second gradient, being identical to the first, further dephases those coherences, which have not changed their coherence order after the second r.f. pulse, but rephases those which changed the sign of the coherence order. Since, by definition, the NMR instruments detect only the I^- level, we have with this experiment selected the I^+ pathway shown in the diagram above.

The chemical shift information during t_1 can be written for the I^+ pathway as in Equation (3).

$$I^+ \xrightarrow{\Omega\, t_1 I_z} I^+\exp(-i\Omega t_1) = I^+ (\cos\Omega t_1 + i\, \sin\Omega t_1) \tag{3}$$

Therefore, both cosine and sine components are retained and added together as in the standard N-type COSY experiment, leading to phase-skewed lineshapes and requiring complex Fourier transformation in the 2D processing.

8. Own Observations

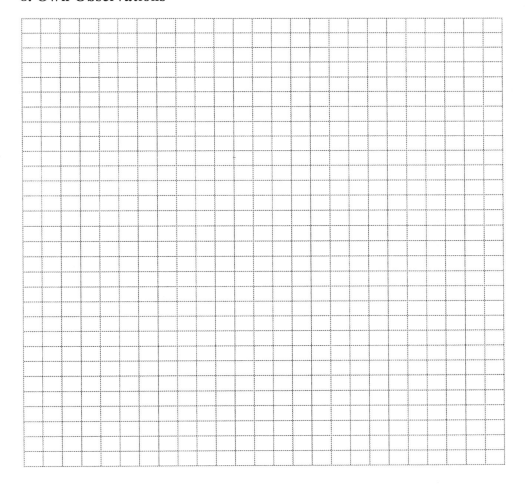

Experiment 11.4

Gradient-Selected Phase-Sensitive DQF-COSY

1. Purpose

The normal gs-COSY experiment (11.3) solves the problem of distinguishing the sign of the frequencies in F_1 without phase cycling, but gives 2D spectra with phase-skewed line-shapes. The double quantum filtered (DQF) COSY experiment can also be performed using gradient pulses, where the gradients serve as the double quantum filter. In contrast to the normal gs-COSY, this experiment can be carried out in the phase-sensitive mode, thus giving 2D spectra with correct line-shapes, again with only a single scan per time increment. Since in COSY spectroscopy one is usually interested only in cross-peaks, which have at least double quantum character, this variant of the COSY experiment will probably become the most popular one in future. Furthermore, due to the gradient double quantum filter one can achieve good solvent suppression.

2. Literature

[1] R. E. Hurd, *J. Magn. Reson.* **1990**, *87*, 422–428.
[2] I. M. Brereton, S. Crozier, J. Field, D. M. Doddrell, *J. Magn. Reson.* **1991**, *93*, 54–62.
[3] A. L. Davis, E. D. Laue. J. Keeler, D. Moskau, J. Lohman, *J. Magn. Reson.* **1991**, *94*, 637–644.

3. Pulse Scheme with Phase Cycle

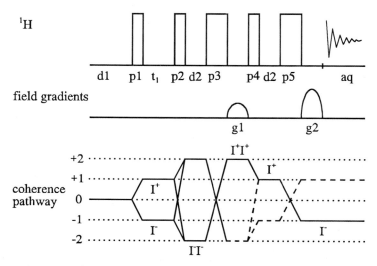

p1: x, -x   phase cycle for p1 incremented according to TPPI
p2, p3, p4, p5: x   aq: x, -x

4. Acquisition

Time requirement: 1 h

Sample: 10% strychnine in CDCl$_3$

Record a normal ^{1}H NMR spectrum of the sample and optimize the spectral width. Change to the 2D mode of the spectrometer software and load the pulse program for gradient selected double quantum COSY. You have to set:

td2: 2 k data points in F_2
td1: 512 data points in F_1
sw2: 10 ppm
sw1: 10 ppm
o1: middle of ^{1}H NMR spectrum
p1, p2, p4: 90° ^{1}H transmitter pulse
p3, p5: 180° ^{1}H transmitter pulse
d1: 2 s
d2: equal to effective length of gradient used, here 2 ms
initial value for t_1 evolution: 3 μs
increment for t_1 evolution: 1/[2·sw1]
g1, g2: sinusoidal shaped field gradients with 1% truncation, 2 ms duration and 0.01 T/m strength, with gradient loop counters, ringdown delays (100 μs), lock blanking and gradient coil blanking switches according to actual instrumentation used. Gradient strength ratio: 1 : 2.
rg: One must be very careful by setting the receiver gain for this experiment. The gradient filter allows only the desired coherences to pass into the receiver, however, the double quantum coherences develop only at higher t_1 increments. The receiver gain must therefore be set using a high t_1 increment to avoid overloading.
ds: 4
ns: 4

5. Processing

Apply zero filling in F_1 to 1 k words in order to have a symmetrical matrix of 1024·1024 data points. Use exponential or Gaussian windows in both dimensions corresponding to the point/Hz resolution of your data set. Apply real Fourier transformation in both dimensions. Phase correction in F_2 can be performed after the 2D transformation in order to get clean up/down patterns of the cross peaks. Zero order phase correction of 90° has to be applied in the F_1-dimension.

6. Result

The figure on page 358 shows the expansion of a 2D spectrum obtained on an AMX-500 spectrometer with an inverse multinuclear gradient probe-head and a BGU (10 A) gradient unit. Note that dotted contours represent negative signals.

7. Comments

As the normal DQF-COSY procedure (see Exp. 10.7) this experiment uses three 90°
pulses where the first two generate double quantum magnetization, whereas the last
(reading) pulse transfers it back into observable magnetization. Instead of phase cycling as in Experiment 10.7 the two gradients act as the double quantum filter. The two
180° pulses correct the phase problems introduced by the final length of the gradients;
therefore d2 should be set exactly equal to the total gradient length including ring-
down time.

As can be seen from the coherence pathway diagram above, the first gradient g1
acts during a period when double quantum magnetization I^+I^+ is present (coherence
level +2) , whereas the second acts at during a period when single quantum coherence
$-I^-$ is present, thus g2 must have twice the gradient strength of g1. All other coherences are further dephased and are not observable. Note that during t_1 both I^+ and I^-
are developing chemical shift information; thus the full phase information is retained
and can be stored separately for different time increments e.g. using the TPPI mode of
phase cycling for the first pulse. Of course, due to the double quantum filter there is a
sensitivity loss compared with the gs-COSY procedure described in Experiment 11.3.

8. Own Observations

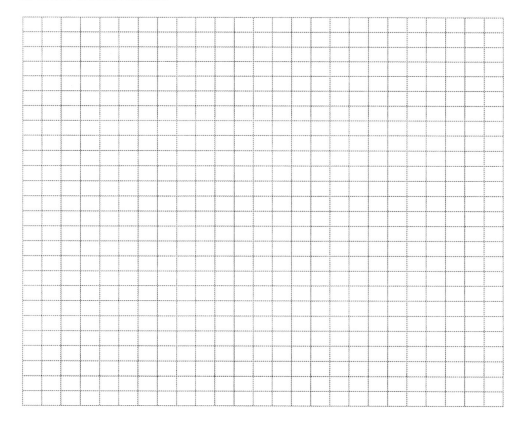

Experiment 11.5

Gradient-Selected HMQC

1. Purpose

The normal HMQC experiment (see Exp. 10.11) uses the BIRD filter and phase cycling to suppress the undesired signals of protons bound to ^{12}C. With pulsed field gradients the selection of the desired coherences can be drastically improved. This yields artefact free H,C correlation spectra in a fraction of the time needed previously, since the receiver gain of the proton channel can be set to a very high value. The version shown here is not phase-sensitive.

2. Literature

[1] R. E. Hurd, B. K. John, *J. Magn. Reson.* **1991**, *91*, 648–653.
[2] J. Ruiz-Cabello, G. W. Vuister, C. T. W. Moonen, P. van Gelderen, J. S. Cohen, P. C. M. van Zijl, *J. Magn. Reson.* **1992**, *100*, 282–303.
[3] W. Wilker, D. Leibfritz, R. Kerssebaum, W. Bermel, *Magn. Reson. Chem.* **1993**, *31*, 287–292.

3. Pulse Scheme and Phase Cycle

4. Acquisition

Time requirement: 10 min

Sample: 10% strychnine in $CDCl_3$

Record normal ^1H and ^{13}C NMR spectra of the sample and optimize the spectral width for CH_n signals. Change to the 2D mode of the spectrometer and load the gs-HMQC pulse program. You have to set:

td2: 1 k data points in F_2
td1: 256 data points in F_1
sw2: 10 ppm
sw1: 165 ppm
o1: middle of ^1H NMR spectrum
o2: middle of ^{13}C NMR spectrum
p1: 90° ^1H transmitter pulse
p2: 180° ^1H transmitter pulse
p3, p4: 90° ^{13}C decoupler pulse
d1: 2 s
d2: $1/[2J(C,H)] = 3.57$ ms, calculated from $^1J(C,H) \approx 140$ Hz
d3: set equal to d2 minus gradient length
start increment for t_1 evolution: 3 μs
increment for t_1 evolution: $1/[2 \cdot sw1]$
g1, g2, g3: sinusoidal shaped field gradients with 5% truncation, 2 ms duration and ca. 0.01 T/m strength, with gradient loop counters, ring-down delays (100 μs), lock blanking and gradient coil blanking switches according to actual instrumentation used. Gradient strength ratio: 5 : 3 : 4
^{13}C decoupler attenuation and 90° pulse for GARP (19 dB, 70 μs)
ns: 1

5. Processing

Apply zero filling in F_1 to 512 words in order to have a matrix of 512·512 real data points. Before Fourier transformation use an exponential window in F_2 with lb = 5 Hz and $\pi/3$ shifted squared sine window in F_1. Phase correction is unnecessary, since the spectrum is displayed in the magnitude mode.

6. Result

The figure on page 362 shows the 2D spectrum obtained on an AMX-500 spectrometer with an inverse multinuclear gradient probe head and a BGU (10 A) gradient unit. Note that ^{13}C nuclei with attached diastereotopic protons show two different correlation signals.

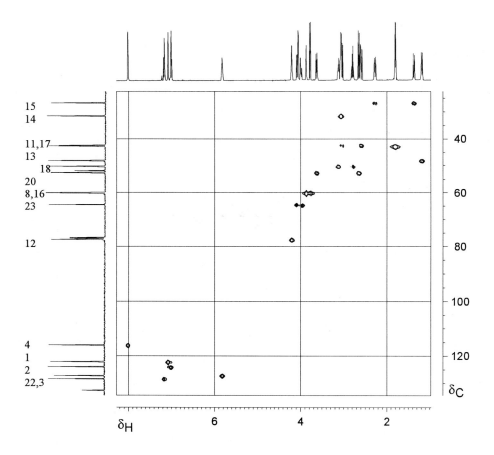

7. Comments

The r.f. pulses are the same as in the normal HMQC sequence, where the first two generate double quantum magnetization, which in the coherence pathway diagram is labeled as $I_H^+ I_C^+$. The relative gradient strength 5 of the dephasing gradient g1 corresponds to this coherence, since $\gamma_H \approx 4\gamma_C$, and the sum of the γ values is the relevant quantity. The 180° pulse in the proton channel transforms the coherence into $I_{\overline{H}} I_C^+$. At this stage the relative sum of γ values is −3. During acquisition, only $I_{\overline{H}}$ is present with a relative γ value of −4. Thus, with the gradient strength used, Equation (1) yields zero only for the selected pathway, whereas all other coherences are effectively dephased. Of course, there are other gradient ratios for which Equation (1) is also fulfilled.

$$g1\,(\gamma_H + \gamma_C) + g2\,(-\gamma_H + \gamma_C) + g3\,(-\gamma_H) = 0 \tag{1}$$

8. Own Observations

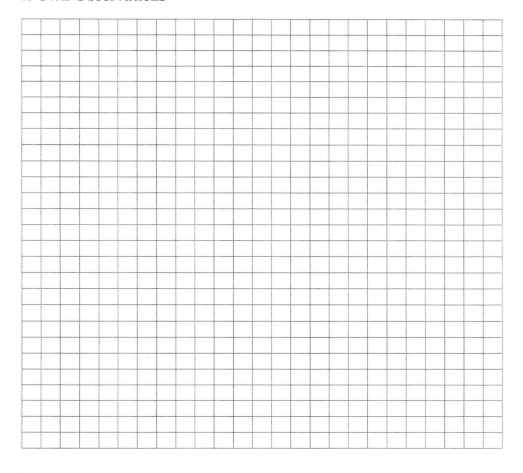

Experiment 11.6

Gradient-Selected HMBC

1. Purpose

To obtain H,C correlations via $^2J(C,H)$ and $^3J(C,H)$ the HMBC pulse sequence was developed which contains a low-pass filter to suppress correlations via $^1J(C,H)$ (see Exp. 10.13). Here we describe the gradient-selected version [2] which is not phase-sensitive. The experiment is usually performed without GARP ^{13}C decoupling. The sequence allows one to set the receiver gain considerably higher than in the normal HMBC experiment, which leads to far better results in a fraction of the time.

2. Literature

[1] A. Bax, M. F. Summers, *J. Am. Chem. Soc.* **1986**, *108*, 2093–2094.
[2] W. Wilker, D. Leibfritz, R. Kerssebaum, W. Bermel, *Magn. Reson. Chem.* **1993**, *31*, 287–292.
[3] J. Ruiz-Cabello, G. W. Vuister, C. T. W. Moonen, P. van Gelderen, J. S. Cohen, P. C. M. van Zijl, *J. Magn. Reson.* **1992**, *100*, 282–303.

3. Pulse Scheme and Phase Cycle

4. Acquisition

Time requirement: 0.5 h

Sample: 10% strychnine in CDCl$_3$

Record normal ^{1}H and ^{13}C NMR spectra of the sample and optimize the spectral width. Change to the 2D mode of the spectrometer and load the gs-HMQC pulse program. You have to set:

> td2: 1 k data points in F_2
> td1: 256 data points in F_1
> sw2: 10 ppm
> sw1: 165 ppm
> o1: middle of ^{1}H NMR spectrum
> o2: middle of ^{13}C NMR spectrum
> p1: 90° ^{1}H transmitter pulse
> p2: 180° ^{1}H transmitter pulse
> p3, p4, p5: 90° ^{13}C decoupler pulse
> d1: 2 s
> d2: 1/[2J(C,H)] = 3.57 ms, calculated from ^1J(C,H) ≈ 140 Hz
> d3: 1/[2J(C,H)] = 60 ms, calculated from ^nJ(C,H) ≈ 8 Hz
> start increment for t_1 evolution: 3 µs
> increment for t_1 evolution: 1/[2·sw1]
> g1, g2, g3: sinusoidal shaped field gradients with 5% truncation, 2 ms duration and ca. 0.01 T/m strength, with gradient loop counters, ring-down delays (100 µs), lock blanking and gradient coil blanking switches according to actual instrumentation used. Gradient strength ratio: 5 : 3 : 4
> ^{13}C decoupler attenuation and 90° pulse for GARP (ca. 70 µs)
> ns: 2

5. Processing

Apply zero filling in F_1 to 512 words in order to have a matrix of 512·512 real data points. Before Fourier transformation use an exponential window in F_2 with lb = 5 Hz and π/3 shifted squared sine window in F_1. Phase correction is unnecessary, since the spectrum is displayed in the magnitude mode.

6. Result

The figure on page 366 shows the 2D spectrum obtained on an AMX-500 spectrometer with an inverse multinuclear gradient probe-head and a BGU (10 A) gradient unit. Note the wealth of information obtainable from ^2J(C,H) and ^3J(C,H) couplings in this molecule.

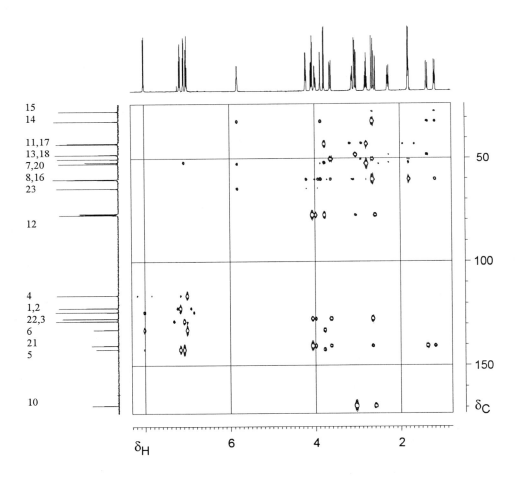

7. Comments

The first ^{13}C pulse serves as a low pass filter, by phase cycling of this pulse the signals of protons experiencing a one-bond coupling ^1J(C,H) shall be suppressed. Therefore the action of this pulse is not considered in the coherence pathway diagram. However, this suppression does not work equally well for all proton signals, and despite this low pass filter some correlation signals via ^1J(C,H) can be seen in any HMBC spectrum. In order to distinguish these signals from the desired correlations it is advisable not to use GARP decoupling. The second ^{13}C pulse selects proton signals experiencing a long-range C,H coupling. The rest of the sequence is identical to the gs-HMQC sequence as described in Exp. 11.5. Thus the discussion of the coherence pathway diagram is not repeated here.

8. Own Observations

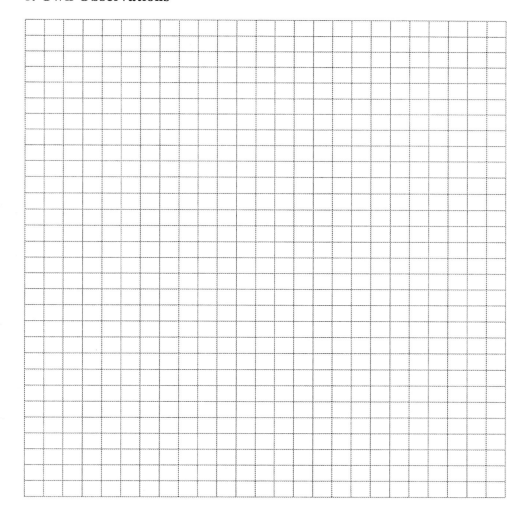

Experiment 11.7

Phase-Sensitive Gradient-Selected HSQC

1. Purpose

The two gradient-selected heteronuclear correlations given in Experiments 11.5 and 11.6 are not phase-sensitive. Gradient selected experiments can also be performed in such a way as to yield pure absorption spectra, which gives better resolution of signals in crowded regions due to the Lorentzian lineshape. The experiment shown here uses the echo/anti-echo selection method [1], which is one of the many possible approaches. Another feature of this experiment is a sensitivity enhancement by a factor of $\sqrt{2}$; however, this occurs only for CH groups [2,3].

2. Literature

[1] L. E. Kay, P. Keifer, T. Saarinen, *J. Am. Chem. Soc.* **1992**, *114*, 10663–10665.
[2] A. G. Palmer III, J. Cavanagh, P. E. Wright, M. Rance, *J. Magn. Res.* **1991**, *93*, 151–170.
[3] G. Kontaxis, J. Stonehouse, E. D. Laue, J. Keeler, *J. Magn. Res. Ser. A* **1994**, *111*, 70–76.

3. Pulse Scheme and Phase Cycle

—————   coherence pathway for N type signals
----------   coherence pathway for P type signals
....   coherence pathway for signals leading to sensitivity enhancement

4. Acquisition

Time requirement: 20 min

Sample: 10% strychnine in CDCl$_3$

Record normal ^{1}H and ^{13}C NMR spectra of the sample and optimize the spectral width for CH$_n$ signals. Change to the 2D mode of the spectrometer and load the phase sensitive gs-HSQC pulse program with echo/anti-echo acquisition. You have to set:

td2: 1 k data points in F_2
td1: 2 times 64 data points in F$_1$
sw2: 10 ppm
sw1: 165 ppm
o1: middle of ^{1}H NMR spectrum
o2: middle of ^{13}C NMR spectrum
p1, p4, p6, p8, p10: 90° ^{1}H transmitter pulse
p2, p5, p7, p9, p11: 180° ^{1}H transmitter pulse
p13, p15, p17: 90° ^{13}C decoupler pulse
p12, p14, p16, p18: 180° ^{13}C decoupler pulse
p3: 2 ms ^{1}H trim pulse
d1: 2 s
d2: $1/[4J(C,H)] = 1.8$ ms, calculated from $^1J(C,H) \approx 140$ Hz
d3: same length as gradient pulse, 1.6 ms used
initial value for t_1 evolution: 3 μs
increment for $t1$ evolution: $1/[2 \cdot sw1]$
^{13}C decoupler attenuation and 90° pulse for GARP (19 dB, 70 μs)
g1, g2: sinusoidal shaped field gradients with 5% truncation, 1.6 ms duration and ca.0.01T/m strength, with gradient loop counters, ring-down delays (100 μs), lock blanking and gradient coil blanking switches according to actual instrumentation used. Gradient strength ratio: $4 : 1 : -4 : 1$
ds: 8
ns: 1

For the phase sensitive echo/antiecho scheme in F_1 use simultaneous data mode in F_2. The pulse sequence uses one scan within the go loop. The echoes (gradients: +4,+1) and the anti-echoes (gradients: −4, +1) are stored in different blocks and are sampled with the 180° phase shift of p17. Two further loops cycle the acquisition phase and the phases of p15 and p4. Thus, the experiment shown was performed with 4 scans of 64 echo and 4 scans of 64 anti-echo accumulations.

5. Processing

Apply zero filling in F_1 to 512 words in order to have a matrix of 512·512 real data points. Use an exponential window in F_2 with lb = 3 Hz and a Gaussian window in F_1. Choose the echo/anti-echo FT mode of the software corresponding to the acquisition technique. Phase correction is usually only necessary in the F_2 dimension.

6. Result

The figure on page 370 shows an expansion of the spectrum obtained on an AMX-500 spectrometer with a BGU (10 A) gradient unit. Note that the correlation signals of CH groups (e.g. H-12, H-13, H-16) have higher intensities than those of the CH_2 groups. This is of importance in protein research, where the CH_α signals are important for the determination of the backbone structure.

7. Comments

There are several modifications to the basic HSQC procedure as described in Experiment 10.14. A proton trim pulse p3 removes unwanted coherences during the first INEPT transfer which arise from imperfect pulses. The two gradients are applied within [delay, 180° pulse, gradient] sandwiches to avoid phase errors due to the finite duration of the gradients. After the first gradient, which acts at a time, when single quantum carbon coherences $2I_{Hz}I_{Cy}$ and $2I_{Hz}I_{Cx}$ are present, a reverse INEPT sandwich transfers the $2I_{Hz}I_{Cy}$ part to in-phase magnetization I_{Hy}. However, $2I_{Hz}I_{Cx}$, is transformed into double quantum magnetization $2I_{Hy}I_{Cx}$ as shown by the dotted line of the coherence pathway diagram. The second reverse INEPT sandwich stores I_{Hy} as z-magnetization and transforms $2I_{Hy}I_{Cx}$ to I_{Hx} in-phase magnetization. The proton pulse p10 reconverts the stored z-magnetization; thus both components of the proton magnetization which are modulated with carbon chemical shift during t_1 can be observed. The final gradient rephases only the desired coherences. This sequence combines echo/anti-echo selection with the sensitivity enhancement as given by Ref. [2].

8. Own Observations

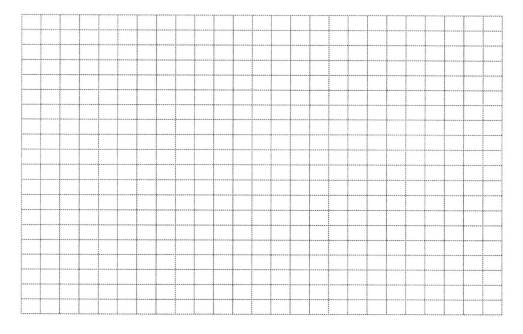

Experiment 11.8

Gradient-Selected TOCSY

1. Purpose

The TOCSY sequence as described in Experiment 10.15 uses phase cycling to achieve frequency discrimination in F_1. With the necessary suppression of axial peaks it therefore needs a minimum of four transients for each t_1 increment. The gradient-selected method shown here requires only one transient and produces a spectrum which is not phase-sensitive. Since the TOCSY experiment leads to in-phase cross-signals, the magnitude spectrum obtained here is usually sufficient to quickly provide connectivity information.

2. Literature

[1] R. E. Hurd, *J. Magn. Reson.* **1990**, *87*, 422–428.
[2] A. Bax, D. G. Davis, *J. Magn. Reson.* **1985**, *65*, 355–360.

3. Pulse Scheme and Phase Cycle

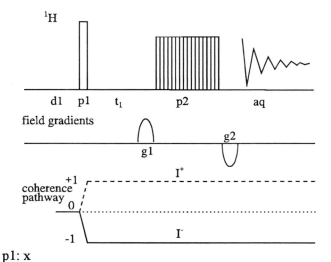

p1: x
p2: spinlock of composite 180° pulses (90°, 180°, 90°)
    using the MLEV16 sequence:
      [90(ph1), 180(ph2), 90(ph1)]$_2$ ph1: x, ph2: y
      [90(ph3), 180(ph4), 90(ph3)]$_3$ ph3: -x, ph4: -y
      [90(ph1), 180(ph2), 90(ph1)]$_2$
      [90(ph3), 180(ph4), 90(ph3)]$_3$ aq: x
      [90(ph1), 180(ph2), 90(ph1)]$_3$
      [90(ph3), 180(ph4), 90(ph3)]$_2$
      [90(ph1), 180(ph2), 90(ph1)]$_1$

4. Acquisition

Time requirement: 10 min

Sample: 10% strychnine in $CDCl_3$

Run a normal ^1H NMR of the sample and optimize the spectral width. Change to the 2D mode of the spectrometer and load the gs-TOCSY pulse program. The 90° pulse-width and attenuation of the spin-lock pulses must be calibrated prior to the experiment (see Exp. 2.6). For optimum results one should take into account the phase difference between the hard pulse p1 and the spin-lock pulses either in the pulse program or in the adjustable parameter set if the software allows (see Exp. 7.1). The duration of the spin-lock is an adjustable parameter. You have to set:

td2: 1 k data points in F_2
td1: 256 data points in F_1
sw2: 9 ppm
sw1: 9 ppm
o1: middle of ^1H NMR spectrum
p1: 90° ^1H transmitter pulse
p2: series of composite 180° pulses (90°, 180°, 90°) at transmitter attenuation
    of spin-lock; 90° pulse-width and transmitter attenuation typically in the
    order of 40 µs and 16 dB, corresponding to an effective spin-lock field of
    ca. 7000 Hz (magnetic field dependent). Duration of spin-lock set to 100
    ms by loop parameter of spin-lock sequence. The loop parameter must be
    an even number (38 was used here).
d1: 2 s
initial value for t_1 evolution: 3 µs
increment for t_1 evolution: 1/sw1
g1, g2: sinusoidal shaped field gradients with 5% truncation, 2 ms duration
    and ca. 0.01 T/m strength, with gradient loop counters, ring-down delays
    (100 µs), lock blanking and gradient coil blanking switches according to
    actual instrumentation used. Gradient strength ratio: 1 : −1
ds: 4
ns: 1

5. Processing

Apply zero filling in F_1 to 512 real data points to obtain a symmetrical matrix of 512·512 real data points. Use unshifted sinusoidal windows in both dimensions. Apply complex Fourier transformation corresponding to the quadrature-off mode of data acquisition in F_1. Since magnitude data are calculated, no phase correction is necessary.

6. Result

The figure shows the result obtained on an AMX-500 spectrometer using a BGU (10 A) gradient unit. A short spin-lock (100 ms) was used, in contrast to Experiment 10.15, and since only one transient per t_1 increment is required, twice the number of t_1 increments were recorded in half the time.

7. Comments

The MLEV-16 spin-lock consists of an even number of composite 180° pulses, so that the coherence level is not changed during its action. Since, by convention, $I_{\overline{H}}$ is detected, the pair of oppositely signed gradients selects P type signals during t_1. The signal distortions mentioned in Ref. [1] were not observed. If a MLEV-17 spin-lock sequence is used, the gradient ratio should be 1 : 1. Phase-sensitive versions using the echo/anti-echo procedure are also known.

8. Own Observations

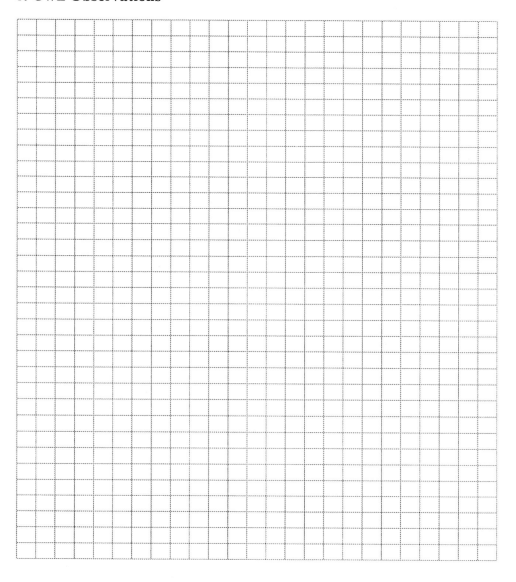

Experiment 11.9

Gradient-Selected HMQC-TOCSY

1. Purpose

The combination of the HMQC method with the TOCSY sequence leads, in principle, to a 3D technique (see Chapter 12). However, if the evolution period of the TOCSY part is omitted, one obtains a 2D sequence which provides a ^{13}C edited TOCSY spectrum. Starting from each HMQC cross-signal one finds in the same row in F_1 additional signals which are caused by a TOCSY transfer. This is very helpful for structural elucidation since normal TOCSY spectra may often be rather crowded. Compared with true 3D sequences the digital resolution is far better using significantly less measuring time. There are many variants known, here we show a non phase-sensitive gradient-selected method, which does not need a BIRD filter.

2. Literature

[1] L. Lerner, A. Bax, *J. Magn. Reson.* **1986**, *69*, 375–380.
[2] T. Domke, *J. Magn. Reson.* **1991**, *95*, 174–177.
[3] G. E. Martin, T. D. Spitzer, R. C. Crouch, J.-K. Luo, R. N. Castle, *J. Heterocyclic Chem.* **1992**, *29*, 577–582.
[4] B. K. John, D. Plant, S. L. Heald, R. E. Hurd, *J. Magn. Reson.* **1991**, *94*, 664–669
[5] W. Wilker, D. Leibfritz, R. Kerssebaum, W. Bermel, *Magn. Reson. Chem.* **1993**, *31*, 287–292.

3. Pulse Scheme and Phase Cycle

p1: x   p2: (x)$_2$, (-x)$_2$ p3: x, -x   p4: (x)$_4$, (-x)$_4$
p5: y   p7: x   aq: (x, -x)$_2$, (-x, x)$_2$
p6: spinlock of composite 180° pulses (90°, 180°, 90°)
  using the MLEV-17 sequence:
  [90(ph1), 180(ph2), 90(ph1)]$_2$ ph1: x, ph2: y
  [90(ph3), 180(ph4), 90(ph3)]$_3$ ph3: -x, ph4: -y
  [90(ph1), 180(ph2), 90(ph1)]$_2$
  [90(ph3), 180(ph4), 90(ph3)]$_3$
  [90(ph1), 180(ph2), 90(ph1)]$_3$
  [90(ph3), 180(ph4), 90(ph3)]$_2$
  [90(ph1), 180(ph2), 90(ph1)]$_1$
  [60(ph2)]

4. Acquisition

Time requirement: 1.2 h

Sample: 10% strychnine in CDCl$_3$

Record normal ^{1}H and ^{13}C NMR spectra of the sample and optimize the spectral width for CH$_n$ signals. Change to the 2D mode of the spectrometer and load the gs-HMQC-TOCSY pulse program. You have to set:

td2: 1 k data points in F_2
td1: 256 data points in F_1
sw2: 10 ppm
sw1: 165 ppm
o1: middle of ^{1}H NMR spectrum
o2: middle of ^{13}C NMR spectrum
p1: 90° [1]H transmitter pulse
p2, p7: 180° [1]H transmitter pulse
p3, p4: 90° [13]C decoupler pulse
p5: 2.5 ms ^{1}H trim pulse
p6: series of composite 180° pulses (90°, 180°, 90°) at transmitter attenuation of spin-lock; 90° pulse-width and transmitter attenuation typically in the order of 40 µs and 16 dB, corresponding to an effective spin-lock field of ca. 7000 Hz (magnetic field dependent). Last pulse 60° according to MLEV-17 scheme. Duration of spin-lock set to 81.8 ms by loop parameter of spin-lock sequence. The loop parameter must be an even number (30 was used here).
d1: 2 s
d2: 1/[2J(C,H)] = 3.57 ms, calculated from [1]J(C,H) ≈ 140 Hz
d3: d2 minus length of gradient pulse
d4: equal to length of gradient pulse
start increment for t_1 evolution: 3 µs
increment for t_1 evolution: 1/[2·sw1]
g1, g2, g3: sinusoidal shaped field gradients with 5% truncation, 2 ms duration and ca. 0.01 T/m strength, with gradient loop counters, ring-down delays

(100 μs), lock blanking and gradient coil blanking switches according to actual instrumentation used. Gradient strength ratio: 5:3:4

[13]C decoupler attenuation and 90° pulse for GARP (19 dB, 70 μs)

ds: 8

ns: 4

5. Processing

Apply zero filling in F_1 to 512 words in order to have a matrix of 512·512 real data points. Before Fourier transformation use sinusoidal windows both in F_2 and in F_1. Phase correction is unnecessary, since the spectrum is displayed in the magnitude mode.

6. Result

The figure on page 378 shows an expansion of the HMQC-TOCSY spectrum obtained on an AMX-500 spectrometer. Since a relative short spin-lock of 82 ms was used, mainly correlations over two bonds, starting from a ^{13}C nucleus, are present. Note e.g. the connectivities C-12 – H-12 – H-11$_\alpha$ and H-11$_\beta$ (δ_C = 78) or C-15 – H-15$_\alpha$ and H-15$_\beta$ to H-14 and H-16 (δ_C = 25).

7. Comments

The HMQC and TOCSY parts of the sequence have been described in Experiments 10.11 and 10.15, their gradient-selected variants in Experiments 11.5 and 11.8. Note that the TOCSY part contains no evolution time as in 3D sequences. The gradients are set similar to Experiment 11.5 for the gradient-selected HMQC, only the final refocusing gradient is set after the spin-lock. As a spin-lock a MLEV-17 sequence is used; the last 180° proton pulse inverts the coherence level once more in order to finally detect I^-. Similar information has been provided earlier by the heteronuclear relayed metods.

8. Own Observations

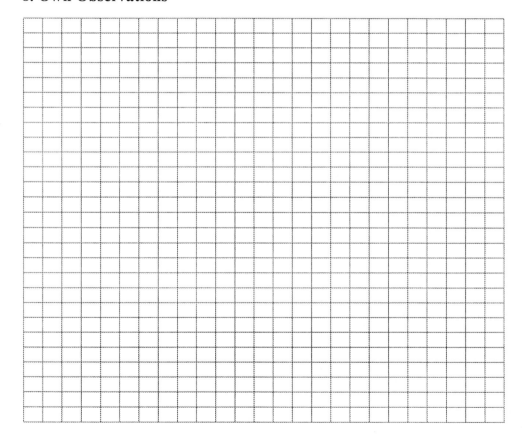

Experiment 11.10

Gradient Selected ^{1}H-Detected 2D INEPT-INADEQUATE

1. Purpose

This experiment detects carbon–carbon connectivities. In contrast to the normal 2D INADEQUATE experiment 10.19, which starts from ^{13}C magnetization and detects ^{13}C magnetization, the experiment described here starts from ^{1}H magnetization and detects ^{1}H magnetization. It is estimated to be about a factor of 13 times more sensitive than Experiment 10.19. The formidable task of suppressing protons bound to ^{12}C (1: 10 000) and protons in molecules containing only one ^{13}C nucleus (1:100) is achieved by the use of pulsed field gradients with additional phase cycling. The method lacks the generality of the normal 2D INADEQUATE since connectivities between two quaternary carbon atoms C_q–C_q cannot be detected, however it is possible to see a C_q–CH_n moiety.

2. Literature

[1] J. Weigelt, G. Otting, *J. Magn. Reson. Ser. A.* **1995**, *113*, 128–130.

3. Pulse Scheme and Phase Cycle

^{1}H   y   x   y x   x   x   x

dl   p1 d2 p2 d2 p3 p4   p5   p6 d2 p7 d2   aq

^{13}C   x   x   x   x   x   GARP

p8   p9 d3 p10 d3 p11 t1/2   t1/2   p12   p13 d3 p14 d3 p15 p16

Pulsed Field Gradients

g1   g2   g3

p8, p9. p10, p11: x, y, -x, -y   aq: x, -x, x, -x

I_H^+

I_C^+

$I_C^+ I_C^+$

$I_C^- I_C^-$

I_H^-

4. Acquisition

Time requirement: 6.5 h

Sample: 2 M sucrose in D_2O

Record normal ^1H and ^{13}C NMR spectra of the sample, note the reqired spectral widths and note the offset of the middle of each spectrum. Change to the 2D mode of the spectrometer and load the required pulse program. You have to set:

td2: 1 k data points in F_2
td1: 2 times 512 data points in F_1
sw2: 3.7 ppm
sw1: 80 ppm (C,C double quantum frequency)
o1: center of ^1H NMR spectrum
o2: center of ^{13}C NMR spectrum
p1, p4, p6: 90° ^1H transmitter pulse
p2, p5, p7: 180° ^1H transmitter pulse
p9, p11, p13, p15: 90° ^{13}C decoupler pulse
p8, p10, p12, p14, p16: 180° ^{13}C decoupler pulse
p3: 2 ms ^1H trim pulse
d1: 1.5 s
d2: $1/[4J(C,H)]$ = 1.8 ms, calculated from $^1J(C,H) \approx 140$ Hz
d3: $1/[4J(C,C)]$ = 5 ms, calculated from $^1J(C,C) \approx 50$ Hz
initial value for t_1 evolution: 3 μs
increment for t_1 evolution: $1/[2 \cdot sw1]$
g1, g2, g3: shaped field gradients with a sinusoidal start reaching a plateau after 32 data points and falling off sinusoidally with 5% truncation, 1 ms duration and ca. 0.02 T/m strength, with gradient loop counters, ring-down delays (200 μs), lock blanking and gradient coil blanking switches according to actual instrumentation used. Gradient strength ratio: 3.97 : −3.97 : 4.0 (exact γ-ratios)
Decoupler attenuation and 90° pulse for GARP (19 dB, 70 μs)
ns: 12 (see below)

For the phase-sensitive echo/anti-echo scheme in F_1 use simultaneous data mode in F_2. The pulse sequence used here for the AMX spectrometer uses one scan within the go loop. The echoes (gradients: 3.97 : −3.97 : 4) and the anti-echoes (gradients: −3.97 : +3.97 : 4) are stored in different blocks. Two further loops cycle the acquisition phase and the phases of p8–p11. Thus, the result shown was obtained with 12 scans of 512 echo and 12 scans of 512 anti-echo accumulations.

5. Processing

Use an exponential window in F_2 with lb = 6.5 Hz and a $\pi/2$ shifted squared sinusoidal window in F_1. Choose the echo/anti-echo FT mode of the software corresponding to the acquisition technique.

6. Result

The figure on page 382 shows the ^1H detected INEPT-INADEQUATE spectrum obtained on an AMX-500 spectrometer with a BGU (10 A) gradient unit. H-3 displays a double quantum signal at δ_{DQ} =182.2 which corresponds to δ_{C-2} = 104.7 + δ_{C-3} = 77.5 and another DQ signal at δ_{DQ} = 152.6 (δ_{C-3} + δ_{C-4}). This connectivity is also seen in F_2 for the signal of H-4 which shows the next DQ signal at δ_{DQ} = 157.5 (δ_{C-4} + δ_{C-5}) leading to H-5. This displays at δ_{DQ} = 145.9 the connectivity C-5–C-6. Thus the solid line gives the carbon-carbon connectivities of the fructose ring. The DQ signal of H-1 appears at δ_{DQ}= 166.0 (δ_{C-2} + δ_{C-1}) and stands alone since C-1 has no further connectivities and C-2 is a quaternary carbon atom. Similarly the glucose ring can be traced (dashed line). Note that the DQ frequencies for C-3' + C-4' and C-4' + C-5' fall together as a strong signal for H-4 at δ_{DQ} = 144.

7. Comments

The sequence starts with an INEPT transfer from protons to ^{13}C. A proton trim pulse p3 removes unwanted coherences, which arise from imperfect pulses during the first INEPT transfer. The antiphase ^{13}C magnetization $2I_{Hz}I_{Cy}$ present after p9 develops C,C spin coupling to a second ^{13}C nucleus yielding a term $4I_{Hz}I_{Cx}I_{Cz}$. This is transformed into double quantum coherence by p11. During t_1 the double quantum chemical shifts of carbon develop and are transformed back in two stages into proton magnetization, and therefore a H–C–C fragment is detected.

The gradients are applied within [delay–180° pulse–gradient] sandwiches to avoid phase errors due to the finite duration of the gradients. The first two gradients act at a time when double quantum carbon coherences $4I_{Hz}I_{Cx}I_{Cy}$ are present. The final gradient therefore rephases only the desired coherences.

8. Own Observations

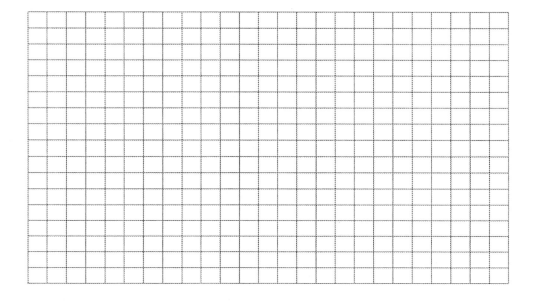

Experiment 11.11

Gradient-Selected SELINCOR

1. Purpose

This experiment yields 1D proton spectra in which the desired proton signal is selected via a selective pulse on the directly bonded ^{13}C nucleus using the $^1J(C,H)$ spin coupling. In comparison to the normal SELINCOR experiment (Exp. 7.6) the HSQC instead of the HMQC principle is used. The elimination of the signals of protons bound to ^{12}C is achieved by pulsed field gradients and is thus better by an order of magnitude. This pulse scheme can thus be used as an initial building block for a variety of subsequent sequences such as SELINCOR-COSY [1], SELINCOR-TOCSY [2], or 2D J-resolved spectroscopy. Here we show the basic gradient-selected SELINCOR building block applied to strychnine as an example.

2. Literature

[1] T. Fäcke, S. Berger, *Magn. Reson. Chem.* **1995**, *33*, 144–148.
[2] T. Fäcke, S. Berger, *Tetrahedron*, **1995**, *51*, 3521–3524.

3. Pulse Scheme and Phase Cycle

4. Acquisition

Time requirement: 1 h

Sample: 10% strychnine in CDCl3

Record both normal ^{1}H and ^{13}C NMR spectra of the sample, and note the offsets of the ^{13}C NMR signals to be irradiated by the selective pulse. You have to set:

td: 32 k
sw: 10 ppm
o1: middle of ^{1}H NMR spectrum
o2: on resonance of chosen ^{13}C NMR signal
p1, p4, p5,: 90° ^{1}H transmitter pulse
p2, p6: 180° ^{1}H transmitter pulse
p10: 90° ^{13}C decoupler pulse
p7, p9, p11: 180° ^{13}C decoupler pulse
p3: ^{1}H spin-lock pulse, same length as p8 [40 ms , 12 dB]
p8: selective 270° ^{13}C decoupler pulse, Gaussian shape, 40 ms [66 dB]
d1: 2 s
d2: 1/[4J(C,H)] = 1.8 ms, calculated from ^1J(C,H) ≈ 140 Hz
^{13}C decoupler attenuation and 90° pulse for GARP (19 dB, 70 μs)
g1, g2, g3, g4, g5: sinusoidal shaped field gradients, 1 ms duration and ca. 0.02 T/m strength for the largest gradient, with gradient loop counters, ring-down delays (100 μs), lock blanking and gradient coil blanking switches according to actual instrumentation used. Gradient strength ratio: 5 : 5 : 60 : −60 : −30.
ns: 128

5. Processing

Use standard 1D processing as described in Experiment 3.1, use an exponential window with lb = 0.5 Hz.

6. Result

The figure on page 386 shows the gs-SELINCOR spectra obtained on an AMX-500 spectrometer with a BGU (10 A) gradient unit. **a** is the normal ^{1}H NMR spectrum. In **b** the selective ^{13}C pulse was adjusted to C-20, in **c** to C-13, and in **d** to C-14. Note that the spectra show correct phases and relative intensities within the multiplets. There are no other signals besides the selected ones.

7. Comments

The sequence starts with an INEPT transfer from protons to carbons. A proton spin-lock pulse p3 decouples the carbon nuclei for the duration of the selective pulse. The selected antiphase ^{13}C magnetization of carbon $2I_{Hz}I_{Cy}$ which is present after p4 is dephased by the two gradient pulses g3 and g4, whereas g1 and g2 only control pulse imperfections. The usual reverse INEPT part of the sequence (see Exp. 6.8) transfers the magnetization back to protons, while the gradient pulse g5 rephases only the de-sired coherences.

8. Own Observations

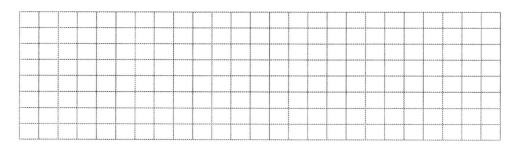

Experiment 11.12

GRECCO

1. Purpose

The GRECCO (**GR**adient **E**nhanced **C**arbon **CO**upling) experiment selectively detects $^2J(C,C)$ and $^3J(C,C)$ carbon carbon couplings, which are useful for a conformational analysis [1]. In principle this task is also performed by SELINQUATE (Exp. 7.7), the selective version of 1D-INADEQUATE (Exp. 6.11). However, whereas the suppression of signals from mono-^{13}C isotopomers is not very important if one is looking for one-bond couplings $^1J(C,C)$, efficient suppression is essential if the small coupling constants $^2J(C,C)$ or $^3J(C,C)$ are to be observed. Otherwise these signals disappear in the foot of the imperfectly suppressed center signal. The method shown here combines three principles of recent NMR developments, namely selective r.f. pulses to choose only the desired carbon signal [1], the use of cross-polarization in liquids for sensitivity enhancement [2], and pulsed field gradients which give efficient suppression of the central signal [3].

2. Literature

[1] T. Fäcke, S. Berger, *J. Am. Chem. Soc.* **1995**, *117*, 9547-9550.
[2] C. Dalvit, G. Bovermann, *J. Magn. Reson. Ser. A* **1994**, *109*, 113–116.
[3] W. Willker, D. Leibfritz, *Magn. Reson. Chem.* **1994**, *32*, 665–669.

3. Pulse Scheme and Phase Cycle

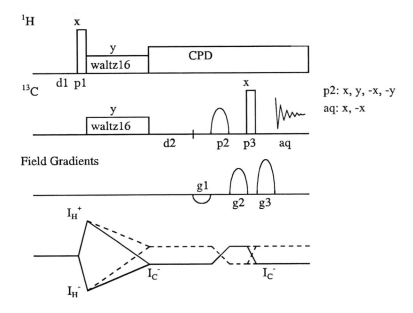

4. Acquisition

Time requirement: 1.5 h

Sample: 90% 2-cyclohexen-1-one in [D$_6$]acetone

Record normal ^{1}H and ^{13}C NMR spectra of the sample, note the offset of the ^{13}C carbonyl signal and the offset of the β-olefinic hydrogen (H-3) signal. You have to set:

> td: 128 k
> sw: 450 ppm to avoid folding
> o1: on resonance of the carbonyl ^{13}C signal
> o2: on resonance of the β-olefinic ^{1}H signal (H-3)
> p1: 90°^{1}H decoupler pulse
> p2: selective 180° ^{13}C transmitter pulse [Gaussian shape, 10 ms, 58 dB]
> p3: 90° ^{13}C transmitter pulse
> ^{1}H spin-lock pulse for cross-polarization [1.8 ms, 50 dB]; carefully adjust the phase difference to p1
> ^{13}C spin-lock pulse for cross-polarization [pulse length must be identical to that of ^{1}H spin-lock pulse]; adjust with ^{13}C transmitter attenuation [1.8 ms, 47 dB]
> duration of spin-lock ≈ 1/J(C,H) = 125 ms, calculated from for ^3J(C,H) ≈ 8 Hz (one cycle of WALTZ-16).
> d1: 10 s
> d2: 1/[2J(C,H)] = 100 ms, calculated from ^nJ(C,H) ≈ 6 Hz
> g1, g2, g3: sinusoidal shaped field gradients 1.5 ms duration and ca. 0.2 T/m strength for the largest gradient, with gradient loop counters, ring-down delays (100 μs), lock blanking and gradient coil blanking switches according to actual instrumentation used. Gradient strength ratio: −5 : 75 : 80.
> decoupler attenuation and 90° pulse for CPD
> ns: 512

5. Processing

Use standard 1D processing as described in Experiment 3.1 with zero filling to 128 k and applying an exponential window with lb = 0.5 Hz.

6. Result

The figure on page 389 shows the GRECCO spectra obtained on an AMX-500 spectrometer with a BGU (10 A) gradient unit using an inverse proton-optimized gradient probe-head. Unfortunately this is not the best choice for this experiment, but ^{13}C-optimized gradient probe-heads are not yet available. **a** is the signal of C-5 (J(C1,C5) = 1.6 Hz) and **b** is the signal of C-4 (J(C1,C4) = 4.8 Hz). Note that the strong signal of the carbonyl ^{13}C atom (not shown) is present in these spectra. Compare the excellent suppression of the center line with the result of Experiment 7.7.

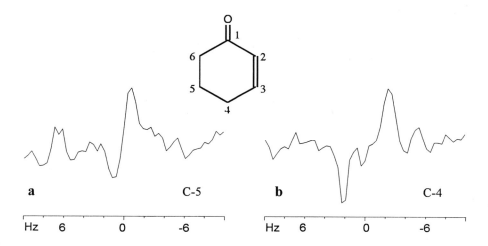

a   C-5   b   C-4

Hz   6   0   -6   Hz   6   0   -6

7. Comments

The sequence starts with cross-polarization from protons to ^{13}C nuclei. For this the spin coupling $^3J(C,H)$ of the carbonyl ^{13}C to the β-olefinic hydrogen is used. Thus, at the end of the spin-lock only enhanced magnetization of the carbonyl ^{13}C is present. During the delay d2, antiphase magnetization $2I_{C1x}I_{C2z}$ to the coupled carbon atoms develops and is dephased by the first gradient g1. The selective 180° carbon pulse inverts this coherence, which is then further dephased by gradient g2. The hard 90° carbon pulse p3 converts $2I_{C1x}I_{C2z}$ into $2I_{C1z}I_{C2y}$ which is rephased by gradient g3. During acquisition in-phase magnetization I_{C2x} develops and is detected. All other signals excited by p3 are dephased by gradient g3. Note that the GRECCO technique does not use a double quantum filter, in contrast to all INADEQUATE methods.

8. Own Observations

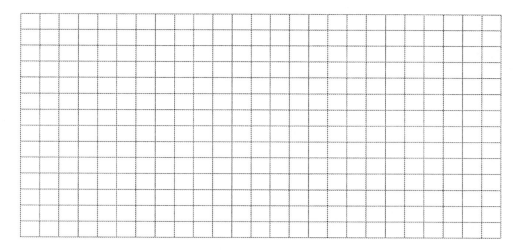

Experiment 11.13

WATERGATE

1. Purpose

The two other water suppression techniques described in this book (see Exps. 6.15 and 6.16) rely on very good shimming. The presaturation technique has the drawback that exchangeable protons may also be saturated. The jump and return method has the disadvantage of the 180° phase shift at the water resonance and the disappearance of signals in the dispersion tail of the residual water peak. The WATERGATE (**WATER** suppression by **GrA**dient **T**ailored **E**xcitation) technique which uses pulsed field gradients is claimed to be independent of line-shape, yielding a superior suppression compared with other methods. Exchangeable protons are not affected and there is no phase jump at the water resonance, although signals very close to the water resonance are also suppressed.

2. Literature

[1] M. Piotto, V. Saudek, V. Sklenar, *J. Biomol. NMR* **1992**, *2*, 661–666.
[2] V. Sklenar, M. Pioto, R. Leppik, V. Saudek, *J. Magn. Reson. Ser. A* **1993**, *102*, 241–245.
[3] L. A. Trimble, M. A. Bernstein, *J. Magn. Reson. Ser. B* **1994**, *105*, 67–72.
[4] T.-L Hwang, A. J. Shaka, *J. Magn. Reson. Ser. A* **1995**, *112*, 275–279.

3. Pulse Scheme and Phase Cycle

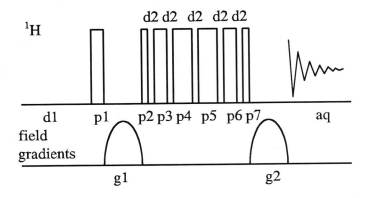

p1, p2, p3, p4: $(x)_2$, $(y)_2$, $(-x)_2$, $(-y)_2$

p5, p6, p7: $(-x)_2$, $(-y)_2$, $(x)_2$, $(y)_2$

aq: $(x)_2$, $(y)_2$, $(-x)_2$, $(-y)_2$

4. Acquisition

Time requirement: 10 min

Sample: 2 mmol sucrose in 90% H_2O/10% D_2O + 0.5 mmol DSS (2,2-dimethyl-2-silapentane-5-sulfonate, sodium salt) + trace of NaN_3 against bacteria growth.

The probe-head must be tuned to the sample used. Record a normal ^{1}H NMR spectrum and center the offset at the water resonance. Load the WATERGATE pulse program. You have to set:

> td : 32 k
> sw: 10 ppm
> o1: on water resonance
> p1: 90° [1]H transmitter pulse
> p2, p7: 0.231·p1
> p3, p6: 0.692·p1
> p4, p5: 1.462·p1
> d1: 1 s
> d2: 300 µs
> g1, g2: sinusoidal shaped field gradients, 2 ms duration and 5% truncation, with gradient loop counters, ring-down delays (100 µs), lock blanking and gradient coil blanking switches according to the actual instrumentation used. Gradient strength must be adjusted experimentally, gradient ratio: 1 : 1.
> ds:4
> ns: 16

5. Processing

Use standard 1D processing as described in Experiment 3.1 with exponential multiplication (lb = 0.5 Hz) and a baseline correction.

6. Result

The figure on page 393 shows the result obtained on an AMX-500 spectrometer with a BGU (10 A) gradient amplifier in a 5 mm inverse gradient probe-head. Compared with Experiment 6.15 the advantages claimed for this experiment are less convincing in our hands due to baseline roll and phasing problems which are adressed in Ref. [4].

7. Comments

The sequence is, in principle, a spin-echo experiment in which the 180° pulse is embedded between two pulsed field gradients. After excitation by the first pulse p1 the field gradient g1 dephases all coherences. The pulses p2 through p7 consist of a binomial sequence (3α, 9α, 19α, 19α, 9α, 3α, with 26α = 180°).

This excites all resonances, excluding those at the offset of the carrier and resonances at positions $k/d2$, where k is an integer. Thus the binomial sequence changes the coherence order of all resonances except that of the water. If d2 is set to 300 µs the next zero excitation of the binomial sequence is outside the spectral range. The second gradient dephases the water signal even further, and rephases all other resonances. The binomial sequence can be replaced by a special selective 180° pulse, which leaves the water resonance unchanged [1]. The advantage of the binomial sequence is that it requires less calibration and can be adjusted even if the carrier frequency is not on the water resonance.

8. Own Observations

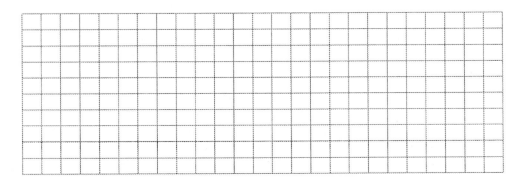

Chapter 12

The Third Dimension

Although 3D NMR experiments cannot be regarded as "basic experiments", we provide in this book three examples as a possible introduction to this exciting field of NMR spectroscopy.

3D experiments are typically constructed from two 2D sequences; thus one has a t_1 period from the first 2D experiment, a t_2 period from the second 2D experiment and the acquisition time, which is often designed as the t_3 period. The detection period of the first 2D sequence is replaced by the evolution part of the second 2D sequence, so that the first pulse of the second sequence is usually missing.

The remarks given in the introduction of Chapter 10 with regard to frequency discrimination and phase-sensitive detection in F_1 and F_2 similarly apply to the 3D case, except that now three time domains have to be considered.

Window functions, Fourier transformation, and phase correction are applied with respect to these three domains to finally yield a cuboid with three frequency axes, which are dependent on the particular experiment. They can be fully heteronuclear (e.g. ^1H, ^{13}C, ^{15}N) or mixed homo- and heteronuclear (e.g. ^1H, ^1H, ^{13}C). Up until now all reported 3D experiments have been proton-detected, which, for sensitivity reasons, has been the only viable option.

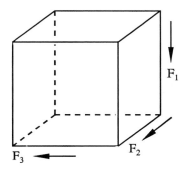

The processing of 3D NMR spectra involves very large data files and is therefore still limited to laboratories which are equipped with reasonably fast work-stations and sufficient data storage capabilities. 3D spectra are inspected by choosing a horizontal or vertical plane through the cuboid which is then treated as a normal 2D spectrum.

Literature

[1] C. Griesinger, O. W. Sørensen, R. R. Ernst, *J. Magn. Reson.* **1989**, *84*, 14–63.
[2] C. Griesinger, H. Schwalbe, J. Schleucher, M. Sattler, in: W. R. Croasmun, R. M. K. Carlson (eds.), *Two-Dimensional NMR Spectroscopy*, VCH, Weinheim, **1994**, 457–580.

Experiment 12.1

3D HMQC-COSY

1. Purpose

HMQC (Exp. 10.11) and H,H-COSY (Exp. 10.3) are the most often used 2D pulse sequences for structure elucidation of organic compounds. However, severe signal overlap can occur in complicated molecules. One alternative is the 3D technique described here, in which the COSY spectra are "edited" via C,H correlation. The 3D spectrum leads to a cuboid in which one axis represents the carbon chemical shift and two axes the proton chemical shift. A C,H correlation signal can be found in a C,H plane of the cuboid for each protonated carbon atom. This signal also forms the diagonal peak of the corresponding COSY plane; thus by moving across between C,H and H,H planes unequivocal assignments are possible, even for very complicated cases. We show here a sequence which is phase-sensitive with respect to all three dimensions and uses the BIRD sandwich to suppress unwanted signals.

2. Literature

[1] C. Griesinger, O. W. Sørensen, R. R. Ernst, *J. Magn. Reson.* **1989**, *84*, 14–63
[2] S. W. Fesik, R. T. Gampe, E. R. P. Zuiderweg, *J. Am. Chem. Soc.* **1989**, *111*, 770–772.

3. Pulse Scheme and Phase Cycle

p1, p2, p4, p5: x   p8: x, -x   Phase of p8 incremented
p3: -x   p9: $(x)_2$, $(-x)_2$ according to TPPI for F_1
p6: y   aq: x, $(-x)_2$, x   Phase of p4 incremented
p7: x   according to TPPI for F_2

4. Acquisition

Time requirement: 24 h

Sample: 10% strychnine in CDCl$_3$

Record normal 1D ^{1}H and ^{13}C NMR spectra, optimize the spectral widths for the aliphatic region only and note the offsets. Narrow spectral windows should be used because of the the the digitization problem in 3D NMR. Switch to the 3D mode of the spectrometer software, and load the 3D HMQC-COSY pulse program. You have to set:

td3: 256 data points in F_3 (^{1}H)
td2: 64 data points in F_2 (^{1}H)
td1: 128 data points in F_1 (^{13}C)
sw3: 3.3 ppm
sw2: 3.3 ppm
sw1: 42 ppm
o1: middle of selected ^{1}H NMR region
o2: middle of selected ^{1}H NMR region
o3: middle of selected ^{13}C NMR region
p1, p3, p4, p6: 90° ^{1}H transmitter pulse
p2, p5: 180° ^{1}H transmitter pulse
p8, p9: 90° ^{13}C decoupler pulse
p7: 180° ^{13}C decoupler pulse
d1: 2 s
d2: 1/[2J(C,H)] = 3.5 ms, calculated from ^1J(C,H) = 145 Hz
d3: BIRD delay to be optimized for minimum FID, ca. 0.4 s (see Exp. 6.11)
^{13}C decoupler attenuation and 90° pulse for GARP
initial values for t_1 and t_2 evolution: 3 µs
increment for t_1 evolution:1/[4·sw1]; increment for t_2 evolution: 1/[2·sw2]
ds: 2
ns: 4

5. Processing

Apply zero filling to 128 real data points in F_2 and to 256 real data points in F_1 to obtain a matrix of 128·128·256 real data points. This will result in 4 MB of processed data. Use an exponential window with lb = 5 Hz line broadening in F_3 and $\pi/2$-shifted squared sinusoidal windows in the other two dimensions. Apply the correct acquisition order parameter (3–1–2) before FT in all three dimensions. Phase correction is best performed after the FT of each dimension. Further details are very dependent on the particular software you use to process such a 3D data file.

6. Result

The figure on page 396 shows a H,H-COSY plane through the 3D cuboid which was obtained on an AMX-500 spectrometer. The plane **a** was chosen at the nearly identical chemical shifts of C-11 and C-17 (δ_C = 42.5). Since protons 11 are attached to the same carbon atom, they reveal a normal COSY pattern; furthermore, the proton 11 at δ_H = 3.05 reveals a cross peak with H-12. The diagonal peak of H-17 leads to two cross-signals of both H-18 protons. In addition, a C,H plane **b** is shown on page 397, chosen at the chemical shift of H-14 (δ_H = 3.05). Nearby are the resonances of one H-18 and one H-11 proton. One observes a C,H correlation signal of C-14 with H-14.

Furthermore H,H correlation signals H-14, H-15 and H-14, H-13 can be seen. The C,H correlation signal of H-11 leads to the signal of the other H-11 and of H-12, and the C,H correlation peak of H-18 leads to the other H-18 and to H-17. Note that these carbon selected COSY spectra are not symmetrical. Under the recording conditions the C,H correlation signal of C-12 ($\delta_C = 78$) is folded and is seen in the lower left corner of the cuboid at about $\delta_C = 53$.

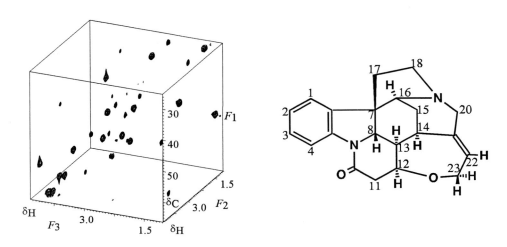

a: H,H plane at $\delta_C = 42.5$

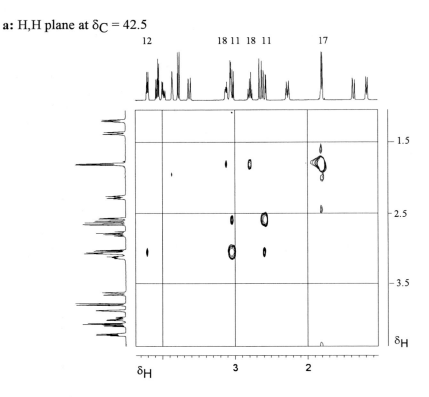

b: C,H plane at $\delta_H = 3.05$

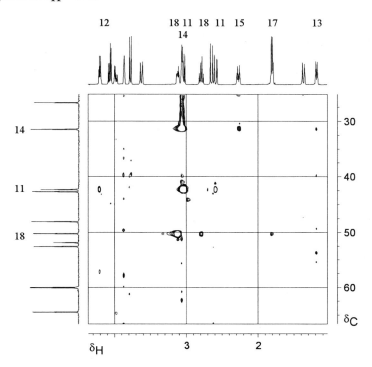

7. Comments

3D sequences are constructed by combining the two corresponding 2D sequences. The last pulse of the first sequence usually replaces the first pulse of the second pulse sequence. Thus, in the case described here, p9 transfers carbon magnetization back to proton magnetization and hence serves as the excitation pulse of the COSY part, so that only a second evolution time t_2 and the COSY read pulse p6 are required. GARP decoupling is switched on after the d2 delay in which the antiphase magnetization of protons with respect to ^{13}C nuclei has developed into in-phase magnetization.

8. Own Observations

Experiment 12.2

3D Gradient-Selected HSQC-TOCSY

1. Purpose

The 3D HMQC-COSY experiment (Exp. 12.1) is very time-consuming because of the required phase cycling. With gradient selection 3D experiments can be considerably shortened. Furthermore, the BIRD sandwich is no longer necessary at the beginning of the sequence and the gradient technique allows a far higher receiver gain. In the experiment described here we replace the HMQC part by the HSQC sequence, which has the advantage that no H,H spin coupling evolves during t_1. The COSY part is replaced by the TOCSY sequence so that only in-phase magnetization is transferred during t_2. This removes the problem of cancelling positive and negative signals due to poor digitization. The length of the spin-lock can be adjusted in order to observe several connectivities in a spin system. The pulse sequence given here is not phase-sensitive. Selective versions are also known [3].

2. Literature

[1] B. K. John, D. Plant, S. L. Heald, R. E. Hurd, *J. Magn. Reson.* **1991**, *94*, 664–669.
[2] W. Wilker, D. Leibfritz, R. Kerssebaum, W. Bermel, *Magn. Reson. Chem.* **1993**, *31*, 287–292.
[3] T. Fäcke, S. Berger, *Tetrahedron* **1995**, *51*, 3521–3524.

3. Pulse Scheme with Phase Cycle

4. Acquisition

Time requirement: 5 h

Sample: 10% strychnine in CDCl₃

Record normal 1D ^{1}H and ^{13}C NMR spectra, optimize the spectral widths for the aliphatic region only, and note the offsets. A narrow spectral window should be used because of the the digitization problem in 3D NMR. Switch to the 3D mode of the spectrometer software and load the gs-HSQC-TOCSY pulse program. You have to set:

td3: 256 data points in F_3 (^{1}H)
td2: 64 data points in F_2 (^{1}H)
td1: 128 data points in F_1 (^{13}C)
sw3: 3.3 ppm
sw2: 3.3 ppm
sw1: 56 ppm
o1: middle of selected ^{1}H NMR region
o2: middle of selected ^{1}H NMR region
o3: middle of selected ^{13}C NMR region
p1, p3, p5: 90° ^{1}H transmitter pulse
p2, p4, p6: 180° ^{1}H transmitter pulse
p8, p9: 90° ^{13}C decoupler pulse
p7, p10: 180° ^{13}C decoupler pulse
90° and 180° ^{1}H pulses within MLEV-16 spin-lock = 40 and 80 µs at transmitter attenuation of 16 dB (see Exp. 11.8); loop counter for length of spin-lock = 40 (must be an even number), giving a spin-lock time of 100 ms
d1: 2 s
d2: $1/[4J(C,H)]$ = 3.5 ms, calculated from $^1J(C,H)$ = 145 Hz
d3: delay to compensate the length of field gradient = 1.5 ms
g1, g2: sinusoidal shaped field gradients with 5% truncation, 1.5 ms duration and ca. 0.01 T/m strength, with gradient loop counters, ring-down delays (100 µs), lock blanking and gradient coil blanking switches according to actual instrumentation used. Gradient strength ratio: 4:1
^{13}C decoupler attenuation and 90° pulse for GARP
initial values for t_1 and t_2 evolution: 3 µs
increment for t1 evolution: $1/[2 \cdot sw1]$; increment for t_2 evolution: 1/sw2
ds: 4
ns: 1

5. Processing

Apply zero filling to 128 real data points in F_2 and to 256 real data points in F_1 to obtain a matrix of 128·128·256 real data points. This will result in 4 MB of processed data. Use an exponential window with lb = 5 Hz line broadening in F_3 and $\pi/2$ shifted squared sinusoidal windows in the other two dimensions. Apply the correct acquisition order parameter (3–1–2) before FT in all three dimensions. Phase correction is not necessary, since a magnitude calculation is performed after the last Fourier transformation in F_1. Further details are very dependent on the particular software you use to process such a 3D data file.

6. Result

The figure on page 400 shows a H,H-TOCSY plane through the 3D cuboid which was obtained on an AMX-500 spectrometer. The plane **a** was chosen at the ^{13}C chemical shifts of C-15 ($\delta_C = 26.7$). Since two protons are bound to this carbon atom their C,H cross-peaks both appear, together with COSY-like H,H cross-peaks. Furthermore, the two cross-signals to neighbour protons H-16 and H-14 are observed.

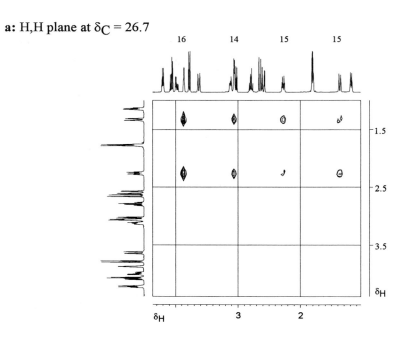

a: H,H plane at $\delta_C = 26.7$

In addition, an expansion of a C,H plane **b** is shown, chosen at the chemical shift of proton 12. The corresponding C,H cross signal can be seen together with cross-peaks to the neighbour protons 11 and 12 and in addition to proton 8, which is a TOCSY result.

b: C,H plane at $\delta_H = 4.2$

7. Comments

The initial part of the sequence uses the basic HSQC method (see Exp. 10.14) while the second part uses the TOCSY technique (see Exps. 10.15 and 11.8). The MLEV-16 pulse train is used as a spin-lock, which consists of an even number of composite 180° pulses and therefore does not change the coherence order. Hence the two positive gradients select the N type pathway during t_1 and P type signals during t_2. The sequence is therefore not phase-sensitive and can be processed in magnitude mode. The overwhelming advantage of this experiment when compared with Experiment 12.1 is that the 3D measurement can be performed with only one transient and, because of the TOCSY part, gives more information in less than a quarter of time. Note, however, that for strychnine the same chemical information is provided by the 2D version of this experiment, as shown in Experiment 11.9.

8. Own Observations

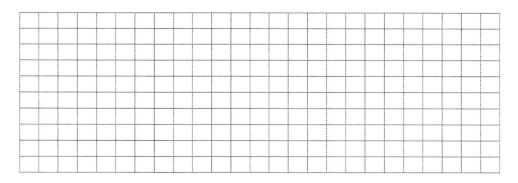

Experiment 12.3

3D H,C,P-Correlation

1. Purpose

In this 3D experiment three different nuclides are correlated with each other, so that one obtains a cuboid in which one axis represents the ^{1}H, the second axis the ^{13}C, and the third axis the ^{31}P chemical shift. Cross-signals appear at points where protons are coupled to ^{13}C nuclei which are in turn coupled to phosphorus. Experiments of this kind, using the spin trio ^{1}H, ^{13}C and ^{15}N, are very important in protein chemistry, whereas the type of experiment described here will find applications in the field of nucleic acids. The very simple example of triphenylphosphane is given here, from which a beginner in this field can gain considerable insight. The experiment is phase-sensitive with respect to all three dimensions.

2. Literature

[1] S. Berger, P. Bast, *Magn. Reson. Chem.* **1993**, *31*, 1021–1023.
[2] H. A. Heus, S. S. Wijmenga, F. J. M. van de Ven, C. W. Hilbers, *J. Am. Chem. Soc.* **1994**, *116*, 4983–4984.
[3] J. P. Marino, H. Schwalbe, C. Anklin, W. Bermel, D. M. Crothers, C. Griesinger, *J. Am. Chem. Soc.* **1994**, *116*, 6472–6473.

3. Pulse Scheme and Phase Cycle

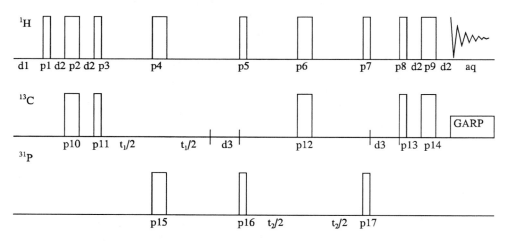

p1, p2, p4, p5, p6, p7, p8, p9, p13, p14, p15, p17: x　　p12: (x)$_4$, (y)$_4$, (-x)$_4$, (-y)$_4$

p3: y, -y　　　　　　　　　　　　　　　　p11: x, incremented according to TPPI during t$_1$

p10: x, -x　　　　　　　　　　　　　　　　aq: x, (-x)$_2$, x, -x, (x)$_2$, -x

p16: (x)$_2$, (-x)$_2$, incremented according to TPPI during t$_2$

4. Acquisition

Time requirement: 6 h

Sample: 10% triphenylphosphane in CDCl$_3$

This experiment requires a three channel spectrometer and a probe-head, which is tunable to ^{1}H, ^{13}C, and ^{31}P. Use appropriate r.f. pass and stop filters in all three channels. Record normal 1D ^{1}H, ^{13}C and ^{31}P NMR spectra, optimize the spectral widths (^{1}H, ^{13}C) for the aromatic region only, and note the offsets. Switch to the 3D mode of the spectrometer software and load the H,C,P correlation pulse program. You have to set:

> td3: 256 data points in F_3 (^{1}H)
> td2: 16 data points in F_2 (^{31}P)
> td1: 64 data points in F_1 (^{13}C)
> sw3: 0.6 ppm
> sw2: 0.5 ppm
> sw1: 12 ppm
> o1: middle of selected ^{1}H NMR region
> o2: middle of selected ^{13}C NMR region
> o3: middle of selected ^{31}P NMR region
> p1, p3, p5, p7, p8: 90° ^{1}H transmitter pulse
> p2, p4, p6, p9: 180° ^{1}H transmitter pulse
> p11, p13: 90° ^{13}C decoupler pulse
> p10, p12, p14: 180° ^{13}C decoupler pulse
> ^{13}C decoupler attenuation and 90° pulse for GARP
> p16, p17: 90° ^{31}P pulse in third channel of the spectrometer
> p15: 180° ^{31}P pulse in third channel of the spectrometer
> d1: 2 s
> d2: 1/[4J(C,H)] = 1.56 ms, calculated from ^1J(C,H) = 160 Hz
> d3: 1/[2J(C,P)] = 38 ms, calculated from ^nJ(C,P) = 13 Hz (average)
> initial values for t_1 and t_2 evolution: 3 µs
> increment for t_1 evolution: 1/[4·sw1]; increment for t_2 evolution: 1/[4·sw2]
> preacquisition delay: as small as possible
> ds: 2
> ns: 8

5. Processing

Apply zero-filling to 32 real data points in F_2 and to 128 real data points in F_1 to obtain a matrix of 128·32·128 real points. This will result in 1 MB of processed data. Use an exponential window with lb = 3 Hz line broadening in F_3 and $\pi/2$ shifted squared sinusoidal windows in the other two dimensions. Apply the correct acquisition order parameter (3–1–2) before FT in all three dimensions. Phase correction is best performed after the FT of each dimension. Further details are very dependent on the particular software you use to process such a 3D data file.

6. Result

The figures **a** and **b** show planes through the 3D cuboid obtained on an AMX-500 spectrometer equipped with an inverse multinuclear probehead containing an additional r.f. channel fixed on the ^{13}C frequency. The plot **a** is a C,H plane chosen at the ^{31}P chemical shift position. Only the signals of the *ortho* and *meta* hydrogen nuclei are seen, since the *para* ^{13}C nucleus does not have a significant C,P spin coupling constant. On page 405 a C,P plane **b** is shown, chosen at the chemical shift of the *ortho* hydrogens.

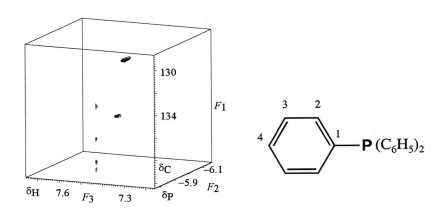

a: C,H plane at $\delta_P = -6$

b: C,P plane at δ_H = 7.48

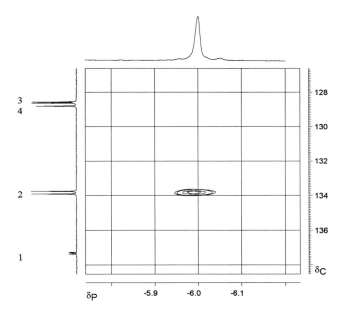

7. Comments

The pulse train begins as for a normal HSQC sequence (see Exp. 10.14). During t_1, when carbon chemical shift develops, a 180° ^{31}P pulse p15 removes any H,P and P,C spin couplings. Antiphase magnetization $4I_{Hz}I_{Cx}I_{Pz}$ of carbon with respect to phosphorus develops during the delay d3, and is subsequently transformed into three-spin coherence $4I_{Hy}I_{Cx}I_{Py}$ by the simultaneous proton and phosphorus 90° pulses p5 and p16. During t_2 phosphorus chemical shift develops. Two simultaneous pulses p7 and p17 create antiphase magnetization $4I_{Hz}I_{Cx}I_{Pz}$ which refocuses to give antiphase magnetization $2I_{Hz}I_{Cy}$ during the second d3 period. This is transferred by the reverse INEPT part of the sequence to protons for detection.

8. Own Observations

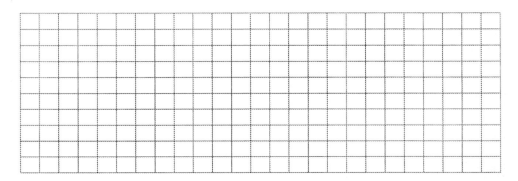

Appendix 1

Instrument Dialects

In recent years the manufacturers of NMR spectrometers have used a variety of instruments, different computers, operating systems, and software. The experiments described in this book are mainly given in the notation of Bruker AMX spectrometers using the UXNMR system. For comparison purposes we give here a glossary which should enable the users of other instruments to find the appropriate parameters to set up the experiments.

Manufacturer	Bruker	Bruker	Bruker	Varian	Varian	Jeol	Jeol
Instrument	AMX ARX	AM AC	DMX DRX DPX	Gemini H/C BB	Gemini-2000 UNITY-plus UNITY-Inova	GX, GSX EX, Alpha, Lambda	Eclipse Delta
Computer	X32, Aspect Station-1	Aspect-3000	SG-Indy	Motoro-la 68000	Sun	DEC-PDP11, VAX Alpha AXP	SG-Indy
Operating System	Unix	Adakos	Irix	VXR-4000	Solaris	RSX11M, VMS, Unix	Irix
time domain data size	td	TD	td	np	np	SAMPO, EX: SPO	x_points
processed data size	si	SI	si	fn	fn	POINT	
time domain in F_2 or F_1	td2 td1	TD2 TD1	td2 td1			F_2: FREQU F_1: CLFRQ	F_2: x_sweep F_1: y_sweep
processed data size in F_2 or F_1	si	SI2/SI1	si	fn fn1	fn fn1	F_2: POINT F_1: CLPNT	
transmitter offset	o1	O1	o1	to	tof	OBSET + OBFIN	x_offset
decoupler offset	o2	O2	o2	do	dof	IRSET + IRFIN	irr_offset
spectral width [ppm]	sw	-	sw	sw	sw		x_sweep

Manufacturer	Bruker	Bruker	Bruker	Varian	Varian	Jeol	Jeol
pulse width	px, x = 0–n	PW, Px, x = 0–9	px, x = 0–n	pw	pw	PWx, x = 1–n	user defined
delay	dx, x = 0–n	Dx, x = 0–n	dx, x = 0–n	dx, x=1–n	dx, x=1–n	PIx, x = 1–n	user defined
receiver gain	rg	RG	rg	gain	gain	RGAIN	recvr_gain
transmitter power level	thi, tlo, tlx, x=0–31	THI, TLO	plx, x = 0–31	tpwr	tpwr	OBATN	obs_attenuator
decoupler power level	dhi dlo,dlx, x=1–31		plx, x = 0–31	dhp,dlp	dpwr	IRATN	irr_attenu-ator
proton trans-mitter power level	hlx, x = 1–4		plx, x = 0–31				module_config(irr.amp_full_pwr)
proton decoupler power level	hlx, x =1–4	Sx, x=1–4	plx, x = 0–31	pplvl	pplvl		normal irr oparation mode
power level for soft pulses on the trans-mitter channel	tpx, x=0–15		spx, x = 0–15		selpwr	OBATN	obs_atte-nuator
power level for soft pulses on the de-coupler	dpx, x=0–15		spx, x = 0–15			IRATN	irr_atte-nuator
number of scans	ns	NS	ns	nt	nt	SCANS	scans
homonuclear decoupling mode	hd	HD	hd	homo	homo	EXMOD =SGHOM IRMOD= HOM	module_config(pulser.time share)
dummy scans	ds	DS	ds	ss	ss	DUMMY INDMY	x_prescans
composite pulse decoupling	cpd	CPD	cpd	w	w	EXMOD =SGCOM IRMOD= COM	irr_noise
continous wave decoupling	cw	CW	cw	c	q	EXMOD =SGSEL IRMOD= SEL	on (irr.gate)
preacquisition delay	de	DE	de	rof2	rof2pad	PREDL	dead_time & delay

Manufacturer	Bruker	Bruker	Bruker	Varian	Varian	Jeol	Jeol
number of incremented periods during t1	nd0	ND0	ndo			CLPNT	
increment for t1 evolution	in0	IN0	in0			PI1	
phase difference between pulses	phcorx, x=0–31		phcorx, x= 0–31				

Appendix 2

Elementary Product Operator Formalism Rules

In the **Comments** section of the experiments the product operator formalism is often used to follow the course of the magnetization. This table provides a summary of the various interrelationships for quick reference.

1. 90° Pulses

$$I_{1z} \xrightarrow{\ 90°\ I_x\ } -I_{1y} \qquad I_{1x} \xrightarrow{\ 90°\ I_x\ } I_{1x} \qquad I_{1y} \xrightarrow{\ 90°\ I_x\ } I_{1z}$$

$$I_{1z} \xrightarrow{\ 90°\ I_y\ } I_{1x} \qquad I_{1x} \xrightarrow{\ 90°\ I_y\ } -I_{1z} \qquad I_{1y} \xrightarrow{\ 90°\ I_y\ } I_{1y}$$

$$I_{1z} \xrightarrow{\ 90°\ I_{-x}\ } I_{1y} \qquad I_{1x} \xrightarrow{\ 90°\ I_{-x}\ } I_{1x} \qquad I_{1y} \xrightarrow{\ 90°\ I_{-x}\ } -I_{1z}$$

$$I_{1z} \xrightarrow{\ 90°\ I_{-y}\ } -I_{1x} \qquad I_{1x} \xrightarrow{\ 90°\ I_{-y}\ } I_{1z} \qquad I_{1y} \xrightarrow{\ 90°\ I_{-y}\ } I_{1y}$$

$$2I_{1x}I_{2z} \xrightarrow{\ 90°\ I_y\ } -2I_{1z}I_{2x}$$

$$2I_{1x}I_{2z} \xrightarrow{\ 90°\ I_x\ } -2I_{1x}I_{2y}$$

2. Chemical Shift

$$I_{1x} \xrightarrow{\ \Omega I_z t\ } I_{1x}\cos\Omega t + I_{1y}\sin\Omega t \qquad\qquad -I_{1x} \xrightarrow{\ \Omega I_z t\ } -I_{1x}\cos\Omega t - I_{1y}\sin\Omega t$$

$$I_{1y} \xrightarrow{\ \Omega I_z t\ } I_{1y}\cos\Omega t - I_{1x}\sin\Omega t \qquad\qquad -I_{1y} \xrightarrow{\ \Omega I_z t\ } -I_{1y}\cos\Omega t + I_{1x}\sin\Omega t$$

$$I_{1z} \xrightarrow{\ \Omega I_z t\ } I_{1z}$$

3. Spin–Spin Coupling

$$I_{1x} \xrightarrow{\ \pi J\, 2I_{1z}I_{2z} t\ } I_{1x}\cos\pi J\, t + 2I_{1y}I_{2z}\sin\pi J\, t$$

$$-I_{1x} \xrightarrow{\ \pi J\, 2I_{1z}I_{2z} t\ } -I_{1x}\cos\pi J\, t - 2I_{1y}I_{2z}\sin\pi J\, t$$

$$I_{1y} \xrightarrow{\pi J\, 2I_{1z}I_{2z}t} I_{1y}\cos\pi J\, t - 2I_{1x}I_{2z}\sin\pi J\, t$$

$$-I_{1y} \xrightarrow{\pi J\, 2I_{1z}I_{2z}t} -I_{1y}\cos\pi J\, t + 2I_{1x}I_{2z}\sin\pi J\, t$$

$$2I_{1x}I_{2z} \xrightarrow{\pi J\, 2I_{1z}I_{2z}t} 2I_{1x}I_{2z}\cos\pi J\, t + I_{1y}\sin\pi J\, t$$

$$-2I_{1x}I_{2z} \xrightarrow{\pi J\, 2I_{1z}I_{2z}t} -2I_{1x}I_{2z}\cos\pi J\, t - I_{1y}\sin\pi J\, t$$

$$2I_{1y}I_{2z} \xrightarrow{\pi J\, 2I_{1z}I_{2z}t} 2I_{1y}I_{2z}\cos\pi J\, t - I_{1x}\sin\pi J\, t$$

$$-2I_{1y}I_{2z} \xrightarrow{\pi J\, 2I_{1z}I_{2z}t} -2I_{1y}I_{2z}\cos\pi J\, t + I_{1x}\sin\pi J\, t$$

$$I_{1z} \xrightarrow{\pi J\, 2I_{1z}I_{2z}t} I_{1z}$$

4. Shift Operators

$$I^+ = I_x + iI_y$$

$$I^- = I_x - iI_y$$

$$I_x = \frac{1}{2}(I^+ + I^-)$$

$$I_y = \frac{1}{2i}(I^+ - I^-)$$

$$2I_{1x}I_{2z} = I_{2z}(I^+ + I^-)$$

$$I^+ \xrightarrow{90°\ I_x} \frac{1}{2}(I^+ + I^-) + iI_z$$

$$I^- \xrightarrow{90°\ I_x} \frac{1}{2}(I^+ + I^-) - iI_z$$

Literature

[1] O. W. Sørensen, G. W. Eich, M. H. Levitt, G. Bodenhausen, R. R. Ernst, *Prog. NMR Spectrosc.* **1983**, *16*, 163–192.
[2] H. Kessler, M. Gehrke, C. Griesinger, *Angew. Chem. Int. Ed. Engl.* **1988**, *27*, 490–536.

Glossary and Index

acquisition time 35, 40
ADC (analog digital converter) 36, 41
alcohol content 231
American Society for Testing and Materials 56
analog digital converter 36, 41
APT (Attached Proton Test) 135
attached proton test 135
ASTM (American Society for Testing and Materials) 56
ASTM sensitivity test for ^{13}C NMR spectroscopy 56
auxiliary reagents 215
baseline correction 36, 37, 42
bilinear rotation decoupling 161, 312, 315, 398, 394
binomial sequence 391, 392
BIRD (BIlinear Rotation Decoupling) 161, 312, 315, 398, 394
Bloch–Siegert shift 69, 80
Born–Oppenheimer approximation 256
boron-11 NMR 269
C,H Correlation by polarization transfer (HETCOR) 299
C,H Correlation via long range couplings (COLOC) 305
calibration of pulsed field gradients 346
CAMELSPIN (Cross relaxation Appropriate for Minimolecules Emulated by Locked Spins) 330
Carr–Purcell–Meiboom–Gill sequence 129
chemically induced dynamic nuclear polarization 240
chiral shift reagent 219
chiral solvating agent 222
CIDNP (Chemically Induced Dynamic Nuclear Polarization) 240
coherence levels 353
COLOC (COrrelation spectroscopy via LOng range Coupling) 305
composite pulse decoupling 20
constant time experiment 305, 307
continous wave decoupling 102, 105
correlation spectroscopy 283, 398
correlation spectroscopy via long range coupling 305
COSY (COrrelation SpectroscopY) 283, 398
COSY-45 292
CPD (Composite Pulse Decoupling) 20
cross-polarization in liquids 257, 387, 389
DANTE (Delays Alternating with Nutation for Tailored Excitation) 186
dB unit 31
dBm unit 32
decoupler
    attenuation 41
    band width 69, 72
    calibration for heteronuclear decoupling 72

calibration for homonuclear decoupling 69
offset 40
pulse-length 20
pulse calibration 180, 183
decoupling techniques 68
delays alternating with nutation for tailored excitation 186
DEPT (Distortionless Enhancement by Polarization Transfer) 150, 248, 251, 257
detection period 273
determination of
a shaped 90° ^{13}C decoupler pulse 183
a shaped 90° ^{1}H decoupler pulse 180
a shaped 90° ^{1}H transmitter pulse 177
long-range C,H coupling constants 206
radiofrequency power 29
the 90° ^{13}C transmitter pulse-length 17
the 90° ^{1}H decoupler pulse-length 20
the 90° ^{1}H transmitter pulse-length 14
the pulse-length 3
deuterium
NMR 264
lock 6
signal 6
diffusion constants 349, 351
digital
filtering 36
lock 7
resolution 36
directional coupler 78
distortionless enhancement by polarization transfer 150, 248, 251, 257
double
INEPT 318
quantum filter 295, 356, 359, 389
quantum filtered COSY 295, 356
quantum magnetization 297, 298, 310, 340
DQF-COSY (Double Quantum Filtered COSY) 295, 356
dummy scans 36, 41
dwell time 80
dynamic NMR spectroscopy 111, 118, 341
dynamic range test for signal amplitudes 65
echo/anti-echo selection 275, 368
editing 124, 132, 141, 144
editing ^{13}C NMR spectra
with APT 135
with DEPT 150
with PENDANT 154
with SEFT 132
enantiomeric excess *ee* 221, 224, 227

enantiomeric purity with Pirkle's reagent 225
evolution period 273
exchangeable protons 118, 341, 390
exchange spectroscopy 341
exponential window function 36, 42
EXSY (EXchange SpectroscopY) 341
external referencing 243
Fellgett principle 176
fluorine lock 7
fluorine-19 NMR 254
food analysis 264
Forsén–Hoffmann method 121
GARP (Globally optimized Alternating-phase Rectangular Pulses) 27, 311, 312
gated ^{1}H-decoupling technique 96
Gauss multiplication 36
globally optimized alternating-phase rectangular pulses 27, 311, 312
Gouy balance 237
gradient
    amplifier 344
    calibration 346
    double quantum filter 356
    enhanced carbon coupling 387
    strength 346
gradient-selected
    COSY 352
    DQF COSY 356
    HMBC 364
    HMQC-TOCSY 376
    HMQC 360
    HSQC 368
    INEPT-INADEQUATE 380
    SELINCOR 384
    TOCSY 372
GRECCO (GRadient Enhanced Carbon Coupling) 387
gs-HSQC-TOCSY 398
gs-COSY 352
gs-DQF COSY 356
gs-HMBC 364
gs-HMQC 360
gs-HMQC-TOCSY 376
gs-HSQC 368
gs-INEPT-INADEQUATE 380
gs-SELINCOR 384
gs-TOCSY 372
H,C,P-correlation 402
helium-refill 1
HETCOR (Heteronuclear Correalation) 299

heteronuclear
    correlation 299
    decoupling 72
    double quantum filter 168
    multiple bond correlation 315, 364
    multiple quantum coherence 308, 312, 360, 376, 398, 394
    NMR 243
    Overhauser effect spectroscopy 334
    single quantum coherence 318, 368, 398, 405
    SPT experiment 84
higher order effects 95
high temperature calibration with 1,2-ethanediol 115
hindered rotation 111
HMBC (Heteronuclear Multiple Bond Correlation) 315, 364
HMQC (Heteronuclear Multiple Quantum Coherence) 308, 312, 360, 376, 398, 394
HMQC-COSY 394 398
HOESY (Heteronuclear Overhauser Effect SpectroscopY) 334
HOHAHA (HOmonuclear HArtmann Hahn) 322
homonuclear
    decoupling 69, 78
    double quantum filter 160
    Hartmann–Hahn 322
    SPT experiment 81
HSQC (Heteronuclear Single Quantum Coherence) 318, 368, 398, 405
HSQC-TOCSY 398
hump test 44, 53
INADEQUATE (Incredible Natural Abundance DoublE QUAntum Transfer Experiment) 157, 337, 380, 387
INAPT 203
incredible natural abundance double quantum transfer experiment 157, 337, 380, 387
INEPT (Insensitive Nuclei Enhanced by Polarization Transfer) 138, 257, 371, 382, 386, 405
INEPT+ 141
INEPT-INADEQUATE 380
insensitive nuclei enhanced by polarization transfer 138, 257, 371, 382, 386, 405
instrument dialect 406
integration 37, 231, 234, 276
inverse
    gated ^{1}H-decoupling 99, 234
    pulse-length 26
    spectrometer configuration 23
isotope effect 256
isotope distribution 264
J-resolved ^{13}C NMR spectroscopy 280
J-resolved ^{1}H NMR spectroscopy 209, 277
JUMP and RETURN sequence 173
lanthanide shift reagent 216, 219

line-shape test for ^{13}C NMR spectroscopy 53
line-shape test for ^{1}H NMR spectroscopy 44
lithium-6 NMR 334
local oscillator 2
lock channel 6
long range COSY 286
long-range C,H correlation by polarization transfer 302
low pass filter 367
low power calibration for heteronuclear decoupling 75
low temperature calibration with methanol 112
LR-COSY (Long-Range COSY) 286
magnet 1
maintenance 3
matching 4
McConnel–Robertson Equation 218
measurement of
        the heteronuclear Overhauser effect 108
        the spin–lattice relaxation time T_1 125
        the spin–spin relaxation time T_2 129
mixing period 273
MLEV-16 374, 401
MLEV-17 321, 375, 378
Mosher ester 224
multiple irradiation 90
multiplet distortion 140, 141
nitrogen NMR 248, 251
NMR time scale 111
NOE difference 87, 90
NOESY (Nuclear Overhauser Enhancement SpectroscopY) 326
nuclear Overhauser difference spectroscopy 87, 90
nuclear Overhauser enhancement spectroscopy 326
ODCB (*ortho*-dichlorobenzene) 47
off-resonance decoupling 90
offset 35, 40
oscilloscope 3
oxygen-17 NMR 270
Overbodenhausen experiment 310
paramagnetic relaxation reagnet 228, 236,
paramagnetic susceptibility 237
peak pickung 37
PENDANT (Polarization ENhancement During Attached Nucleus Testing) 154
Pirkle's reagent 225
PGSE (Pulsed Gradient Spin Echo) 349
phase-sensitive
        COSY 289
        COSY-45 292
        gradient-selected HSQC 368

mode 274, 275

P/N type selection 275

POF (Product Operator Formalism) 22, 43, 139, 152, 155, 159, 162, 165, 168, 285, 297, 310, 320, 340, 353, 371, 409

polarization
    enhancement 144
    enhancement during attached nucleus testing 154
    transfer 138, 146, 299, 302

preacquisition delay 35, 41

preemphasis 344

preirradiation 87

preparation period 273

presaturation 170, 295

principles of an NMR Spectrometer 1

probe-head 3

probe-head ringing 270

product operator formalism 22, 43, 139, 152, 155, 159, 162, 165, 168, 285, 297, 310, 320, 340, 353, 371, 409

pulse calibration 177, 180, 183

pulsed gradient spin-echo 349

pulse-length 13, 14f

pulse repetition time 36

pulse-width 13, 14f

pulsed field gradients 344

pulsed gradient spin-echo experiment 349

quadrature image test 62

quality factor 32

quantitative
    determination 215, 231, 234
    ^{13}C NMR spectroscopy 234
    ^{1}H NMR spectroscopy 231

radiofrequeny power 29

reaction mechanism 215, 240

RE-BURP (REfocused Band selective Uniform Response Pure phase) 206

receiver gain 36, 41

Redfield method 275

reflection meter 3

referencing 37, 42, 243

refocused band selective uniform response pure phase 206

refocused INEPT 144

relaxation measurement 125, 129

relaxation reagent Cr(acac)$_3$ 228

resolution test for ^{1}H NMR spectroscopy 47

reverse INEPT 147, 320, 371, 386

RIDE (RIng Down Elimination) 270

ring-down 272
    delay 344

elimination 270
ROESY (Rotating frame Overhauser Enhancement SpectroscopY) 330
rotating frame Overhauser enhancement spectroscopy 330
routine NMR spectroscopy
Ruben–States–Habercorn procedure 275, 290
saturation transfer experiment 121
SEFT (Spin-Echo Fourier Transform) 132
selective
    COSY 189
    determination of C,H spin coupling 206, 209
    determination of H,H spin coupling 212
    excitation with DANTE 186
    INADEQUATE 195
    INEPT 203
    inverse H,C correlation 192, 384
    population transfer 81, 84
    resolution of C,H Coupling 209
    refocussing 212
    r.f. pulses 387
    TOCSY 196
self shielded gradient coils 344
SELINCOR: (Selective Inverse H,C Correlation) 192, 384
SELINQUATE (Selective INADEQUATE) 195
SELRESOLV (Selective Resolution of C,H Coupling) 209
sensitivity test for ^{13}C NMR spectroscopy 59
sensitivity test for ^{1}H NMR spectroscopy 50
sequential acquisition 274
SERF (SElective ReFocussing) 212
shift operator 410
shim gradients 8
shimming 7
shim gradients 8
shimming procedure 9
signal separation of enantiomers using a chiral shift reagent 219
signal-to-noise ratio 50
sign of spin coupling constants 81, 292
silicon-29 NMR 257
simultaneous acquisition 274
single frequency decoupling of ^{13}C NMR spectra 102
spectrometer console 2
spectroscopy with selective pulses 176
spin-echo 129, 137, 278, 281, 390, 350, 348
spin-echo Fourier transform 132
spin–lattice relaxation 125
spin-lock 183, 199, 322, 324, 330, 333, 329, 397, 401
spin simulation 83, 86, 96, 98
spin–spin relaxation 129

SPT (Selective Population Transfer) 81, 84
standard ^{13}C NMR experiment 39
standard ^{1}H NMR experiment 34
standard tests 33
stereochemical assignment 87, 218
subtraction artefacts 88
symmetrization 278, 281, 284, 287
TANGO (Testing for Adjacent Nuclei with a Gyration Operator) 164
temperature calibration 112, 115
testing for adjacent nuclei with a gyration operator 164
three-dimensional experiments 393
three spin coherence 404
time domain 35, 40
time proportional phase increment 275
tin-119 NMR 261
TOCSY (TOtal Correlation SpectroscopY) 322, 374
total correlation spectroscopy 322, 374
TPPI (Time Proportional Phase Increment) 275
transmitter pulse-length 14
tuning 4
tuning a probe-head 3
tuning and matching
     with a reflection meter 3
     with a wobble generator 5
     with an r.f. bridge and an oscilloscope 4
two-dimensional experiments 273
valence isomerization 111
volume integrals 276
WATERGATE (WATER suppression by GrAdient Tailored Excitation) 391
water suppression
     by presaturation 170
     by gradient tailored excitation 391
     by the jump and return method 173
window function 36, 42, 275
wobble generator 5
work station 3
Ξ-scale 243

Research   p 29.